New Ethics for the Public's Health

Edited by

DAN E. BEAUCHAMP

Professor Emeritus
Department of Health Policy,
Management, and Behavior
School of Public Health
University at Albany
State University of New York

BONNIE STEINBOCK

Professor
Department of Philosophy
University at Albany
State University of New York

New York   Oxford
OXFORD UNIVERSITY PRESS
1999

Oxford University Press

Oxford   New York
Athens   Auckland   Bangkok   Bogotá   Buenos Aires   Calcutta
Cape Town   Chennai   Dar es Salaam   Delhi   Florence   Hong Kong   Istanbul
Karachi   Kuala Lumpur   Madrid   Melbourne   Mexico City   Mumbai
Nairobi   Paris   São Paulo   Singapore   Taipei   Tokyo   Toronto   Warsaw

and associated companies in
Berlin   Ibadan

Library of Congress Cataloging-in-Publication Data
New ethics for the public's health / edited by Dan E. Beauchamp, Bonnie Steinbock.
p.   cm.   Includes bibliographical references and index.
ISBN-13 978-0-19-512438-5—ISBN-10 0-19-512439-2 (pbk.)
ISBN 0-19-512438-3—ISBN 0-19-512439-1 (pbk.)
1. Public health—Moral and ethical aspects.   2. Medical policy—Moral and ethical
aspects.   I. Beauchamp, Dan E.   II. Steinbock, Bonnie.
RA652 .N49   1999
174'.2—dc21   99-23617

9 8 7 6

Printed in the United States of America
on acid-free paper

New Ethics for
the Public's Health

For

Carole

and

Nick, Sarah, and Sam

Preface

New Ethics for the Public's Health is a fresh departure for a textbook on health policy and ethics. For the first time such a book addresses head-on the public health issues that are important for the new century. How do we provide access for all to health care in an era of market forces and managed care? How do we defend the public's health in the midst of old and newly emergent epidemics (drug-resistant tuberculosis and Ebola and Hanta viruses)? How do we create a rational drug policy and health policy, issues that are highly politicized and increasingly complicated in the context of worldwide immigration and crumbling borders? How do we assess the ethics of reproduction in a time of transformation of the family; the meaning of kinship? What are the implications of the burgeoning of genetic information for the treatment of disease and of privacy, for confidentiality, and for discrimination? What are the rights of undocumented aliens and other strangers to Medicaid and of other public health protections in a time of soaring deficits and shrinking budgets? What are the prospects for practicing medicine, nursing, social work and public health when "the patient" is not only individuals but, more and more, whole communities?

New Ethics for the Public's Health aims to be very different from typical medical ethics textbooks. Most texts on medical ethics are edited by philosophers and include articles by philosophers and other health experts who are philosophically inclined. Their readers include students in courses on medical ethics. These courses are offered in departments of philosophy or in schools of medicine and are usually taught by philosophers. Such textbooks have a standard format. After an introductory overview of ethics and philosophy in medicine, the books turn to a long series of topic areas such as the doctor–patient relationship; the definition of death, abortion, and reproductive technology; the new biology; emergent ethical issues; and problems in the just allocation of health care. The focus of the disputes is typically some enduring philosophical question: When does life begin, or end? What is the meaning of a person? What are our obligations to future generations? What is the meaning of autonomy in the doctor–patient relationship? The articles are usually considered to be "classics" or to represent widely admired arguments. The thrust of the text is to expose the student to contrasting and powerfully argued views on problems which are deeply disputed or in perpetual conflict and not likely to be resolved in the near term. Hence the need for (and value in) the philosopher and the instructor to lead the students through the moral thicket and let them choose which arguments they accept, on a reasoned basis.

As we see it, a textbook on ethics and public health needs to be considerably different. In the first place, the ethics of public health concern communities as much as they do individuals. Thus, the focus needs to be on public health's methods and perspective, and a text ought to consider the issues and ethical conflicts that arise from that method or perspective. Philosophers teaching in departments of philosophy may use this text in courses on bioethics or health policy, but it is aimed more directly at public health, social welfare, public policy, and medical schools. Its emphases have been chosen to help students interested in learning about the method and philosophy of public health as viewed from the standpoint of ethics and public health.

This book differs from traditional medical ethics textbooks in another way: It is not based on abstract ethical theory. Unlike modern applied ethics, with roots in utilitarian or contract theory, public health is a pragmatic, somewhat eclectic, approach to real-life problems. Not a philosophy in the same sense as utilitarianism or other ethical theories, public health is more a perspective, one that stresses what practitioners and researchers call the "population" or "community" approach. This approach is built on the communal and contingent bases of knowledge, and on practical and contingent approaches to promoting the common good and social justice. In that it seeks to expand the scope of community health institutions or programs in a liberal democratic society, public health can be viewed as a kind of communitarianism, so long as this is understood as a practical, rather than theoretical, philosophy.

As a perspective, public health is about facing health problems as a group and using organized community approaches to resolve those problems. Its roots lie in the public health campaigns of the 19th and early 20th centuries. Its core method is epidemiology, which is the study of diseases that strike the community or the "people" as a whole. The good it promotes is a common good, one that is aggregate in nature. However, and this is a crucial point for the rest of the text, public health as a method does not *provide first principles*. Public health as a method assumes background principles of community and equality, although these principles are often implicit rather than made explicit in a system of ethics. Its justifications are rooted in legal decisions, in constitutional debates about the state's regulatory powers, and in political debates and controversies on the scope and purpose of democratic government over the individual citizen and the control of markets and the great professions. Protecting the public's health also raises fundamental questions about the duties and obligations owed by citizens to the political community. But the point is that public health must pay careful attention to the larger horizon of community and to the justifications for promoting and protecting the health of the people if it is to prosper and persuade. Empirical methods, even those constructed on a population foundation, are not enough.

The topics in this book differ from other bioethics readers in that they raise fundamental political questions. What is the meaning and scope of community, and the balance between the market and the public realm, in today's modern liberal society, which is so highly individualistic? Does a strong public health policy require a rethinking of the current belief that the market ought to be dominant in most domains to assure an adequate standard of living for all and a high rate of growth? Should safety and the public's health be treated as "market failures," exceptions to the general beneficence of market institutions? Or should the market be captive to the democratic community, subject to oversight by elected and accountable officials? What is the proper balance between the cultural or moral sphere and the public's health given that the former powerfully shapes a community's response to human immunodeficiency virus (HIV), drugs, (including alcohol and tobacco), sex education, and the like? What are the justifications for limiting individual liberty in order to promote the public's health as a common good? And what are the boundaries and limits for free discussion and speech, and for the public's health? Such topics lead the discussion far from the traditional emphases of most applied philosophy and even from its interest in distributive justice. These topics require a consideration of not just what each individual deserves and needs but of what will help whole communities hold together and what will encourage people to consider themselves a community given the powerful forces in health policy (from abortion to national health reform) that tend to pull a community apart.

This book recognizes that not all philosophical issues connected with health are ethical in nature. Social definitions of voluntariness, of risk, and of the causes of public health problems are equally important. Society constantly changes its ways of perceiving public or community problems. Progress is made by changing the perceptions or the "stories" of how drinking and driving, smoking, or HIV and AIDS are caused and prevented. Are our public problems to be conceived of as dominantly individualistic (or market-driven) stories? Are public problems the result of a collapse of morals? Or are these problems rooted in a more complex story about how society is organized and how culture functions? *New Ethics for the Public's Health* seeks to show how the tools of philosophy and analysis are crucial in this process of constructing the new stories of community.

Alcoholism policy provides a good example of this point. For a long time, the prevailing assumption was that excessive drinking is due to the power of alcohol as a societal evil (the Prohibitionist story) or an individual one (whether from a lack of will power, self-deception, or of a "condition" called alcoholism). After Prohibition, alcoholism became defined as a "kind of people" problem, and the locus shifted from the bottle to the person. The simplified version of this story is that alcoholism is located in the person, not the bottle. Today however, most experts acknowledge that both stories—one rooted in moralism and the other in a misguided search for a physiological or psychological explanation for how alcoholism is caused—are seriously defective. A different approach—a public health story—has become more widely accepted despite the fact that it does not seek to answer the question, "What causes alcoholism?" Instead, this new story asks a more practical and answerable question: Can we reduce alcohol problems in society for young people and adults alike through prudent measures such as taxes on alcohol, age limits, and restrictions on advertising?

Of course, new policies that would limit the sale and advertising of alcohol, or tax it more heavily, impose restrictions on the liberty of individuals. Some libertarians will argue that individuals should be free to purchase alcohol at all times, in all places, and at the lowest possible price. For this reason, libertarians are usually at odds with a public health perspective. (This conflict is examined in Chapter 3.) The public health proponent responds that minor infringements on individual liberty that result in significant improvements in aggregate welfare or the common good are justified and are not paternalistic in any objectionable sense.

We attempt to represent differing views and to show how these views clash or agree, but we also attempt to clarify and extend the community perspective on the public's health. Thus, this is a reader with a point of view, yet not one that is devoted exclusively to one view. Our aim is to stimulate students and scholars alike to think about the public's health in a new way, as an issue that requires political and philosophical analysis. We hope that those in epidemiology or health management or medical school working on related issues and facing similar conflicts will find this book both provocative and informative.

Regretfully, for reasons of space, we have eliminated the footnotes to the included articles. Readers who wish to follow up sources should consult the original articles.

We owe thanks to many people. First, we thank our authors and their publishers for graciously allowing us to use their work. We also received generous gifts of time and helpful advice from Lori Andrews (Kent Law School), Mila Aroskar (University of Minnesota), John Arras and Jonathan Moreno (University of Virginia), Ron Bayer (Columbia University), Sissela Bok (Harvard University), Dan W. Brock (Brown University), George Cunningham (California Public Health Department), Signe Dayhoff (Genetic Screening Research Group), Norman Fost (University of Wisconsin), Cynthia Hinton (Emory University), Neil A. Holtzman, Eric Juengst (Case Western Reserve), Erik Parens (The Hastings Center), Karen Rothenberg (Georgetown Law School), and Benjamin Wilfond (National Institutes of Health).

Dan Beauchamp thanks Larry Churchill (University of North Carolina at

Chapel Hill), his colleagues in the New York State Department of Health from 1988 to 1992 during his tenure as a health official, who introduced him to the "real world" of ethical issues in public health, to colleagues in bioethics over the years who have taught him so much, especially Dan Wikler (University of Wisconsin, Madison), Daniel Callahan (The Hastings Center), Ronald Bayer (Columbia University), and to those in the field of alcohol problems and injury, who were instrumental in shaping his ideas about public health, especially James Mosher (the Marin Institute), Larry Wallack (University of California at Berkeley), Robin Room (the Addiction Research Institute, Toronto), Wolfgang Schmidt (formerly of the Addiction Research Institute, Toronto), Alex Wagenaar (University of Minnesota), Steve Teret (Johns Hopkins University), and Milton Terris (*Journal of Public Health Policy*). Finally, a special note of thanks to Bonnie Steinbock for her patience and for making him think harder about the ethics of public health.

Bonnie Steinbock thanks her fellow board members of the now-defunct National Advisory Board of Ethics in Reproduction (NABER); the members of the Hastings Center working groups on maternal–fetal relations, long-term contraceptives, and prenatal testing for disability; and the members of the European Union–sponsored working group on reproductive choice and control of fertility. She has learned much from all of you and had a lot of fun in the process. She also thanks her co-author, Dan Beauchamp, for introducing her to the public health perspective.

Finally, we thank Jeffrey House, our editor at Oxford University Press, who shepherded this book from conception to reality.

Bisbee, AZ   D.E.B.
Albany, NY   B.S.
October 1998

Contents

IV New Technology and the Public's Health

I

THE SCOPE OF PUBLIC HEALTH
AS ETHICS

INTRODUCTION: ETHICAL THEORY AND PUBLIC HEALTH

THE TURN TO APPLIED ETHICS

About 30 years ago, professional philosophers began to become interested in "applied ethics." This was a major shift in academic philosophy. In the 1920s and 30s, logical positivism taught that ethics could not be done at all, since ethical statements were at best expressions of feeling and at worst arrant nonsense. During the 1950s, the teaching of ethics usually was limited to investigating the meaning of such words as *duty, right,* and *ought*. Discussions of particular ethical problems or policies were considered unphilosophical and best left to theologians and policy makers. A sea change occurred partly as a result of the demand of students in the 1960s for education that was "relevant" and partly as a result of advances in medicine that raised new ethical questions and dilemmas. A number of centers and institutes dedicated to ethics and policy were created where philosophers, often working with individuals in other disciplines, could examine the normative and conceptual issues raised in medicine, law, and other professions.

The result of all this activity has been an extensive literature in bioethics. Bioethicists have written on a wide range of issues including the doctor–patient relationship, confidentiality, informed consent, medical experimentation, the definition of death, euthanasia and physician-assisted suicide, genetic testing and manipulation, abortion, assisted reproduction, and many others. Some of these issues, such as genetic screening and assisted reproduction, can be examined from a public health perspective as well as from the more individualistic perspective typical of biomedical ethics. Some issues, such as alcohol and drug policy or domestic violence, are unlikely to be represented in medical ethics texts. Much of the discussion on these various issues is factual. It focuses on the likely consequences of various policies. Equally important are conceptual tools used to assess both consequences and the means to achieve them. This is where ethical theory has a role to play. There are many different ethical theories. The aim of this Introduction is not to provide a thorough depiction or analysis of all of them. The intention is rather to provide students of public health or public policy who have not had courses in ethical theory with enough background to be able to understand and evaluate the ethical arguments made in this book.

MORALITY, ETHICS, AND MORAL PHILOSOPHY

We start with some terminology. The word *ethics* can be used to refer to the set of rules, principles, values, and ideals of a particular group of people. This is called its descriptive sense. Thus, we might contrast the ethics of the Puritans with the ethics of the Hawaiian Islanders. The word *ethics* can also be used to refer to the systematic study of moral concepts and theories, typically in departments of philosophy. Some philosophers use the term *morality* to refer to ethics in its descriptive sense, that is, concerning the beliefs of particular groups of people about right and wrong, reserving the term *ethics* (or *moral philosophy* or *ethical theory*) for the subject taught in departments of philosophy. However, this usage is not universal, and we use the terms *ethics* and *morality* interchangeably. Students will have to examine the context to determine whether the subject is a group's beliefs about right and wrong or the theoretical study of moral beliefs and concepts.

Theories of morality can be divided roughly into two kinds. *Normative ethics* is primarily concerned with providing a theoretical or foundational basis for how people ought to behave, while *metaethics* is primarily concerned with analyzing the meanings of central ethical terms like *good, right, duty,* and *obligation.* The two are not as rigidly separate as it might at first seem, because normative issues often turn on our interpretation of difficult concepts. For example, an issue in population policy is whether coercive means of reducing population growth are permissible. Clearly, forced abortions and the mandatory contraception of unwilling women are coercive means. But is coercion limited to threats of inflicting harm or can offers and incentives in some contexts also be coercive? For example, it has been charged that laws increasing the welfare payments of women who agree to have Norplant, a long-acting contraceptive, implanted, are a form of coercion. Others reject this label, saying that women who prefer to have more children are not deprived of the payments they would have received. Therefore, they are not harmed or made worse off because of their choice. Nor are they forced to choose the higher welfare payments. The critics of such statutes respond that the "choice" to receive higher payments or have more children is really "no choice," given the poverty in which welfare recipients live. This issue cannot be resolved without a persuasive analysis of the concept of coercion. (Of course, even if incentives are determined not to be coercive, they may be objectionable on a number of other grounds. By the same token, the mere fact that a policy is coercive is not a conclusive reason for regarding it as morally impermissible. Most laws are coercive, but they are not for that reason wrong.)

We see, then, that conceptual analysis is part of ethical and policy analysis. Equally important are normative ethical theories: theories about what makes right actions right (and wrong actions wrong). Such theories are not simply descriptions of what is conventionally considered right or wrong behavior in a particular society or group. Instead, normative ethics attempts to identify and justify basic moral principles and to derive from them guidance for what we ought to do and what kind of people we should strive to become. The basic principles, values, character traits, and so forth can then be applied to specific ethical issues, such as whether there should be mandatory acquired immuno-deficiency syndrome (AIDS) testing in hospitals, when to begin population screening for genetic diseases, and what sort of alcohol and drug policies we should have.

THEORY AND PRACTICE

As we will see, different ethical theories provide different basic principles for deciding what is right or wrong, what should be done or avoided. However, ethical decision making is almost never a matter of automatically applying principles and generating an answer. There are several reasons why this is so. One reason is that the right thing to do often depends on the facts of the case, and these may be difficult to ascertain. For example, at the beginning of the HIV-AIDS epidemic there was much discussion about whether public health officials should close gay bathhouses. Those who argued in favor said that the bathhouses, which were places where men could engage in sex with dozens of partners, were breeding grounds for the spread of disease. Those who opposed said that closing the bathhouses would not change behavior. Men would continue to have multiple partners in more private settings, and the opportunity to educate people about safe sex would be lost. Both sides made a plausible case and it was not obvious which strategy would reduce the spread of AIDS.

Another reason why principles cannot be used to generate solutions in any straightforward way is that they sometimes conflict with one another as well as with other values or goals. For example, an important principle or goal of public health is to reduce the incidence of disease. Genetic diseases can be prevented by screening people to find out who are carriers and then attempting to influence them not to reproduce and thereby pass on genes that cause disease. But it can be argued that any attempt to influence individuals' reproductive decision making violates another important principle, namely, self-determination or autonomy. Which value—the reduction of disease or respect for autonomy—should take precedence? The answer is not obvious. Thus, even if we could decide which ethical theory is the correct one, the application of that theory to specific practical issues will often be indeterminate or controversial. In any event, there is no consensus about the right ethical theory. This fact is often discouraging to students, who may become cynical about the value of studying moral philosophy. What's the point, if no one can say whether utilitarianism is superior to Kantian ethics, or if both are superseded by contractarianism or virtue ethics or feminist approaches?

We maintain that this disillusionment is unwarranted. The purpose of studying moral philosophy is not to discover which ethical theory "has it right"; rather, different ethical theories provide insight into a range of important considerations. Utilitarians are right to insist on the relevance of consequences and the importance of securing happiness and well-being, but their critics (nonconsequentialists) are equally right in insisting that there are other important values, such as justice and self-determination, which cannot be reduced to happiness. It seems increasingly likely that no one moral theory is the whole story. Rather, each represents a partial contribution to an extraordinarily complex moral reality.

ETHICS AND RELIGION

For many people, morality is identified with religion. The reasons for this are fairly obvious: All major religions—Judaism, Christianity, Islam, Hinduism, and Buddhism—have ethical teachings associated with them, and the fundamental ethical tenets of virtually all societies are based on religious teachings. Moreover, many people receive their moral training in religious institutions, such as church, synagogue, or Sunday school. This may lead them to think that ethics *must* be based in religious teaching. However, there is no necessary connection between religion and ethics. A person can be ethical and a nonbeliever. A completely secular ethics is perfectly possible, although it undoubtedly will coincide with the teachings of most religions in certain respects.

Moreover, religious tenets themselves can be subjected to moral assessment. For example, the doctrine of purgatory in Christianity was developed in response to the feeling of many Christians that it was cruel and unfair to commit unbaptized infants to eternal damnation. More recently, some Christian churches have rejected the traditional teachings of Christianity regarding homosexuality or the ordination of women, based on moral arguments. Such moral evaluations of religious teachings would be literally impossible if morality were merely a function of religion.

ETHICS AND LAW

Another source of guidance regarding how we should behave is the law. The law may reflect a society's moral consensus on issues such as abortion, surrogate motherhood, or physician-assisted suicide. Interpretation of what the law is often requires normative ethical analysis, as evidenced by legal writings, such as judicial decisions, amicus briefs, and articles by law professors. For example, in the landmark case of *Brown* v. *Board of Education* (347 U.S. 483, 1954), the Supreme Court was faced with the question of whether racially segregated public schools are constitutionally permissible. The Supreme Court decided that segregated schools violate the Constitution, even if the facilities in white and black schools are (as they never were in fact) equal. They are inherently unequal, and so violate the equal protection clause of the Fourteenth Amendment, because the intention and effect of racial segregation is to degrade, stigmatize, and deny equal opportunity to Negro children. The Court's decision was not a narrowly legalistic one, but was based on substantive moral analysis of the concept of equality as it has evolved in the context of American institutions, traditions, and history.

The law may also be viewed as providing limits on what can and cannot be done. For example, federal rules governing medical experiments forbid the use of human subjects without their informed consent or that of a court-appointed surrogate. The rules settle the question of whether an experiment may be done; any study that uses people without their informed consent is impermissible. However, although legal considerations sometimes determine what may or may not be done, and legal considerations are often relevant to moral decisions, the law, no more than religion, does not determine morality. For one thing, just as religious teachings can be criticized on moral grounds, so too can the law. Sometimes this results in changes in the law. For another, it may sometimes be right to violate the law, although determining when this would be justified is obviously a complex ethical issue.

ETHICS AND POLICY

Because of its concern with populations, public health tends to have a macro focus, that is, it tends to be concerned with institutions and policies rather than relations between individuals. To put it another way, public health is a species of public policy. Public policy certainly includes ethical considerations, but it must also consider nonethical factors, such as politics. For example, a single-payer system of health care, such as is found in Canada and Europe, might be the fairest and most efficient system, but it may not be politically feasible in the United States, at least at the present time. Policy makers who ignore political realities do so at their peril. At the same time, existing policies and institutions (like religion and the law) can be criticized on moral grounds. National advisory bodies, such as the President's Commission for the Study of Ethical Problems in Medicine and Biomedical and Behavioral Research or the more recent National Bioethics Advisory Commission, offer recommendations on a range of issues, stressing such moral principles as respect for persons and justice.

As we have seen, ethics is related to, but separate from, religion, law, and policy. Before turning to some of the most influential ethical approaches, we will consider some challenges to ethics.

ETHICAL NIHILISM AND RELATIVISM

A source of cynicism about moral philosophy comes from the conviction—or suspicion—that there is no such thing as *moral reality*. This is known as *ethical nihilism* and it can take several forms. One version of ethical nihilism maintains that morality is simply an illusion, like religion, and something we should get over. This implies that there's nothing really wrong with raping, torturing, and murdering a child. While it is difficult to know how to go about disproving this extreme nihilist claim, it is so far from the experience of virtually everyone that it is even more difficult to take it seriously.

A more plausible version of nihilism claims that morality simply reflects the interests of those in power. This view, originally stated by Thrasymachus in Plato's *Republic*, is also reflected in Marxist theory, as well as in contemporary critical legal theory and postmodernism. It must be admitted that not only the laws and institutions of society, but its moral beliefs, are typically formulated and propagated by people in positions of power. They may impose what promotes their own self-interest on the downtrodden masses while hoodwinking the masses into believing that they are morally required to do what they are told to do. This sort of cynicism about morality seems most plausible in totalitarian regimes. However, even if power is more widely dispersed, as in a democracy, a variation of the criticism can be made. That is, it can be objected that what is claimed to be "objective morality" is nothing but disguised self-interest. Thus, people with well-paying jobs or other sources of income—the *haves*—may view their economic status as something they have worked for, and therefore morally deserve, while the *have-nots* may regard the more fortunate as beneficiaries of an unjust economic system which profits from the existence of an underclass. There is no objectively correct moral answer, according to this version of moral nihilism, but only the self-interest of the respective parties.

We can certainly acknowledge the ability of those in power to control behavior, ideology, and even the interpretation of history. We can also recognize that self-interest may skew people's moral beliefs. It does not follow, however, that morality is *nothing but* the expression of the interests of those in power. An important distinction can be drawn between *conventional morality* or the rules and values currently accepted and promulgated, and *critical* or *ideal* morality, which can be used to assess conventional morality. If morality were just the interests of the powerful, as Marxist theory alleges, it would be literally impossible to condemn on *moral* grounds the behavior and policies of those in power. Yet this is exactly what Marxist and other critics of capitalism attempt to do! The very existence of intelligible social criticism rests on the possibility of a critical or ideal morality which is not identified with the interests of those in power.

A related form of nihilism is *ethical relativism.* Ethical relativism does not say that morality is merely an illusion or something to get over. Nor does it identify morality with the interests of the powerful. Rather, it claims that morality is relative to the mores, values, standards, or rules of a particular culture. What is right for one culture may be wrong for another. Thus, in one culture, premarital sex may be regarded as normal and healthy, while in another it may be regarded as sinful. There is no way to determine which culture is correct about the morality of premarital sex. Indeed, the question does not even make sense because morality is always relative to a particular culture. There is no right and wrong independent of culture.

A major advantage of ethical relativism is its ability to explain the variation in moral beliefs and customs throughout the world. Ethical relativism seems superior to an absolutist conception of morality which maintains that there is one true moral code and that any divergence from that code is immorality. Such a view seems arrogant and presumptuous in the face of the moral diversity of different cultures. Another point in favor of relativism is its recognition that moral beliefs and practices can only be understood within the context of a culture. A practice that at first sight appears irrational or abhorrent may come to make sense when we understand both the material conditions in which it occurs and its symbolic significance. The more we understand a culture, the less likely we are to misinterpret its moral beliefs.

At the same time, ethical relativism has consequences that are difficult to accept. For example, the Nazis thought that Aryans were a superior people and that certain groups—Jews, gypsies, Slavs, etc.—should be deported, enslaved, or exterminated. If ethical relativism is true, then the fact that they believed that it is morally right to exterminate Jews makes it morally right—for them. Ethical relativism rules out the possibility of saying that their behavior was immoral, wicked, and wrong. Is there a way to acknowledge legitimate variations in moral beliefs without proclaiming that whatever people think is right is right—for them?

A first step might be to challenge the seemingly obvious claim that morality differs among cultures. While this may be true in relation to views about (permissible) sex and marriage arrangements, it is less clear that such variation exists as regards basic or fundamental principles of morality, such as the wrongness of lying, stealing, assault, and murder. These acts seem to be universally condemned, undoubtedly because no group can continue to exist where distrust and aggression are the norm. Thus, despite initial appearances, there may be some universal norms due to the very nature of morality as a mechanism enabling people to live together in groups. A second important point is that it does not follow from the mere fact that people in different cultures have different beliefs about morality that their beliefs are correct or justifiable, any more than it follows from the fact that people have different beliefs about the physical world that all their beliefs are equally correct. The mere fact that some people think the world is flat or that disease is caused by devils doesn't make it so (or even "true for them"). It means only that they sincerely (and mistakenly) believe it.

However, ethical relativists may argue that this is precisely the point. While we can offer objective evidence that the world is round, not flat, or that disease is caused by microorganisms, not devils, it is impossible to offer objective evidence about morality. But is this in fact the case? Consider the 19th-century claim that slavery was morally justified. This rested in part on a belief in the intrinsic inferiority of the Africans who were captured and enslaved. It was said that they were incapable of taking care of themselves, incapable of learning, incapable of the emotions their masters felt (such as anguish at the sale of their spouses or children). Not only is this clearly nonsense in hindsight, but it seems that at some level even those who made the claims must have known them to be false. After all, why make teaching a slave to read illegal if slaves are incapable of learning to read?

The point here is that objective, scientific facts play a significant role in moral judgments and constitute a basis for accepting or rejecting moral beliefs. The practice of clitoridectomy or female circumcision provides a good example. This practice, common to certain groups in Africa, is usually performed at puberty, although it may be done on very young children. The girl is held down by older women while her clitoris, or a portion of it, is removed. Anesthesia is not used, and the procedure is done with unsterilized razor blades or knives. In the more radical versions of the procedure, the entire genitalia are removed. The lips of the vulva are sewn up, with only a small hole for urination and menstrual blood. The purpose of clitorectomy is to reduce sexual pleasure and remove the temptation to sexual activity; the vulva is sewn up to ensure that the young woman will remain a virgin until her marriage. In cultures in which the practice is widespread, it may be difficult or impossible for an uncircumcised girl to marry.

Public health professionals and women's health activists around the world have condemned the practice, calling it "female genital mutilation." Not only is it extremely painful when performed, it can have repercussions throughout the woman's life, especially for those subjected to the radical surgery where the entire external genitalia is cut off. Intercourse is more difficult and painful, and childbirth more dangerous. Ironically, those who engage in the practice believe that it is necessary for cleanliness and conducive to fertility. In fact, circumcised women are more susceptible to infection and sexually transmitted diseases and are often rendered infertile. Insofar as the justification for the practice rests on incorrect factual beliefs, it can be rejected without challenging the moral beliefs of those who accept it.

However, the objection to female genital mutilation is not solely based on its adverse health consequences. Feminists also reject the set of beliefs which underlie the practice: that it is wrong for women to experience sexual pleasure, that female virginity must be preserved, that women's bodies are the property of their husbands, that it is permissible to mutilate the bodies of women to keep them meek, submissive, and sexually pure. The contribution of feminism has been to show that such beliefs are endemic to patriarchy and inconsistent with the recognition of women as full human persons entitled to equality and justice.

To summarize, ethical relativism has something to teach us, namely, that human cultures have diverse moral beliefs, many of which are equally valid. Moreover, to understand beliefs that differ from our own, it is necessary to understand them in the context of an entire culture and belief system. But it does not follow that *whatever* people believe is right or immune from moral criticism. Moreover, our own cherished beliefs can also be challenged, something which ethical relativism rules out on principle. In fact, it is only if we *reject* relativism that we can learn from other cultures. For example, we can criticize our own materialistic and wasteful attitudes in contrast with those of most American Indian tribes. Such criticism implies an objective, nonrelativistic standpoint from which we can critically examine our own attitudes and habits as well as those of other cultures.

METHODS FOR RESOLVING OR UNDERSTANDING ETHICAL QUESTIONS

Once we free ourselves from the thrall of ethical relativism, the next question is, How can ethical disagreements be resolved? If ethical progress is possible, how is it possible? On what basis can we arrive at solutions to the problems we face?

An obvious component of understanding and resolving ethical issues in public health is factual information. For example, recombinant DNA technology expands the possibility of screening for genetic disease. A recent issue has been whether there should be mandatory newborn screening for cystic fibrosis (CF).

A host of factual questions arises. For example, what is the accuracy of the proposed test? Will routine or mandatory screening help to identify affected children earlier and improve the treatment of affected newborns? Or will parents become unduly protective of children shown to be affected by pre-symptomatic tests? How much will presymptomatic screening cost and will there be adequate counseling for the parents of affected newborns? Would this be the most effective use of funds to improve the lives of those who have CF?

Sometimes these factual questions are not resolved or even addressed before a policy is put into place. For example, a pilot study of newborn screening for CF was begun in Colorado in 1982, but mandatory screening was legislated even before it was completed! And where a prospective controlled study was done (in Wisconsin), the benefits of routine screening were not demonstrated.[1] This suggests that mass screening programs of newborns and others are some-times driven by political considerations rather than solidly based on scientific evidence. Politicians have an understandable if not always creditable desire to be seen as "doing something," even if that "something" has not been shown to be valuable and could turn out to be harmful. In addition, the role of profit in screening decisions cannot be ignored. As Benjamin Wilfond notes:

> Within weeks of the announcement of the cloning of the cystic fibrosis gene in September 1989, biotechnology companies began marketing the DNA-based test to physicians. Because the initial charge for cystic fibrosis carrier testing was over $200, a mass screening program of pregnant women could have translated into a billion-dollar-a-year industry.[2]

Facts—scientifically based evidence—are crucial to determining good public policy, but facts by themselves cannot indicate which policies should be implemented. Facts can influence policy only when the goals to be achieved are delineated. Despite a recognition that goals may differ in different cultures and different communities, there are some goals and principles that have widespread acceptance. These include benefiting individuals (for example, by decreasing disease and improving their health), respect for self-determination, equality, and justice. Of course, the interpretation of these goals and principles is varied, as are beliefs about which policies are most likely to promote them. Moreover, sometimes goals and principles can conflict. When they do, a strategy for prioritizing them is useful. This is a major reason for the appeal to ethical theory.

ETHICAL THEORIES

Philosophers are often interested in ethical theory as providing a single key to morality. Classical utilitarians regard the maximization of happiness or pleasure as the ultimate goal, and everything else as reducible to happiness. Kantians regard happiness as relatively insignificant morally, and in any event deny that principles like justice or respect for autonomy can be reduced to happiness. Virtue theorists maintain that there has been an overemphasis on right actions and too little attention paid to the kinds of people we should strive to become, while feminists and Marxists claim that power relations are essential to an adequate moral theory. Communitarians deplore the excessively individualistic turn in modern moral philosophy, whether utilitarian or Kantian, and emphasize the importance of shared traditions, values, and goals, as well as the impact of actions and policies on the community considered as a whole rather than as a collection of individuals with separate interests.

Our aim here is not to determine the "correct" moral theory. Indeed, we are dubious that any one moral theory has a monopoly on truth. Probably all of them have something to contribute to the understanding of something as complex and multifaceted as morality. Two of them, utilitarianism and Kantian moral theory, have been dominant in both moral thinking and public policy. At least a rudimentary acquaintance with these theories is essential for understanding the readings in this anthology. However, a third, communitarianism, is particularly appropriate for the aggregate approach to policy exemplified by public health.

UTILITARIANISM

Classical utilitarianism was formulated in the 19th century by Jeremy Bentham and John Stuart Mill, although it built on ideas that go back at least as far as the ancient Greeks. The heart of utilitarianism is "the greatest happiness principle," which holds that actions are right insofar as they tend to promote the greatest happiness of the greatest number, wrong as they tend to promote the reverse.[3]

The first thing to note about the utilitarian tradition is its emphasis on the likely consequences of whatever is under consideration. Actions, policies, motives, and so forth are all judged to be right or wrong, good or bad in terms of their expected consequences. Thus, utilitarianism is a form of consequentialism. Not all consequentialists are utilitarians, but since utilitarianism is the most familiar and influential consequentialist theory, it is the one on which we will focus. Second, the overarching goal to be achieved is pleasure or happiness, where pleasure and happiness are understood, not as transient states of mind or feelings, but rather as total well-being. The theory of value that maintains that pleasure or happiness is the ultimate good is known as *hedonism*. According to hedonism, pleasure is the only thing that is intrinsically good; all other good things—health, knowledge, friendship, love, for example—are desirable because of the happiness they bring. Pain is intrinsically bad, although pain may be good if the experience of pain ultimately brings more pleasure or avoidance of pain. Thus, vaccination is good, even though it hurts, because it avoids the greater harm of serious disease.

Contemporary utilitarians have by and large rejected hedonism, for several reasons. First, happiness is hard to define and even harder to measure. If it is equated to pleasure, considered as episodic sensations, then happiness can be quantified, but it is hard to believe that a life of pleasant sensations is the ultimate good. Happiness is more plausible as the ultimate end if we conceive of it as not limited to pleasant sensations but more globally as the satisfaction of goals contributing to well-being. However, this conception makes quantification and interpersonal comparison, which are essential to utilitarianism, extremely difficult.

Another reason for the rejection of hedonism is that the reduction of all goals and values to happiness, even on the broader interpretation of happiness, is implausible. Knowledge, art, and meaningfulness are all values, and it is far from clear either that these reduce to an aspect of happiness or that these things are valued because they contribute to happiness. They may be valued for themselves, independent of how happy they make people. For these reasons, contemporary utilitarians are more likely to think of the ultimate end not as happiness or pleasure but rather as the satisfaction of individual preferences.

An important question for any moral theory is how it determines which individuals or entities are entitled to moral consideration or moral status. Utilitarians generally consider *sentience,* or the ability to experience pain and pleasure, to be the important feature in deciding who counts or who has moral status. Given a hedonist theory of value, the emphasis on sentience is not surprising. But even preference utilitarians tend to consider sentience an important marker for moral status. This is because nonsentient beings (plants, rocks, buildings) do not have preferences and cannot be happy or unhappy. Thus, sentience is a necessary condition for inclusion in the utilitarian calculus. It is also considered a sufficient condition. That is, if a being suffers, there is no justification for ignoring that suffering, whatever other characteristics it may have or lack. As Bentham said, "The question is not can they reason? Nor can they talk? But can they suffer?"[4] The principle of utility is to be applied not only to all human beings but also, as Mill said, to all sentient creation, as far as is possible.[5] (Some contemporary utilitarians think that it is a good deal more possible than Bentham or Mill were willing to acknowledge. Peter Singer, for example, has argued not merely that animals count, but that they count as much as human beings.[6])

The third point about utilitarianism is that it is a maximizing theory. That is, the right action or policy is the one that achieves the greatest happiness possible. There is only one right action in any situation: the one that maximizes happiness or welfare. Fourth, utilitarianism is an egalitarian theory insofar as it insists that everyone's happiness is to be considered equally.

There are several features that make utilitarianism an attractive theory. One is that it provides a method for deciding which is the right action or policy, namely, the one that produces more good (however this is defined) than other alternatives. Another is that its goals are clearly important ones. What is the point of morality, it may be asked, if not to promote happiness and reduce misery? Surely rules have no intrinsic value unless they achieve good results. Even someone who bases his conception of right and wrong on what God wants must ask *why* God wants us to do certain things and abstain from others. Following the Ten Commandments and the Golden Rule is likely to result in a happier world; this certainly was the way Mill regarded it.[7]

The possibility remains, however, that in certain situations actions which maximize happiness could conflict with other values, such as honesty and fairness. A major objection to utilitarianism is that it could countenance great injustice, such as knowingly condemning an innocent person to prevent mob violence that would result in the deaths of many more innocent persons. Utilitarians respond by saying that this objection fails to consider the total, long-term effects of unjust or dishonest actions. Mill emphasized the destructive effects lying has on trust, saying that these bad effects could rarely, if ever, be outweighed by the good effects to be achieved by deception.[8] Moreover, the temptation to lie is often motivated by self-interest rather than a dispassionate and accurate assessment of the general utility. Recognition of this tendency requires us to adhere in most cases to what Mill called *secondary principles,* such as the rule against lying, as our best bet for achieving the greatest happiness. At the same time, Mill acknowledged that there may be rare instances in which it is justified to break a moral rule—for example, to lie to save a life.

In creating social policy, we often rely on utilitarian reasoning and the notion of the greatest good for the greatest number. For example, a policy requiring that all persons be immunized, with few exceptions, is likely to be most effective in combating communicable diseases. At the same time, it might expose a few, rare, susceptible individuals to vaccine-related damage or even death. Most people would find this acceptable, because the good of universal vaccination outweighs the harm to a few. Nevertheless, the idea that the good of the majority can cancel out the welfare of the few has led to the criticism that utilitarianism devalues individuals and individual rights.

Resistance to utilitarian reasoning can be seen in other examples. Should society compel people to participate in genetic screening or even abortion in order to reduce the number of people born with serious genetic defects? Such a policy would reduce the costs of caring for such individuals and might be rational from a utilitarian standpoint. There is widespread agreement that even if such a policy did promote "the greatest happiness of the greatest number," it would nonetheless be morally unacceptable. As the President's Commission said in *Genetic Screening and Counseling:*

> The chief objection to this argument is that it rests upon a general principle that few, if any, would wish to see consistently implemented—namely, that a person's freedom to make the most intimate choices, and even a person's very existence, depends upon the degree to which social utility is maximized. . . . Rather than finding utilitarianism particularly appropriate in determining social policy on genetics programs, the contrary appears to be the case, in light of the especially strong reasons to preserve individual liberty on matters of medical treatment and reproduction.[9]

It is likely that most utilitarians would opt for a principle of voluntariness with regard to reproductive decisions and try to justify such a principle on utilitarian grounds. Their argument would be that a society in which people's most intimate choices were regulated by state interference would be unlikely to be one that promoted the greatest happiness. Mill himself argued in *On Liberty* that a society that allowed for the greatest amount possible of individual liberty would be the happiest. However, there is no guarantee that this coincidence between the greatest liberty and the greatest happiness will obtain. Policies that are justified on grounds of social utility might conflict with other equally important principles, such as liberty, autonomy, equality, or justice.

KANTIAN ETHICS

Although Immanuel Kant (1724–1804) lived before the classical utilitarians, Kantian ethics is best understood as a critique of the utilitarian approach (which after all was not entirely new with Bentham and Mill).[10] Kant rejected both the theory of value associated with utilitarianism (hedonism) and its consequentialism. In contrast to the utilitarian emphasis on sentience as the basis for moral status, Kant regards the capacity for experiencing pain and pleasure as morally fairly insignificant. Instead, he emphasizes the connection between morality and reason. Reason is what separates man (human beings) from the rest of the animals and what makes us subject to the moral law. Our capacity for rational thought both entitles us to treatment and rights to which animals are not entitled and imposes on us obligations that animals do not have. Animals are not morally required to refrain from murder, theft, and deception. Indeed, these concepts cannot even be applied to animal behavior. Only rational creatures, capable of knowing the difference between right and wrong, can be responsible moral agents.

Of course, the fact that normal adult human beings are capable of rational thought (and thus are moral agents) does not entail that they will always behave morally, that is, in a morally correct fashion. To call people moral agents is not to deny that they may be immoral but rather to say that they are *responsible for* their behavior, that they can be *blamed* for acting wrongly. By contrast, infants, severely retarded individuals, and most animals are not capable of understanding the difference between right and wrong. Whether some primates, such as gorillas and chimpanzees, and perhaps other mammals, such as dolpins, have a moral sense is a debatable point. Nevertheless, even if these animals behave altruistically and reciprocally, it is unlikely that they can be considered moral agents in the way that most humans are. Certainly most animals, like babies and very young children, are not responsible, nor would it be appropriate to blame them for any harm they might cause. Animals can often be trained to act in certain ways by rewards and punishments, but they are not capable of being motivated by moral reasons (such as, "You wouldn't like it if he did that to you").

Kant also objected to consequentialism. It is not the consequences of an act that make it right or wrong. For what happens as the result of what you do is not wholly within your control. It is perfectly possible that doing the right thing will have disastrous consequences and that wrong actions may result in unexpected good results. Basing morality on the consequences makes it altogether too contingent, depriving it of the necessity which Kant regarded as essential to the possibility of morality and a moral law.

Does this mean that Kantian ethics tells us to ignore consequences? If that were the case, we would have to reject Kantian ethics as absurd. In deciding which course of action to take, of course we need to think about the impact on others. Rather, consequences are relevant for Kant only if the proposed action is morally permissible. And the permissibility of an action is not determined by the consequences.

If the permissibility of an action is not determined by its consequences, how is it determined? Or to put the question another way, What makes right actions right and wrong actions wrong? There is widespread agreement that certain actions are wrong, such as lying, stealing, cheating, and harming others. The fundamental question for Kant is *why* these things are wrong. The utilitarian answer is that such actions predictably lead to human misery. Kant considers this answer to be inadequate. He would say that even if no one gets hurt by a wrong action, even if it promotes more happiness than unhappiness, that does not make it right. Lying, stealing, murder are intrinsically wrong; they cannot be made right by their creation of happiness.

Take cheating on examinations, for example. The utilitarian objection is based on the expected bad consequences. Would you want someone who graduated from law school or medical school by cheating to be your lawyer or doctor? Of course not. In addition, cheating quickly becomes insidious and demoralizes those who do not cheat. If "everyone is doing it" and getting away with it, why put the effort into actually learning the material? The negative consequences of cheating are easily demonstrated.

However, these utilitarian objections to cheating could be met in certain circumstances. What if only a few people cheat while most remain honest? It is far from obvious that an isolated instance of cheating will necessarily have more bad effects than good. Nor is it always the case that successful cheating results in an unqualified person posing a risk to others. Imagine, for example, a very good student in a college with an honor code who accidentally comes across the answers to his physical anatomy exam. This gives him the opportunity to "ace" what will certainly be a very difficult exam and improve considerably his chances of getting into a top medical school. Should he use the answers? It seems obvious that this would be wrong but it is not clear that the wrongness stems from the consequences. It cannot be said that cheating in this situation will enable an unqualified student to go on to practice medicine, since we are assuming that the student is qualified. Yet this will not guarantee him a place in medical school, given the competition for admission. Of course, there is the chance that he will be found out, in which case he may be expelled. But what if the chances of anyone finding out that he has seen the answers are extremely low? If no one finds out, then the subsequent demoralization and widespread cheating that are often alleged to be the consequences of particular acts of cheating will not occur. From a consequentialist perspective, the likelihood of the bad effects actually occurring is all-important. Yet most of us do not base the judgment that he should not use the answers on how probable it is that he will be caught, or what the effect on other students will be, or whether he will go on to a brilliant medical career. Instead, if asked *why* it is wrong for him to use the answers even if none of these bad consequences will occur, we are likely simply to say, "It's still cheating." This captures the Kantian idea that the morally relevant consideration is not the consequences of the act but the kind of act it is. An act can have the best consequences—for example, save the most lives, make the greatest number of people happiest—and still be morally wrong.

If consequences do not determine the rightness or wrongness of actions, what then is the mark of right and wrong for Kant? Kant suggests that when we want to know if a proposed action (like cheating on an exam) is morally permissible, the question to ask ourselves is not What are the likely consequences of doing this act? but rather Can I, as a rational agent, consistently will that everyone should act as I am now proposing to act? If we turn this question into an action-guiding principle (what Kant calls a *command* or an *imperative*), we get, "Act only on the maxim of an action that you can consistently will universally." Kant calls this principle the *Categorical Imperative*. What does it mean?

The intuitive idea is that morality requires us not to make exceptions of ourselves. We are not morally permitted to do things that we would regard as wrong if done by others. It does not matter that no one gets hurt as a result. An action is wrong if you cannot consistently will that everyone in this situation act in the way you propose to act.

How is this applied to the example of cheating? A typical misunderstanding is that universalizing the maxim (from "I should cheat" to "Everyone should cheat") would have bad results. If everyone cheated, then exams would be useless, and that would be unfortunate, since exams are a good way to determine who is most qualified. However, this interpretation is not Kantian, but utilitarian, specifically rule-utilitarian, since it is based on the advantage to society of having exams. Kant's point is importantly different. The wrongness of cheating is not based on the social utility of having an examination system. Rather, Kant notes that there is an inherent contradiction in the idea of cheating being adopted as a universal policy. It is this feature that makes it impossible for a rational agent to will such a policy.

What makes cheating as a universal policy self-contradictory? When I consider cheating, I am thinking of acting on something like the following maxim: I should cheat whenever that will enable me to get a better grade. If I apply this universally, it becomes: Everyone should cheat when cheating will enable him or her to get a better grade. In willing this, I am willing two contradictory things:

1. That there be examinations. For if there weren't, I couldn't get a better grade, or indeed any grade at all. Whatever advantage accrues to me from doing well on examinations requires that there be examinations in the first place.

2. That there be no examinations. For if everyone cheated, an examination system could not exist. The very existence of an examination system depends on most people not cheating. If everyone cheated, there would be no point to examinations, and the system would self-destruct.

Someone who refrains from cheating, not out of fear of getting caught, and not even because she thinks that cheating will have bad consequences for everyone, but simply because she recognizes that it is wrong (that is, that it contravenes the Categorical Imperative), acts from the motive of duty. For Kant, only those acts done from the motive of duty have genuine moral worth. Acts done out of sympathy, for example, lack real moral worth, although they are certainly not wrong and indeed should be encouraged.

This is perhaps the hardest aspect of Kantian ethics to understand. Why should not feelings be a source of moral behavior? Why should not an action that derives from sympathy be as morally praiseworthy as one done out of a sense of duty? Kant's answer is that our feelings are not something we can control, and therefore they are not something for which we can be held responsible. Rational agents can be expected to act rightly (that is, consistently with the Categorical Imperative), but not to have certain feelings. Indeed, doing the right thing (sharing one's possessions, helping others) is more praiseworthy if one does it even when one is feeling antisocial and misanthropic.

A central Kantian idea is that persons are ends in themselves, who have values and goals and make choices and decisions. As rational agents, persons have dignity and are entitled to respect. To treat individuals as persons is to respect their values and choices, insofar as these are morally permissible. This means that people must never be treated merely as the means to others' ends. This notion is used to explain the importance of obtaining informed consent from patients and human subjects used in medical and scientific experiments. One of the most blatant examples of the violation of the principle of informed consent occurred in the Tuskegee Syphilis Experiment.

Between 1932 and 1972 the United States Public Health Service (PHS) conducted an investigation into the natural history of untreated syphilis on 399 black men from Macon County, Alabama. The purpose of the experiment was to find out if racial differences affected the course of the disease. The men were led to believe that they were part of a select group receiving special medical care. In fact, they were receiving no care at all for their syphilis.

In 1932, when the study began, there was no effective treatment for syphilis. Victims were usually given arsenic, which had little if any ameliorative, and no curative, effect. It was not until after World War II that penicillin became available as a treatment for syphilis. Therefore, at least at the beginning of the experiment, the men were not deprived of treatment that might have cured them or lessened their symptoms. Indeed, the health of some of the men was undoubtedly improved due to their participation because they got medical care for other conditions that would have gone untreated.

However, the Tuskegee Syphilis Experiment continued until 1972, long after the discovery of penicillin. Men who could have been cured of a devastating disease were allowed to go blind and mad and ultimately die. They were certainly harmed by the withholding of penicillin, and thus the experiment can be condemned on purely utilitarian grounds. It might be countered that, prior to the establishment of Medicaid, the government had no obligation to provide syphilis sufferers with medical treatment, but even if this is true, it certainly had an obligation not to deceive individuals about effective medical treatment in order to get them to participate in the experiment. The Tuskegee Syphilis Experiment is a shameful episode in the history of the Public Health Service, as was acknowledged by President Clinton on May 16, 1997, when he apologized to the few remaining survivors and their relatives.[11] The wrongness was compounded by the harmful effects that occurred when penicillin was available and withheld, but the experiment was wrong from its inception, even before a cure was available. This judgment is best explained in Kantian terms. It is wrong to conduct medical experiments, regardless of their potential social value and independent of the harm that may be inflicted, on persons who have not given their free and informed consent. To use people in this way is to treat them as mere means, rather than ends in themselves.

Public health has a clear utilitarian or consequentialist component. It aims to promote human welfare and reduce human misery, and is solidly based on factual evidence. At the same time, it is limited by Kantian or deontological considerations, such as respect for persons and their rights. The hard questions arise when individual rights clash with the general welfare. Rights-theorists maintain that rights "trump" consideration of the general welfare, but surely this depends on the nature and significance of the right claimed as well as the magnitude of risk to the general population. This issue is particularly important when considering such topics as genetic screening, reproductive decision making, AIDS, and alcohol and drug policy.

COMMUNITARIAN ETHICS

Despite their differences, utilitarianism and Kantian ethics share some presuppositions. Both regard the individual as the focal point of moral concern. Although utilitarianism seeks to promote the greatest happiness of the greatest number, it determines what that is by reference to individual preferences. Kantian ethics also focuses on individuals in its insistence that the rights and dignity of the individual should never be sacrificed for the welfare of the whole. Both ethical approaches also share the idea that since different individuals have different values and different conceptions of the good life, society should remain neutral between these conceptions and not adopt any particular conception to the exclusion of others. The Categorical Imperative, for example, is consistent with many different ways of life. It gives very little positive guidance on how best to live. And while the Principle of Utility instructs us to maximize welfare, it leaves the determination of what constitutes an individual's welfare up to the individual. Mill was particularly insistent that the individual is best positioned to know what is in his or her own interest.

Recently, there has been a reaction to the emphasis on the individual in the dominant ethical theories by a somewhat disparate group of theorists who can be labeled "communitarians." Communitarians reject the notion of timeless, universal ethical truths based on reason. Instead they maintain that our moral thinking has its source in historical traditions of particular communities. Communities are not simply collections of individuals who happen to inhabit the same geographical area. Rather, they are composed of people who share customs, institutions, and values. These provide the starting point from which attempts to solve ethical problems must begin.

Perhaps the most important feature of communitarian ethics for our purposes is its idea of a *common good*. Whereas utilitarianism seeks to promote the welfare of all individuals taken together, communitarianism looks to the *shared* values, ideals, and goals of a community. It asks what kind of community we want to live in and uses this, rather than individual welfare exclusively, as guidance in determining social policy.

A problem for communitarians is that the individuals who make up communities may have very different ideas of what the community should be like. Which vision of "the good life" or "the good society" should prevail? Does not communitarianism, like utilitarianism, threaten a "tyranny of the majority"? In response, communitarians argue that even people with very different values will have shared values. Education is a good example of a shared value. That is, over and above each person's interest in becoming educated, the community as a whole has an interest in seeing that its citizens are educated. This is essential if the society is to be healthy economically, and also for democracy (another shared value of our community) to operate. Undoubtedly, different individuals and groups will have different ideas as to what and how the schools should teach, and these differences will have to be worked out in democratic fashion, which includes private schools, religious schools, and home schooling. Nevertheless, the commitment of the society to educating the young is a shared value.

The health of the public is another shared value. Not only does each individual have an interest in staying healthy, but all of us together share an interest in having a healthy population. Again, we may disagree about the best ways to promote the public's health and over how to weigh individual liberty against the welfare of the whole. Nevertheless, reducing disease, saving lives, and promoting good health are shared values, part of the common good. As public health is fundamentally an effort to promote these shared goals, public health is a species of communitarianism.

Communitarianism challenges the libertarian or market model, which places the highest value on liberty. Liberty here means the absence of restraint, not the liberty to accomplish certain goals, which is often called *positive liberty*. Libertarians see the government as the biggest threat to liberty in the modern state because government controls the means of violence and coercion. They regard the market as the most efficient way to expand liberty for all citizens.

Like libertarians, liberals also place a high value on individual liberty. However, liberty is not the sole value for liberals: Social and economic equality is also a desirable end. Furthermore, liberals do not embrace the market with the same enthusiasm as libertarians. Liberals believe that the government has a significant role to play in regulating the market and offering some form of social safety net which includes health care for the needy, employment and education programs, and pensions to protect the elderly.

Communitarians share with liberals the view that the market needs to be controlled and regulated in order to protect people. But where liberals tend to think solely in terms of harms and benefits to individuals and to insist that individuals determine their own ends and goods, communitarians stress goods that are held or enjoyed in common: clean air and water, the environment, education, and the public's health and safety. These goods cannot be achieved by individual effort alone but must be obtained by collective action and new institutions. Moreover, such collective action and new institutions not only promote the common good but can also strengthen the allegiance of individuals to the community.

Many philosophers have seen the principal issue of public health as that of paternalism, or the intrusion of the state upon individual liberty in order to promote health and safety, such as with requirements that individuals wear seat belts while using automobiles. These kinds of issues were not seen as inherently exciting or as illuminating of the future that was coming for medicine and ethics. Yet the ethical disputes in public health are far more extensive than the debates over paternalism would suggest. What is the nature of the population? Of the community? Does the community share a common good? Who bears the burdens of prevention? Should public health turn away from moralism, the use of the law to promote a specific morality, altogether, even when that morality might reduce the risks of contracting a dread disease? What do all Americans deserve when it comes to health care, and can the market provide affordable health care for all? Should we provide health care for all in a way that recognizes its character as a common good, and in a way that promotes a sense of sharing something in common? What is the ethical relevance of emergent new epidemics and ecological threats, worldwide? These are the issues we turn to in the readings that follow.

NOTES

1. Benjamin S. Wilfond, "Screening Policy for Cystic Fibrosis: The Role of Evidence," Special Supplement, *Hastings Center Report* 25, No. 3 (1995), p. S22.
2. Ibid.
3. John Stuart Mill, Chapter II, "What Utilitarianism Is." *Utilitarianism (1861)*. Edited by George Sher (Indianapolis, IN: Hackett 1979, p. 7).
4. Jeremy Bentham, "An Introduction to the Principles of Morals and Legislation," Chapter XVII, paragraph 4 in Burns and Hart, eds., *The Collected Works of Jeremy Bentham* (London, 1970, p. 283).
5. Mill, *supra* note 3, p. 11.
6. Peter Singer, *Animal Liberation* (New York: Avon Books, 1975).
7. Mill, *supra* note 3, p. 17.
8. Ibid, p. 22.
9. President's Commission for the Study of Ethical Problems in Medicine and Biomedical and Behavioral Research, 1983. Screening and Counseling for Genetic Conditions (Washington, D.C.: Government Printing Office. Chapter 2, pp. 47–48).
10. Kant's best known work on ethics is *Groundwork of the Metaphysic of Morals*.
11. "Clinton Regrets 'Clearly Racist' U.S. Study," *New York Times*, May 17, 1997, A10.

1

POPULATION PERSPECTIVE

Everything in public health ethics begins with the population perspective and with the effort to measure and improve the health status of populations. By "population perspective" we mean the effort to understand the occurrence of disease from a group or community perspective. Whereas in medicine, the patient is an individual person, in public health, the "patient" is the whole community or population. The goal of public health is to reduce disease and early death in populations. Its methodology is epidemiology, a science which uses strategies and methods to determine that which causes the levels, patterns, and etiology of health and disease in communities.

Another facet of the population perspective is that public health measures save *statistical* lives and reduce *rates* of disease within populations. These savings are of real lives and real disease, but the savings cannot be linked to specific persons. No politician can send postcards to particular individuals and claim credit for saving their lives through public health programs they have advocated. What they can and will do is claim credit for improving the health and safety of the whole community, much as they can claim that a new school building or a new bridge benefits the whole community.

The population's health is in this sense a construct of our methods, something built out of the various statistical measures we have developed over time: births, deaths, reports of disease, numbers of people who live in cities, in rural areas, the age distribution of a population, and so forth. When we speak of the health of the population, we are speaking of something real but it is a reality constructed from our methods, abstracted from other elements of our common world.

It is widely appreciated that death and disease are social harms that require governmental action, as with immunization. Less appreciated is the need to understand disease and health risks in different groups in the community: who smokes and who does not, which groups suffer high rates of heart disease and which groups have much lower rates, and why these differences exist. Such information is essential for the prevention of disease.

Still less understood is the way in which health benefits to communities diverge from health benefits to individuals. This central point is made in Geoffrey Rose's classic article, "Sick Individuals and Sick Populations," the first selection in this chapter. As Rose puts it, "A preventive measure which brings much benefit to the population offers little to each participating individual."[1] Rose calls this *the preventive paradox.*[2] It is a paradox because populations are made up of individuals; how, then, can one benefit a population without benefiting the individuals who compose it? Rose is not saying, of course, that populations are made up of anything other than individuals. He *is* saying that improving the health of populations results in disappointingly small improvements to the health of any given individual. For example, the finding that elevated cholesterol levels measured in a population produce elevated rates of coronary artery disease and premature death is a finding about relationships between aggregate or widespread risks and associated rates of disease. Lowering the average level of cholesterol for an entire population would presumably lower the rates of disease and early death and would save thousands of lives. It does not follow, however, that measures to lower the average level of cholesterol would significantly reduce the risk of heart attack for any particular person who is at risk of coronary heart disease. The reason is that there are millions of people who have high levels of cholesterol in their blood. Lowering the average level of cholesterol in the whole population can save thousands of lives while having only disappointingly small reductions of risk for the average individual.

Another example is state and federal seat-belt laws. This legislation clearly saves lives, possibly in the neighborhood of 10,000 lives a year, nationally. This is a lot of lives saved and a significant benefit to the community as a whole. However, this result comes from the wearing of seat belts by well over a hundred million drivers and passengers, each of whom is at a relatively low risk of dying in a highway crash. Wearing a seat belt decreases only marginally any particular person's chance of dying in an automobile accident, which is already low. This does not mean, of course, that there is no reason to wear a seat belt, but rather that the rationale comes from the collective good obtained, the saving of a substantial number of lives, rather than from the benefit to any individual personally.

The social and ecological causes of disease are many and varied, including, for example, nutrition, clean water, the genetic makeup of subgroups, safe housing, access to medical care, and exposure to pathogens. Among other things, epidemiology seeks to explain how the health of populations develops and how disease manifests itself across populations. It asks questions such as, Why has health improved over the past 100 years? Why has tuberculosis reemerged as a serious threat? Why do the Chinese and Japanese have lower rates of heart disease and cirrhosis than, say, Europeans or North Americans?

A fundamental question is how major divisions in the population like race and class shape the health of the total population. Ill health is concentrated among those with low incomes and few social advantages, and these characteristics in turn are concentrated among minority groups like African Americans, Hispanics, and Native Americans. As Vincente Navarro points out in "Race or Class Versus Race and Class," it is hard to distinguish whether the primary factor in producing ill health is race or class; it is likely a combination of both. For example, rates of infant mortality are much higher in the United States than in other industrialized countries, largely due to the existence of a large underclass composed of minorities and poor whites. Understanding institutionalized inequity is part of the effort to understand risks to health and how the public's health can be improved.

Epidemiology is also supposed to develop theories about how the population's health can be explained and improved. In the third selection, Nancy Krieger and Sally Zierler criticize those epidemiologists so focused on the scientific side, on making more accurate and reliable methods for sampling the occurrence of disease and early death, that they neglect the goal of epidemiology—improving the public's health.

Another aspect of causal inference has to do with the way we determine "the cause" of an event. Commonly we ask: Why did this person get sick at this time? Why did this person die of heart disease? But from a population perspective, we have a different purpose. We want to know why this population (or community) has a higher rate of disease than other societies, or why disease rates in a society are on the rise. Which conditions we identify as "the cause" depends in large measure on our purposes.[3] For example, alcoholism has often been viewed as the result of an individual failure to control one's drinking. Those who take a population perspective, however, are more likely to focus on the conditions in society that make excessive drinking likely, from the availability of alcohol to the social practices that encourage heavy or frequent use of alcohol. Similarly, highway crashes have in the past been seen as the result of careless or reckless driving on the part of individuals. After three decades of public health crusades, led by Ralph Nader and others, we now focus more on the safety of automobiles or highways. Individual responsibility is not forgotten, but hazardous driving conditions that affect whole populations are given far more attention than before. The population perspective constructs a new story about how highway injuries occur in society.

NOTES

1. Geoffrey Rose, "Sick Individuals and Sick Populations," *International Journal of Epidemiology* 14 (1985), p. 38.
2. Ibid.
3. For an excellent discussion of the way causes are identified, see H.L.A. Hart and A. M. Honore, *Causation in the Law* (Oxford: Clarendon Press, 1959).

Sick Individuals and Sick Populations

GEOFFREY ROSE

THE DETERMINANTS OF INDIVIDUAL CASES

In teaching epidemiology to medical students, I have often encouraged them to consider a question which I first heard enunciated by Roy Acheson: 'Why did *this* patient get *this* disease at *this* time?'. It is an excellent starting-point, because students and doctors feel a natural concern for the problems of the individual. Indeed, the central ethos of medicine is seen as an acceptance of responsibility for sick individuals.

It is an integral part of good doctoring to ask not only, 'What is the diagnosis, and what is the treatment?' but also, 'Why did this happen, and could it have been prevented?'. Such thinking shapes the approach to nearly all clinical and laboratory research into the causes and mechanisms of illness. Hypertension research, for example, is almost wholly preoccupied with the characteristics which distinguish individuals at the hypertensive and normotensive ends of the blood pressure distribution. Research into diabetes looks for genetic, nutritional and metabolic reasons to explain why some people get diabetes and others do not. The constant aim in such work is to answer Acheson's question, 'Why did *this* patient get this disease at this time?'.

The same concern has continued to shape the thinking of all of us who came to epidemiology from a background in clinical practice. The whole basis of the case-control method is to discover how sick and healthy individuals differ. Equally the basis of many cohort studies is the search for 'risk factors', which identify certain individuals as being more susceptible to disease; and from this we proceed to test whether these risk factors are also causes, capable of explaining why some individuals get sick while others remain healthy, and applicable as a guide to prevention.

To confine attention in this way to within-population comparisons has caused much confusion (particularly in the clinical world) in the definition of nor-

From the *International Journal of Epidemiology*, 14 (1985), 32–38. Reprinted by permission of Oxford University Press.

mality. Laboratory 'ranges of normal' are based on what is common within the local population. Individuals with 'normal blood pressure' are those who do not stand out from their local contemporaries; and so on. What is common is all right, we presume.

Applied to aetiology, the individual-centered approach leads to the use of relative risk as the basic representation of aetiological force: that is, 'the risk in exposed individuals relative to risk in non-exposed individuals'. Indeed, the concept of relative risk has almost excluded any other approach to quantifying causal importance. It may generally be the best measure of aetiological force, but it is no measure at all of aetiological outcome or of public health importance.

Unfortunately this approach to the search for causes, and the measuring of their potency, has to assume a heterogeneity of exposure within the study population. If everyone smoked 20 cigarettes a day, then clinical, case-control and cohort studies alike would lead us to conclude that lung cancer was a genetic disease; and in one sense that would be true, since if everyone is exposed to the necessary agent, then the distribution of cases is wholly determined by individual susceptibility.

Within Scotland and other mountainous parts of Britain there is no discernible relation between local cardiovascular death rates and the softness of the public water supply. The reason is apparent if one extends the enquiry to the whole of the UK. In Scotland, everyone's water is soft; and the possibly adverse effect becomes recognizable only when study is extended to other regions which have a much wider range of exposure. Even more clearly, a case-control study of this question within Scotland would have been futile. Everyone is exposed, and other factors operate to determine the varying risk.

Epidemiology is often defined in terms of study of the determinants of the distribution of the disease; but we should not forget that the more widespread is a particular cause, the less it explains the distribution of cases. The hardest cause to identify is the one that is universally present, for then it has no influence on the distribution of disease.

THE DETERMINANTS OF POPULATION INCIDENCE RATE

I find it increasingly helpful to distinguish two kinds of aetiological question. The first seeks the causes of cases, and the second seeks the causes of incidence. 'Why do some individuals have hypertension?' is a quite different question from 'Why do some populations have much hypertension, whilst in others it is rare?'. The questions require different kinds of study, and they have different answers.

[We can show] the systolic blood pressure distributions of middle-aged men in two populations—Kenyan nomads and London civil servants. The familiar question, 'Why do some individuals have higher blood pressure than others?' could be equally well asked in either of these settings, since in each the individual blood pressures vary (proportionately) to about the same extent; and the answers might well be much the same in each instance (that is, mainly genetic variation, with a lesser component from environmental and behavioural differences). We might achieve a complete understanding of why individuals vary, and yet quite miss the most important public health question, namely, 'Why is hypertension absent in the Kenyans and common in London?'. The answer to that question has to do with the determinants of the population mean; for what distinguishes the two groups is nothing to do with the characteristics of individuals, it is rather a shift of the whole distribution—a mass influence acting on the population as a whole. To find the determinants of prevalence and incidence rates, we need to study characteristics of populations, not characteristics of individuals.

A more extreme example is provided by the population distributions of serum cholesterol levels in East Finland, where coronary heart disease is very common, and Japan, where the incidence rate is low: the two distributions barely overlap. Each country has men with relative hypercholesterolaemia (although their definitions of the range of 'normal' would no doubt disagree), and one could research into the genetic and other causes of these unusual individuals; but if we want to discover why Finland has such a high incidence of coronary heart disease we need to look for those characteristics of the national diet which have so elevated the whole cholesterol distribution. Within populations it has proved almost impossible to demonstrate any relation between an individual's diet and his serum cholesterol level; and the same applies to the relation of individual diet to blood pressure and to overweight. But at the level of populations it is a different story: it has proved easy to show strong associations between population mean values for saturated fat intake *versus* serum cholesterol level and coronary heart disease incidence, sodium intake *versus* blood pressure, or energy intake *versus* overweight. The determinants of incidence are not necessarily the same as the causes of cases.

HOW DO THE CAUSES OF CASES RELATE TO THE CAUSES OF INCIDENCE?

This is largely a matter of whether exposure varies similarly within a population and between populations (or over a period of time within the same population). Softness of water supply may be a determinant of cardiovascular mortality, but it is unlikely to be identifiable as a risk factor for individuals, because exposure tends to be locally uniform. Dietary fat is, I believe, the main determinant of a population's incidence rate for coronary heart disease; but it quite fails to identify high-risk individuals.

In the case of cigarettes and lung cancer it so happened that the study populations contained about equal numbers of smokers and non-smokers, and in such a situation case/control and cohort studies were able to identify what was also the main determinant of population differences and time trends.

There is a broad tendency for genetic factors to dominate individual susceptibility, but to explain rather little of population differences in incidence. Genetic heterogeneity, it seems, is mostly much greater within than between populations. This is the contrary situation to that seen for environmental factors. Thus migrants, whatever the colour of their skin, tend to acquire the disease rates of their country of adoption.

Most non-infectious diseases are still of largely unknown cause. If you take a textbook of medicine and look at the list of contents you will still find, despite all our aetiological research, that most are still of basically unknown aetiology. We know quite a lot about the personal characteristics of individuals who are susceptible to them; but for a remarkably large number of our major non-infectious diseases we still do not know the determinants of the incidence rate.

Over a period of time we find that most diseases are in a state of flux. For example, duodenal ulcer in Britain at the turn of the century was an uncommon condition affecting mainly young women. During the first half of the century the incidence rate rose steadily and it became very common, but now the disease seems to be disappearing; and yet we have no clues to the determinants of these striking changes in incidence rates. One could repeat that story for many conditions.

There is hardly a disease whose incidence rate does not vary widely, either over time or between populations at the same time. This means that these causes of incidence rate, unknown though they are, are not inevitable. It is possible to live without them, and if we knew what they were it might be possible to control them: But to identify the causal agent by the traditional case-control and cohort methods will be unsuccessful if there are not sufficient differences in exposure within the study population at the time of the study. In those circumstances all that these traditional methods do is to find markers of individual susceptibility. The clues must be sought from differences between populations or from changes within populations over time.

PREVENTION

These two approaches to aetiology—the individual and the population-based—have their counterparts in prevention. In the first, preventive strategy seeks to identify high-risk susceptible individuals and to offer them some individual protection. In contrast, the 'population strategy' seeks to control the determinants of incidence in the population as a whole.

The 'High-Risk' Strategy

This is the traditional and natural medical approach to prevention. If a doctor accepts that he is responsible for an individual who is sick today, then it is a short step to accept responsibility also for the individual who may well be sick tomorrow. Thus screening is used to detect certain individuals who hitherto thought they were well but who must now understand that they are in effect patients. This is the process, for example, in the detection and treatment of symptomless hypertension, the transition from healthy subject to patient being ratified by the giving and receiving of tablets. (Anyone who takes medicines is by definition a patient.)

What the 'high-risk' strategy seeks to achieve is something like a truncation of the risk distribution. This general concept applies to all special preventive action in high-risk individuals—in at-risk pregnancies, in small babies, or in any other particularly susceptible group. It is a strategy with some clear and important advantages (Table 1).

Its first advantage is that it leads to intervention which is appropriate to the individual. A smoker who has a cough or who is found to have impaired ventilatory function has a special reason for stopping smoking. The doctor will see it as making sense to advise salt restriction in a hypertensive. In such instances the intervention makes sense because that individual already has a problem which that particular measure may possibly ameliorate. If we consider screening a population to discover those with high serum cholesterol levels and advising them on dietary change, then that intervention is appropriate to those people in particular: they have a diet-related metabolic problem.

The 'high-risk' strategy produces interventions that are appropriate to the particular individuals advised to take them. Consequently it has the advantage of enhanced subject motivation. In our randomized controlled trial of smoking cessation in London civil servants we first screened some 20 000 men and from them selected about 1500 who were smokers with, in addition, markers of specially high risk for cardiorespiratory disease. They were recalled and a random

TABLE 1 Prevention by the 'High-Risk Strategy': Advantages

1. Intervention appropriate to individual
2. Subject motivation
3. Physician motivation
4. Cost-effective use of resources
5. Benefit:risk ratio favourable

half received anti-smoking counselling. The results, in terms of smoking cessation, were excellent because those men knew they had a special reason to stop. They had been picked out from others in their offices because, although everyone knows that smoking is a bad thing, they had a special reason why it was particularly unwise for them.

There is, of course, another and less reputable reason why screening enhances subject motivation, and that is the mystique of a scientific investigation. A ventilatory function test is a powerful enhancer of motivation to stop smoking: an instrument which the subject does not quite understand, that looks rather impressive, has produced evidence that he is a special person with a special problem. The electrocardiogram is an even more powerful motivator, if you are unscrupulous enough to use it in prevention. A man may feel entirely well, but if those little squiggles on the paper tell the doctor that he has got trouble, then he must accept that he has now become a patient. That is a powerful persuader. (I suspect it is also a powerful cause of lying awake in the night and thinking about it.)

For rather similar reasons the 'high-risk' approach also motivates physicians. Doctors, quite rightly, are uncomfortable about intervening in a situation where their help was not asked for. Before imposing advice on somebody who was getting on all right without them, they like to feel that there is a proper and special justification in that particular case.

The 'high-risk' approach offers a more cost-effective use of limited resources. One of the things we have learned in health education at the individual level is that once-only advice is a waste of time. To get results we may need a considerable investment of counselling time and follow-up. It is costly in use of time and effort and resources, and therefore it is more effective to concentrate limited medical services and time where the need—and therefore also the benefit—is likely to be greatest.

A final advantage of the 'high-risk' approach is that it offers a more favourable ratio of benefits to risks. If intervention must carry some adverse effects or costs, and if the risk and cost are much the same for everybody, then the ratio of the costs to the benefits will be more favourable where the benefits are larger.

Unfortunately the 'high-risk' strategy of prevention also has some serious disadvantages and limitations (Table 2).

TABLE 2 Prevention by the 'High-Risk Strategy': Disadvantages

1. Difficulties and costs of screening
2. Palliative and temporary—not radical
3. Limited potential for (a) individual
                        (b) population
4. Behaviourally inappropriate

The first centres around the difficulties and costs of screening. Supposing that we were to embark, as some had advocated, on a policy of screening for high cholesterol levels and giving dietary advice to those individuals at special risk. The disease process we are trying to prevent (atherosclerosis and its complications) begins early in life, so we should have to initiate screening perhaps at the age of ten. However, the abnormality we seek to detect is not a stable lifetime characteristic, so we must advocate repeated screening at suitable intervals.

In all screening one meets problems with uptake, and the tendency for the response to be greater amongst those sections of the population who are often least at risk of the disease. Often there is an even greater problem: screening detects certain individuals who will receive special advice, but at the same time it cannot help also discovering much larger numbers of 'border-liners', that is, people whose results mark them as at increased risk but for whom we do not have an appropriate treatment to reduce their risk.

The second disadvantage of the 'high-risk' strategy is that it is palliative and temporary, not radical. It does not seek to alter the underlying causes of the disease but to identify individuals who are particularly susceptible to those causes. Presumably in every generation there will be such susceptibles; and if prevention and control efforts were confined to these high-risk individuals, then that approach would need to be sustained year after year and generation after generation. It does not deal with the root of the problem, but seeks to protect those who are vulnerable to it; and they will always be around.

The potential for this approach is limited—sometimes more than we could have expected—both for the individual and for the population. There are two reasons for this. The first is that our power to predict future disease is usually very weak. Most individuals with risk factors will remain well, at least for some years; contrariwise, unexpected illness may happen to someone who has just received an 'all clear' report from a screening examination. One of the limitations of the relative risk statistic is that it gives no idea of the absolute level of danger. Thus the Framingham Study has impressed us all with its powerful discrimination between high and low risk groups, but when we see the degree of overlap in serum cholesterol level between future cases and those who remained healthy, it is not surprising that an individual's future is so often misassessed.

Often the best predictor of future major disease is the presence of existing minor disease. A low ventilatory function today is the best predictor of its future rate of decline. A high blood pressure today is the best predictor of its future rate of rise. Early coronary heart disease is better than all the conventional risk factors as a predictor of future fatal disease. However, even if screening includes such tests for early disease, our experience in the Heart Disease Prevention Project (Table 3) still points to a very weak ability to predict the future of any particular individual.

TABLE 3 Five-Year Incidence of Myocardial Infarction in the UK Heart Disease Prevention Project

ENTRY CHARACTERISTIC	% OF MEN	% OF MI CASES	MI INCIDENCE RATE %
Risk factors alone	15	32	7
'Ischaemia'	16	41	11
'Ischaemia' + risk factors	2	12	22
All men	100	100	4

This point came home to me only recently. I have long congratulated myself on my low levels of coronary risk factors, and I joked to my friends that if I were to die suddenly, I should be very surprised. I even speculated on what other disease—perhaps colon cancer—would be the commonest cause of death for a man in the lowest group of cardiovascular risk. The painful truth is that for such an individual in a Western population the commonest cause of death—by far—is coronary heart disease! Everyone, in fact, is a high-risk individual for this uniquely mass disease.

There is another, related reason why the predictive basis of the 'high-risk' strategy of prevention is weak. It is well illustrated by some data from Alberman which relate the occurrence of Down's syndrome births to maternal age (Table 4). Mothers under 30 years are individually at minimal risk; but because they are so numerous, they generate half the cases. High-risk individuals aged 40 and above generate only 13% of the cases.

The lesson from this example is that *a large number of people at a small risk may give rise to more cases of disease than the small number who are at a high risk.* This situation seems to be common, and it limits the utility of the 'high-risk' approach to prevention.

A further disadvantage of the 'high-risk' strategy is that it is behaviourally inappropriate. Eating, smoking, exercise and all our other life-style characteris-

TABLE 4 Incidence of Down's Syndrome According to Material Age

MATERNAL AGE (YEARS)	RISK OF DOWN'S SYNDROME PER 1000 BIRTHS	TOTAL BIRTHS IN AGE GROUP (AS % OF ALL AGES)	% OF TOTAL DOWN'S SYNDROME OCCURRING IN AGE GROUP
< 30	0.7	78	51
30–34	1.3	16	20
35–39	3.7	5	16
40–44	13.1	0.95	11
> 45	34.6	0.05	2
All ages	1.5	100	100

tics are constrained by social norms. If we try to eat differently from our friends it will not only be inconvenient, but we risk being regarded as cranks or hypochondriacs. If a man's work environment encourages heavy drinking, then advice that he is damaging his liver is unlikely to have any effect. No one who has attempted any sort of health education effort in individuals needs to be told that it is difficult for such people to step out of line with their peers. This is what the 'high-risk' preventive strategy requires them to do.

The Population Strategy

This is the attempt to control the determinants of incidence, to lower the mean level of risk factors, to shift the whole distribution of exposure in a favourable direction. In its traditional 'public health' form it has involved mass environmental control methods; in its modern form it is attempting (less successfully) to alter some of society's norms of behaviour.

The advantages are powerful (Table 5). The first is that it is radical. It attempts to remove the underlying causes that make the disease common. It has a large potential—often larger than one would have expected—for the population as a whole. From Framingham data one can compute that a 10 mm Hg lowering of the blood pressure distribution as a whole would correspond to about a 30% reduction in the total attributable mortality.

The approach is behaviourally appropriate. If nonsmoking eventually becomes 'normal', then it will be much less necessary to keep on persuading individuals. Once a social norm of behaviour has become accepted and (as in the case of diet) once the supply industries have adapted themselves to the new pattern, then the maintenance of that situation no longer requires effort from individuals. The health education phase aimed at changing individuals is, we hope, a temporary necessity, pending changes in the norms of what is socially acceptable.

Unfortunately the population strategy of prevention has also some weighty drawbacks (Table 6). It offers only a small benefit to each individual, since most of them were going to be all right anyway, at least for many years. This leads to the *Prevention Paradox:* 'A preventive measure which brings much benefit to the population offers little to each participating individual'. This has been the history of public health—of immunization, the wearing of seat belts

TABLE 5 Prevention by the 'Population Strategy': Advantages

1. Radical
2. Large potential for population
3. Behaviourally appropriate

TABLE 6 Prevention by the 'Population Strategy': Disadvantages

1. Small benefit to individual ('Prevention Paradox')
2. Poor motivation of subject
3. Poor motivation of physician
4. Benefit:risk ratio worrison

and now the attempt to change various life-style characteristics. Of enormous potential importance to the population as a whole, these measures offer very little—particularly in the short term—to each individual; and thus there is poor motivation of the subject. We should not be surprised that health education tends to be relatively ineffective for individuals and in the short term. Mostly people act for substantial and immediate rewards, and the medical motivation for health education is inherently weak. Their health next year is not likely to be much better if they accept our advice or if they reject it. Much more powerful as motivators for health education are the social rewards of enhanced self-esteem and social approval.

There is also in the population approach only poor motivation of physicians. Many medical practitioners who embarked with enthusiasm on anti-smoking education have become disheartened because their success rate was no more than 5 or 10%: in clinical practice one's expectation of results is higher. Grateful patients are few in preventive medicine, where success is marked by a non-event. The skills of behavioural advice are different and unfamiliar, and professional esteem is lowered by a lack of skill. Harder to overcome than any of these, however, is the enormous difficulty for medical personnel to see health as a population issue and not merely as a problem for individuals.

In mass prevention each individual has usually only a small expectation of benefit, and this small benefit can easily be outweighed by a small risk. This happened in the World Health Organization clofibrate trial, where a cholesterol-lowering drug seems to have killed more than it saved, even though the fatal complication rate was only about 1/1000/year. Such low-order risks, which can be vitally important to the balance sheet of mass preventive plans, may be hard or impossible to detect. This makes it important to distinguish two approaches. The first is the restoration of biological normality by the removal of an abnormal exposure (eg, stopping smoking, controlling air pollution, moderating some of our recently-acquired dietary deviations); here there can be some presumption of safety. This is not true for the other kind of preventive approach, which leaves intact the underlying causes of incidence and seeks instead to interpose some new, supposedly protective intervention (eg, immunization, drugs, jogging). Here the onus is on the activists to produce adequate evidence of safety.

CONCLUSIONS

Case-centred epidemiology identifies individual susceptibility, but it may fail to identify the underlying causes of incidence. The 'high-risk' strategy of prevention is an interim expedient, needed in order to protect susceptible individuals, but only for so long as the underlying causes of incidence remain unknown or uncontrollable; if causes can be removed, susceptibility ceases to matter.

Realistically, many diseases will long continue to call for both approaches, and fortunately competition between them is usually unnecessary. Nevertheless, the priority of concern should always be the discovery and control of the causes of incidence.

Race or Class Versus Race and Class:
Mortality Differentials in the United States

VICENTE NAVARRO

The latest annual report of the US federal government about the health of the US population has created enormous concern about the mortality differentials between whites and blacks. For example, in 1988 life expectancy at birth was 75·5 years for whites but only 69·5 years for blacks. For most causes of death, the death rate in blacks is higher than that in whites, and for many causes of death mortality differentials are increasing rather than decreasing. Alarming reports about these differences have appeared in both the lay press and medical publications. Consequently, it makes sense that the federal government has chosen the reduction of these differentials as one of its top objectives and has called for a "decrease [of the] disparity in life expectancy between white and minority populations to no more than four years."

Although this emphasis on reducing race differentials is undoubtedly very important, another component of the nation's health that is highly relevant to race differentials in mortality has passed unnoticed. The stark fact is that these differentials cannot be explained merely by looking at race. After all, some blacks have better health indicators (including mortality rates) than some whites, and not all whites have similar mortality indicators. Thus we must look at class differentials in mortality in the US, which are also increasing rather than declining. Class is harder to define than race, but the most frequent indicators of social class used for morbidity and mortality statistics in the western industrialised world are occupation, education, and income.

IMPORTANCE OF CLASS DIFFERENTIALS

The US is the only western developed nation whose government does not collect mortality statistics by class. The federal report on health indicators in the

From *The Lancet*, 336 (1990), 1238–1240. Copyright © by The Lancet Ltd. Reprinted by permission of the publisher.

US—*Health, United States, 1989*—tabulates mortality statistics by age, sex, and race but not by class indicators such as income, education, or occupation. With the active encouragement of the European office of the World Health Organisation, most European countries have chosen as the top target in their health policies a reduction, by the year 2000, of the differentials in health status among classes. By contrast, the US is alone among major industrialised nations in not aiming for this goal—in the US, race is used as a *substitute* for class. What the US government seems to ignore is that even if there were no race differentials in mortality, most blacks would still have higher mortality rates than the median or the mean rate in the US population. To understand this point, one has to appreciate that the US has classes as well as races.

How people live, die, and get sick depends not only on their race, gender, and age but also on the class to which they belong. There is empirical information to sustain this position. On one of the few occasions (in 1986) that the US government collected information on mortality rates (for heart and cerebro-vascular disease) by class, the results showed that, by whatever indicators of class one might choose (level of education, income, or occupation), mortality rates are related to social class. People with less formal education, with lower income, and belonging to the working class (eg, labourers in the US Census categories of operator and services) are more likely to die of heart disease than are people with more formal education, with higher income, and belonging to the upper classes (eg, managerial and professional).

Mortality Differentials

Figure 1 shows mortality rates for heart disease by occupation. Managerial and professional groups had lower mortality rates for heart disease than did major components of the working class, such as operators and service workers.

Data from the same survey (1986 National Mortality Followback Survey) also show that most of those who died of cerebrovascular disease and all other causes had family incomes of less than $25 000 in 1985 and less than a high school education; the largest proportion of the deceased had worked in techni-cal, sales, and operator occupations—the main occupational groups in the working class. Similar class mortality differentials have been found for breast cancer and for all causes of death.

For both causes of mortality—heart disease and cerebrovascular disease—the class differentials in mortality were larger than the race differentials. The mortality rate for heart disease in blue-collar workers (operators) was 2·3 times higher than the rate in managers and professionals (Figure 1).

Table 23 (age-adjusted death rates for selected causes of death according to sex and race: United States, selected years, 1950–87) of *Health, United States, 1989* shows that for 1986, the heart disease mortality rate for black males was

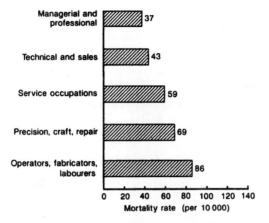

FIGURE 1 Mortality rate for heart disease by occupation, 1986. This figure has been calculated with data from (a) numerator in table 4, ref 7, and (b) denominator in table 627, *Statistical abstract of the United States,* 1988: 376–77 (published by the US Department of Commerce, Bureau of the Census, Washington, DC).

1·2 times higher than for white males, and for black females was 1·5 times higher than for white females.

Morbidity Differentials

Although there are no published data to show mortality rates by class and race, it is likely that the mortality rates for white service workers, for example, are closer to those of black service workers than to those of white professionals. Since there are no data to establish this point, we can look instead at data on morbidity. Morbidity differentials by class are much larger than differentials by race. In 1986, those making $10 000 or less per year reported 4·6 times more morbidity than those making over $35 000, while blacks reported 1·9 times more morbidity than whites. The race differentials were less than half the class differentials. The same report shows that race differentials within each income group are less pronounced than those between income groups. Figure 2 shows the average annual percentage of persons assessing themselves to be in fair or poor health, classified by race and family income. Morbidity rates for blacks making less than $20 000 were much closer to those for whites in the same income group than to those for blacks in income groups greater than $20 000. Similarly, morbidity rates for whites with incomes below $20 000 were closer to those of blacks in the same income group than to those of whites in income groups over $20 000. Whites making under $20 000 had higher morbidity rates than blacks earning over $20 000.

A similar pattern is observed when occupation is used rather than income. Thus blue-collar workers (operators) reported a morbidity rate (9·5%) that was

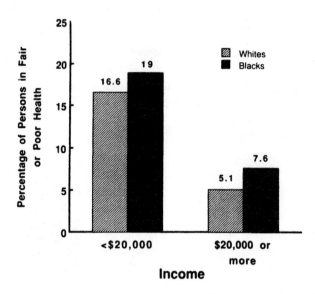

FIGURE 2 Average annual percentage of persons self-assessed to be in fair or poor health, by race and income, 1985–87.

2·9 times higher than that of professionals (3·2%), while blacks reported a morbidity rate 1·9 times higher than that of whites.

Consideration of the annual percentage of persons with limited activity due to chronic conditions rather than self-reported morbidity provides further confirmation. Figure 3 shows, again, that class differentials (measured by income differentials) are larger than race differentials. Moreover, these class differentials have grown larger during the 1980s—even larger than race differentials (figure 4).

DISPARITY OF WEALTH AND INCOME BY CLASS

Within each class (measured by education, income, or occupation), blacks often have worse health indicators than whites. These are the differentials that the US government is targeting for reduction, an important and much-needed task. But the overwhelming majority of blacks (and other minorities) are members of the low-paid, poorly educated working class that have higher morbidity and mortality rates than high-earning, better educated people. The growing mortality differentials between whites and blacks cannot be understood by looking only at race; they are part and parcel of larger mortality differentials—class differentials. In the 1980s, the US witnessed an increased class polarisation of the population, with a reduction of the middle class, a slow growth of the upper and upper-middle classes, and a rapid growth of the low-paid, unskilled working

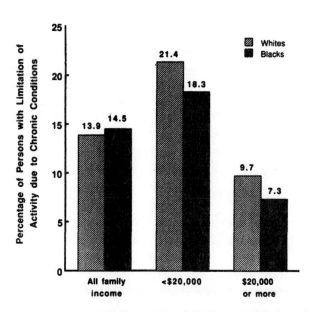

FIGURE 3 Average annual percentage of persons with limitation of activity due to chronic conditions, by race, age, and family income: United States, 1985–87.

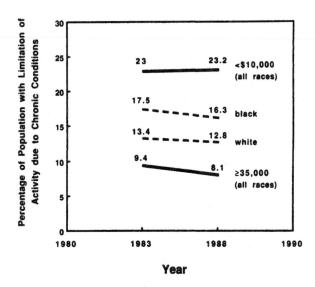

FIGURE 4 Limitation of activity caused by chronic condition, according to income and race, US, 1983 and 1988.

class. Members of the working class are increasingly non-unionised, poorly paid, and part-time, and with a preponderance of minorities and women. The low-earners comprise a heterogeneous group—blacks, Hispanics, whites, men, and women—whose standards of living are rapidly deteriorating because of the growing wealth and income differentials between the upper and lower classes. These social groups belong to the 40% of the population who received only 15·7% of the total income in 1984, the lowest figure since data collection was initiated in 1947. By contrast, the wealthiest 20% received 42·9% of total income, the highest ever. This growing disparity of wealth and income by class mainly, but not exclusively, explains the race differentials in morbidity and mortality.

The growing class differential in mortality rates is not unique to the US. Other countries have noticed that these differentials are not only persistent but growing, and a large national and international debate about the reasons for these class differentials has been initiated. However, in the US there is a deafening silence on this topic. If a prerequisite for finding the right answer is to ask the right question, then it is unlikely that by concentrating solely on race differentials we will ever be able to understand why the health indicators of our minorities are getting worse.

What Explains the Public's Health?—A Call for Epidemiologic Theory

NANCY KRIEGER and SALLY ZIERLER

MR. JORDAN: Is there nothing then but prose, or verse?

PHILOSOPHY-MASTER: No, sir, whatever is not prose, is verse! and whatever is not verse, is prose.

MR. JORDAN: And when one talks, what may that be then?

PHILOSOPHY-MASTER: Prose.

MR. JORDAN: How? When I say, Nicola, bring me my slippers, and give me my nightcap, is that prose?

PHILOSOPHY-MASTER: Yes, sir.

MR. JORDAN: On my conscience, I have spoken prose above these forty years without knowing anything of the matter. . . .

(Jean Baptiste Molière. *Le bourgeois gentilhomme.* 1670)

Epidemiology is a wonderfully ambitious science. It provides a basis for understanding and altering societal patterns of health and disease. These patterns reflect a complex interplay of people's social and biological experience. This interplay integrates the richness and poverty of human life with mechanisms of disease pathogenesis. Understanding this interplay is the fundamental challenge facing epidemiologists. Since our work is to explain what shapes population patterns of disease rather than what makes an individual ill, we have to think consciously about these links. Such thinking we would call the stuff of epidemiologic theory.

Although epidemiologic theory drives much of the work epidemiologists do, we rarely recognize it as such. What we call theory in epidemiology today typically refers to study methodology. Communication of our ideas is explicit about methodologic underpinnings of our study design and analysis. We distinguish multiple ways that error could explain our study results. Assuming that the role of error is not too great, we explain our findings in light of other knowledge about biological, and sometimes social, processes. But where ex-

From *Epidemiology,* 7, January 1996, 107–109. Reprinted by permission of Williams & Wilkins.

plicitly do we name theory to understand the interplay between social and bio-logical processes that shape the public's health?

Our discipline's inattention to epidemiologic theory is relatively new. When epidemiology was first taught in the early 1900s as a self-consciously defined discipline, the first U.S. professor of epidemiology, Wade Hampton Frost, urged development of theories to explain the distribution of disease in populations. Moving away from the more usual focus on natural history of disease in individuals, in 1927 he argued:

> In collecting facts about the distribution of disease, the purpose and view is always to arrive at a better understanding of its nature, sources, means of spread and eventually its control. This implies that the facts must be related to each other in such an orderly way as to establish a theory or philosophy of the disease. . . .

Similar calls for elaborating epidemiologic theory were made in the 1930s in two landmark texts: Major Greenwood's *Epidemics and Crowd Diseases: An Introduction to the Study of Epidemiology,* and Edgar Sydenstricker's *Health and Environment.* These works, synthesizing the epidemiologic knowledge of their times, underscored the importance of social inequalities as determinants of disease in conjunction with biological factors.

In contrast to these researchers, epidemiologists today emphasize creative and effective approaches to modeling causation and explaining effects of error. These approaches have been interpreted as the substance of our field. Notably, as others have observed, we rarely ask: what is the theoretical and ideological basis for conceptualizing and articulating meaningful explanations of the public's health?

EPIDEMIOLOGIC THEORY *vs* THEORIES OF CAUSATION AND OF ERROR

We believe it is useful to distinguish three contexts for theory in our field: (1) epidemiologic theories that frame our etiologic questions, (2) causal theories that form the basis for mathematical models for disease causation, and (3) theories of error that guide our study design, analysis, and interpretation.

What do we mean here by epidemiologic theories *vs* theories of causation and of error? By epidemiologic theories, we refer to interconnected ideas about what explains population health. These theories, by definition, incorporate interdependent social and biological parameters. They organize a complex body of knowledge into coherent interrelations across disease outcomes and make explicit philosophical and ideological assumptions about why, in the words of the noted British epidemiologist Geoffrey Rose, some populations—and not simply some individuals—are sicker than others. Examples of such theories include biomedical, life-style, cultural, behavioral, and social production of disease.

Alternatively, by theories of causation, we refer to interconnected ideas that explain relations among causal effects. These causal relations typically are expressed in the form of schematic or mathematical models that are used in many scientific disciplines. Examples of theoretical constructs relevant to these models include necessary, sufficient, and component causes, and additive and multiplicative effects. And, by theories of error, we refer to interconnected ideas that explain the distribution of error in the design, conduct, and analysis of scientific studies. Operative theoretical concepts include confounding, selection and information bias, misclassification, and random error. The application of these theories of causation and of error to epidemiologic research constitutes the methodologic core of our science.

WHY EPIDEMIOLOGIC THEORY MATTERS

We offer the following example to illustrate the importance of epidemiologic theory. We contrast two distinct theories—life-style and social production of disease—as frameworks for generating hypotheses regarding the single question: what explains the distribution of human immunodeficiency virus (HIV)/AIDS?

A life-style theory explains determinants of population disease occurrence as behavioral clusters or cultural factors that are shared among individuals. This theory has dominated epidemiologic research on HIV, as well as much of the public health agenda for preventing HIV transmission. The first Centers for Disease Control report of unexplained immune suppression that was later named as AIDS proposed a life-style hypothesis: "The fact that these patients were all homosexuals suggests an association between some aspect of a homosexual lifestyle or disease acquired through sexual contact and Pneumocystis pneumonia in this population." Other life-style risk factors named in the epidemiologic literature include "promiscuity", injection drug use, prostitution, or in the case of women not fitting into these categories, "sexual partners of" men who are in defined HIV risk groups. Yet, although the term "life-style" may be used, rarely is the life-style theory named as such. Scholars in other disciplines, however, explicitly identify life-style theory as a major conceptual framework driving epidemiologic knowledge about HIV.

What does it mean to attribute life-style as an explanation for the distribution of HIV within and across populations? Life-style implies that individuals make choices among options, and that these choices are amenable to change given sufficient incentive. Prostitution, for example, is treated as an activity that women choose to engage in, even though the motivation for this choice is rarely ascribed (but is sometimes implied to be a drug habit or desire for "easy money"). Thus, the interconnected explanatory ideas named as life-style theory posit: (1) individuals choose ways of living that have health consequences; (2) what epidemiologists measure on a population level are aggregates of these individual choices, and (3) individualized interventions can alter the distribution of these choices, and ultimately, of disease. These unstated but powerful assumptions are rife within the epidemiologic literature on HIV (and other diseases). Investigators base their study hypotheses, designs, and interpretations on these assumptions. For example, research premised on a life-style framework focuses on inadequate use of condoms (and of sterile needles) as the principal explanation for patterns of HIV incidence within and across different geographic regions.

By contrast, a theory of social production of disease conceptualizes determinants of disease distribution as economic and social relationships forged by a society's political and economic structure. Social groups defined by these relationships are differentially helped or harmed by their position relative to each other. Terms used to convey these relationships include social class, gender and sexism, and race/ethnicity and racism. The imposition of inequalities inherent in these relationships unevenly affects each group's health and well-being.

What would it mean to attribute economic and social relationships as an explanation for the distribution of HIV within and across populations? Surveillance of HIV based on this approach emphasizes the link between increased risk of HIV infection and membership in groups defined by economic deprivation and racial discrimination. Related research explicitly names social policies and political priorities (for example, availability of low-income housing, employment, and affordable education) as critical cofactors in the geographic spread of AIDS in the United States. And, in the case of women and AIDS, theories of social production of disease lead epidemiologists to investigate how gender-based economic inequalities may affect women's ability to determine sexual uses of their bodies. This theory also explains prostitution as an economic survival strategy that has its own political economy. Studies of prostitution and HIV recognize prostitution's complex occupational structure, which includes a range of working conditions affecting risk of exposure to HIV. Reflecting prostitutes' relative material or social deprivation, these conditions include the location of work (on the street, in clubs, brothels, or privately owned homes), characteristics of clients, worker control over agreement to provide services, worker control over what services she or he will provide, and options for protection from physical and sexual violence, as well as from sexually transmitted diseases.

Thus, social production of disease theories provide interconnected explanatory ideas that posit: (1) the relative social and economic positioning of people shapes their exposures, including behaviors; (2) what epidemiologists measure on a population level are attributes of this positioning, and (3) population level interventions shift structural conditions that cause material and social deprivation, and thus alter societal distribution of disease. Hypotheses emerging from this theory propose explanations of HIV transmission in relation to: social class, access to health-related resources, work place conditions, and discrimination based on gender, race/ethnicity, sexual orientation/identity, or other attributes.

EPIDEMIOLOGY AND SOCIETY

As these two contrasting examples suggest, ideas for studies, formation of hypotheses, and emergence of knowledge begin within a theoretical framework. This framework, which we are naming epidemiologic theory, largely determines what we know, what we consider knowable, and what we ignore. We thus argue that epidemiologic theory should be fully acknowledged and debated in our research and training. It is, after all, epidemiologic theory, and not methodology, that distinguishes our discipline from other population-based sciences (for example, demography, quantitative sociology) equally concerned about valid study design, data analysis, and causal inference. Epidemiologic theory also distinguishes our field from other biomedical disciplines because their focus is solely on biological processes (for example, disease pathogenesis), whereas ours is on social and biological pathways that explain the distribution of disease in populations.

And it is the population experience of disease, in actual societies, that is the subject of our investigations. Epidemiologic theory reminds us that our work has a context, and that this context is human society. Ultimately, we are accountable for the knowledge we produce and its effects on the public's welfare.

II

PUBLIC HEALTH AS COMMUNITY PERSPECTIVE

2

COMMUNITY

The science of public health arose when methods of collecting data and statistical analysis for examining the health of populations were developed. But public health is not simply methods of determining rates of disease in populations. Public health must also be seen as collective action to improve the health of the community. This raises the question: What do we mean by "community"?

Community is one of the most important words in our democratic lexicon, perhaps second only to the idea of the individual. In its most basic meaning, *community* refers to our life together, and the attachments which sustain that life together. A community is not simply a group of people living in close proximity. A community has a life in common which stems from such things as a shared history, language, and values. The term *community* can apply to small groups, such as self-help groups, which share a common goal, or groups formed because of some shared crisis (like AIDS). It can also apply to very large groups, such as a nation which, despite the diversity of its members, has in common political institutions, symbols, and memories.

The term *community* has often been used as part of a critique of the conditions of contemporary life—a critique of industrial capitalism and its world of factories, mines, urban squalor, disease, and social injustice; this sort of generic critique was later broadened in the 20th century to include the scale of mass society and its lack of meaning and shared purpose. For these ills, many blamed the market and the aimlessness of consumer society; others blamed government and its projects, or liberalism and the freedom granted individuals to reject traditional values and go their own way.

Amongst the more egalitarian, *community* became a call to secure a dignified, safe existence for all, including the conditions which make people and communities healthy. Community also serves to unify the political community. The political community is seen as existing to provide security for its members, and security against disease and avoidable death is seen as unifying and making more cohesive the political community. Public health for the past 150 years has constantly altered and expanded its sense of just which health and safety challenges should be viewed as affecting the whole community and deserving of a collective response, including new institutions to guide that response. From the perspective of public health, community involves three closely related ideas:

1. Seeing health risks as common problems that effect the whole community. Seeing health risks as group threats rather than individual ones often results in challenges to the way in which market models of justice view these problems, which range from occupational risks to highway safety to class and race.

2. Using collective measures like regulation, policy, and new institutions to solve those problems. Building new regulation and institutions helps to "institutionalize" health and safety as permanently the responsibility of government at all levels, but especially at the national and state levels.

3. Finding solutions to common problems that strengthen and reaffirm our attachments to the community as a whole and that forge a more cohesive and more meaningful political community.

We have in recent political history in the United States an excellent example of this process of transforming our perception of our public problems and a more meaningful sense of ourselves as a national community. During the 1960s and early 1970s, advocates like Ralph Nader persuaded Congress to pass legislation that made automobiles safer and also made mines and factories safer and water and air cleaner. The success of this legislation caught many by surprise. Politics was supposed to be driven by the actions of organized, powerful interest groups. Advocates speaking on behalf of the whole community were not supposed to represent a real or influential constituency. James Q. Wilson argued that most public policies, before the health and safety legislation of the period, provided benefits to tightly organized and influential groups or powerful, cohesive majorities.[1] The new public health legislation seemed different, however. It conferred benefits on a large, diffuse, and poorly organized group—often the nation as a whole (as with air pollution controls or highway safety). Wilson found this puzzling because, in his words, the public *does not* usually think of itself as a community with common purposes or interests, and because public health legislation usually means painful cost imposed on powerful interests like the automobile industry or the steel industry (air pollution controls in these two examples), it is a wonder that legislation like this ever gets passed at all.

Jack Walker offered a different and more optimistic account of the rise of health and safety legislation. Walker argued that the victory of the public health legislation occurred *because* it expressed a powerful interest of the whole community.[2] Walker argued that such legislation makings cars, highways, mines, and smokestacks safer was attractive to elected officials *precisely because* they affect large numbers of people. Walker believes that the passage of health and safety legislation and the big victory over the automobile industry (the most powerful industry in the United States) constituted the breakthrough that opened the door to public health legislation for the next ten years. While the public that benefits from the policies is large and diffuse, it can be viewed, and can see itself, as possessing shared interests and purposes; in other words, it can see itself as a community that contains all segments of American society, including the most influential and active segments. Today, despite several decades of well-organized opposition to this legislation by business and others, there is little sentiment for making health and safety an entirely local or state issue.

The three selections for this chapter provide different but complementary approaches to the idea of community. In the first selection, Beauchamp argues that the field of public health represents an important if neglected tradition of community: the republican tradition. A republic (like the government of the United States) is a form of democracy that employs representative institutions to achieve common purposes and the common good. The republican tradition in the United States is reflected in our long legal and Constitutional traditions surrounding the development of the regulatory power to promote and protect the public's health. Laws requiring that people wear seat belts, that children be vaccinated before entering school, and that cars have antipollution devices are possible largely because of a republican legacy which permits limits to the rights of property and to individual liberty in order to protect the common good.

In the selection from his book, *Spheres of Justice: A Defense of Pluralism and Equality,* Michael Walzer provides a different but related argument about community. Walzer argues that measures like medical care and public health protections, which promote individual well-being, have another important function, namely, to strengthen individuals' attachment to the community. On this conception of community, a national health plan, for example, not only secures needed medical treatment to individuals but also reaffirms our collective identity as members of a society. In other words, when we face problems as a group and use group methods to solve our problems, we achieve both security for individuals and a stronger sense of community.

In the third selection in the chapter, Jonathan Mann advocates a human rights perspective for public health. A rights perspective is usually seen as individualistic and thus seemingly opposed to a community approach. However, Mann argues in favor of viewing public health as a human rights problem, in part to give it the urgency it deserves. At the same time, taking a public health approach helps to rectify the tendency among medical ethicists to ignore the social foundations of health, including divisions of race and class. While Mann employs a more individualistic discourse than does Walzer or Beauchamp, all three seek to develop health care as a communal responsibility that demands communal action.

NOTES

1. James Q. Wilson, ed., *The Politics of Regulation* (New York: Basic Books, 1980).
2. Jack L. Walker, "Setting the Agenda in the U.S. Senate: A Theory of Problem Selection," *British Journal of Political Science,* 7 (1977), pp. 423–445.

Community: The Neglected Tradition of Public Health

DAN E. BEAUCHAMP

What are the limits of government in protecting the health and safety of the public? As more and more states regulate personal behavior to protect the public health and safety, this question again becomes central. Can there be good reasons for public health paternalism in a democracy? Are health and safety individual interests, or also common and shared ends? . . .

THE MEANING OF THE COMMON GOOD

In one version of democratic theory, the state has no legitimate role in restricting personal conduct that is substantially voluntary and that has little or no direct consequence for anyone other than the individual. This strong antipaternalist position is associated with John Stuart Mill. In his essay, "On Liberty," which has deeply influenced American and British thought for over one hundred years, Mill wrote: "[t]he only purpose for which power can be rightfully exercised over any member of a civilized community, against his will, is to prevent harms to others." The exceptions are children and the incompetent. In this view the common good consists in maximizing the freedom of each individual to pursue his or her own interests, subject to a like freedom for every other individual. In the words of Blackstone, "The public good is in nothing more essentially interested than the protection of every individual's private rights."

In a second version, health and safety remain private interests but some paternalism is accepted, albeit reluctantly. As Joel Feinberg argues, common sense makes us reject a thoroughgoing antipaternalism. Many restrictions on liberty are relatively minor and the savings in life and limb extremely great. Further, often voluntary choices are not completely so; many choices are impaired in some sense. But, as Dennis Thompson contends, even where choices are not

From *The Hastings Center Report*, 15 (1985), 28–36. Copyright © The Hastings Center. Reproduced by permission.

impaired, as in the choice not to wear seatbelts or to take up smoking, paternalism might still be accepted, because the alternative would be a great loss of life and a society in which each citizen was, for many important decisions, left alone with the consequences of his or her choice.

This reluctant acceptance of paternalism leaves many democrats uneasy. Another alternative is to redefine voluntary risks to an individual as risks to others. Indeed, many argue that all such risks have serious consequences for others, and that the state may therefore limit such activities on the basis of the harm principle. Others challenge the category of voluntariness head on, arguing that most such risks, like cigarettes and alcohol use, have powerful social determinants.

The constitutional basis for the protection of the public health and safety has largely been ignored in this debate. This tradition, and particularly the regulatory power (often called the police power), flows from a view of democracy that sees the essential task of government as protecting and promoting *both* private and group interests. Government is supposed to defend both sets of interests through an evolving set of practices and institutions, and it is left to the legislatures to determine which set of interests predominate when conflicts arise.

In the constitutional tradition, the common good refers to the welfare of individuals considered as a group, the public or the people generally, the "body politic" or the "commonwealth" as it was termed in the early days of the American Republic. The public or the people were presumed to have an interest, held in common, in self-protection or preservation from threats of all kinds to their welfare. The commonwealth idea was widely influential among New England states during the first half of the nineteenth century.

The commonwealth doctrine helped shape the regulatory power in Massachusetts and throughout the U.S. The central principles underlying the police or regulatory power were the treatment of health and safety as a shared purpose and need of the community and (aside from basic constitutional rights such as due process) the subordination of the market, property, and individual liberty to protect compelling community interests.

This republican image of democracy was a blending of social contract and republican thought, as well as Judeo-Christian notions of covenant. In the republican vision of society, the individual has a dual status. On the one hand, individuals have private interests and private rights; political association serves to protect these rights. On the other hand, individuals are members of a political community—a body politic.

This common citizenship, despite diversity and divergence of interests, presumes an underlying shared set of loyalties and obligations to support the ends of the political community, among which public health and safety are central. In this scheme, public health and safety are not simply the aggregate of each private individual's interest in health and safety, interests which can be pursued more effectively through collective action. Public health and safety are community or group interests (often referred to as "state interests" in the law), interests that can transcend and take priority over private interests if the legislature so chooses.

The idea of democracy as promoting the common or group interest is captured in Joseph Tussman's classic work on political obligation: "Familiar as it is, there is something fundamentally misleading about the slogan that the aim of government is 'the welfare of the individual' . . . [T]he government's concern for the individual is not to be understood as special concern for *this* or *that* individual but rather as concern for all individuals. Government, that is to say, serves the welfare of the community."

This emphasis on the *public's* health has never meant that the state's power to protect health and safety is unlimited. It has meant that individual liberty and the institutions of the market and private property, operating in the public world, are subject to a developing set of practices designed to defend the common life and the community. Although we call markets "private," all markets operate within the public or common world shared by individual members of the community.

Beyond this public world, which includes the market and collective spheres, there is the private or personal sphere where each individual is devoted to his own. As Hannah Arendt noted, "Throughout his life man moves constantly within what is his *own,* and he also moves in a sphere that is *common* to him and his fellow men. The 'public good,' the concerns of the citizen, is indeed the common good because it is localized in the *world* which we have in common *without* owning it."

It is the private sphere that is problematic for public health. Public health sometimes intrudes into this private sphere in the interest of the health and safety of the community. But, as we shall see in the development of the regulatory or police power, the main thrust has been to focus on the controlling conditions in the public world, particularly by shaping the institutions of the market and private property.

EMERGENCE OF POLICE POWER

In 1850, the Massachusetts Sanitary Commission presented its *Report* to the state legislature. Lemuel Shattuck, a member of the legislature, was the chief author. The guiding definition of public health was set out in the opening pages:

> The condition of perfect *public health* requires such laws and regulations, as will secure to man associated in society, the same sanitary enjoyments that he would have as an isolated individual; and as will protect him from injury from any influ-

ences connected with his locality, his dwelling-house, his occupation, or those of his associates or neighbors, or from any other social causes. It is under the control of public authority, and public administration; and life and health may be saved or lost, and they are actually saved or lost, as this authority is wisely or unwisely exercised.

Shattuck's report clearly accepts the existence of a public realm that is the legitimate object of government intervention to protect the public health, and that requires the alteration of the existing system of property rights and the regulation of the marketplace for its protection.

In Massachusetts, during the same period when the Sanitary Commission's *Report* was issued, a parallel development in legislation and in law sought to alter the system of rights surrounding private property. The goal was to facilitate rapid economic development on the one hand, and at the same time to permit the state to control and monitor that development in order to protect the public's health and safety.

The commonwealth idea was a direct legacy of eighteenth-century American and English radical republican opposition to the Crown, a body of political thought that powerfully shaped the American revolutionary tradition. The primacy of the public or the common good over private interests and the use of the powers of legislation to regulate the economy and protect the health and safety of the community were central to this body of republican thought.

Our root ideas about health and safety policy can be traced to these early state policies. As a leading constitutional scholar, Leonard Levy, has argued: "[T]he police power may be regarded as the legal expression of the Commonwealth idea, for it signifies the supremacy of public over private rights. To call the police power a Massachusetts doctrine would be an exaggeration, though not a great one. [I]t is certainly no coincidence that in Massachusetts, with its Commonwealth tradition, the police power was first defined and carried to great extremes from the standpoint of vested interests."

Apparently, Chief Justice John Marshall was the first to coin the term "police power" in referring to the powers of the states to regulate public health and safety matters in the classic case of *Gibbons v. Ogden* in 1824. Marshall was attempting to clarify the boundary between these powers and the powers of Congress over interstate commerce: "[Police] powers form a portion of that immense mass of legislation which embraces everything within the territory of the state, not surrendered to the general government; all which can advantageously be exercised by the states themselves. Inspection laws, quarantine laws, health laws of every description . . . are component parts of this mass."

The classic definition of the police power was established in *Commonwealth v. Alger* (1851), a decision written by Chief Justice Shaw of the Massachusetts Supreme Court. In this case, Shaw established the basic premises of the police power of the states. His broad definition of this power remains the most influential to this date: "The power we allude to is . . . the police power, the power vested in the legislature by the constitution, to make, ordain and establish all manner of wholesome and reasonable laws, statutes and ordinances, either with penalties or without, not repugnant to the constitution, as they shall judge to be for the good and welfare of the commonwealth, and of the subjects of the same."

In this decision Justice Shaw was ruling on what might seem a minor issue. The case involved a man who owned property on Boston Harbor and who built a wharf that extended beyond a boundary to the public right of way established by the legislature. When the state ordered him to take it down, he went to court, arguing that the legislature had interfered with his property, and that it had not been demonstrated or even argued that his wharf constituted a nuisance or a harm to anyone.

As Levy noted (in referring to another case), great principles are often decided in cases of little factual interest. In the *Alger* decision, Shaw set out the basic premise underlying the police power: "We think it is a settled principle, growing out of the nature of a well ordered civil society, that every holder of property, however absolute and unqualified may be his title, holds it under the implied liability that his use of it may be so regulated, that it shall not be injurious to the equal enjoyment of others having an equal right to the enjoyment of their property in this commonwealth."

To Shaw, the idea of the "common good" implied the health, safety, or welfare of the citizens of Massachusetts. This common interest in health and safety was not adequately protected by common law principles governing the use of property. The common interest in health and safety could only be adequately protected through legislation and regulations affecting the whole people. The common law doctrine regulating the use of property was: *Sic utere tuo ut alienum non laedas* ("Use your own property in such a manner as not to injure that of another").

In *Alger,* Shaw greatly broadened this principle from a case-by-case investigation of whether each citizen had harmed the interest of another, to a broad instrument for the control of property potentially injurious to the interests of the community. As Shaw argued, "Things done may or may not be wrong in themselves, or necessarily injurious and punishable as such at common law, but laws are passed declaring them offenses, and making them punishable, because they tend to injurious consequences."

According to Levy, Shaw "believed that the general welfare required the anticipation and prevention of prospective wrongs from the use of private property." As Ernest Freund argued decades later, the common law of nuisance could deal with evils only after they came into existence: "The police power endeavors to prevent evil by checking the tendency toward it, and it seeks to place a margin of safety between that which is permitted and that which is sure to lead to injury or loss. This can be accomplished . . . by establishing positive standards and limitations which must be observed, although to step beyond them would not necessarily create a nuisance at law."

In perhaps the second most influential police power decision of the nineteenth century, *Munn v. Illinois* (1876), the Supreme Court affirmed these basic principles. The case involved the state of Illinois and its regulation of grain operators' rates in Chicago. Justice Field, arguing for the minority, stated that the market was essentially a private institution: "The business of a warehouseman was, at common law, a private business, and is so in its nature. It has no special privileges connected with it, nor did the law ever extend to it any greater protection than it extended to all other private business."

But Chief Justice Waite, arguing for the majority, disagreed: "Property does become clothed with a public interest when used in a manner to make it of public consequence, and affect the community at large. When, therefore, one devotes his property to a use in which the public has an interest, he, in effect, grants to the public an interest in that use, and must submit to be controlled by the public for the common good, to the extent of the interest he has thus created."

All authorities agree that the police power is very extensive and checked only by express grants of the Constitution to protect basic rights. There is still recurring disagreement on the underlying principle of the regulatory power. Some scholars argue that the basic principle of the regulatory power remains *sic utere*. But other scholars reject this view. For example, Ernest Freund, in one of the most thorough studies of the regulatory power of any period, argues that "[N]o community confines its care of the public welfare to the enforcement of the principles of the common law . . . it exercises its compulsory powers for the prevention . . . of wrong by narrowing common law rights . . . and [through] positive regulations which are not confined to wrongful acts. It is this latter kind of state control which constitutes the essence of the police power."

THE RELEVANCE OF COMMUNITY

This is a crucial issue because on it turns the relevance of the category of the community for the regulatory power. If the regulatory power is simply the enforcement—writ large—of the law that no one should use his or her property in a manner that offends another individual's interests, then the category of community is rendered meaningless. But as W. G. Hastings, another leading scholar of the police power, pointed out, if this power was limited only to prevent harms to others, this doesn't explain why courts uniformly supported the drastic regulation of alcohol by the states. Although judges often pointed to the evil that drinking causes for others than themselves (such as their families or their employers), it was plain to everyone that regulating the "liquor traffic" involved limiting actions that harmed mostly the drinkers themselves. The temperance and prohibition campaigns, first in the 1950s and later at the turn of the century, to control legally and even destroy the alcohol trade provided some of the strongest and clearest rulings of the courts on the police powers.

Perhaps the most significant case testing the constitutionality of state prohibition was *Mugler v. Kansas* (1887). *Mugler* concerned a brewery owner charged with making beer after a state constitutional amendment forbade the manufacture, sale, and use of alcoholic beverages. Plaintiff's counsel argued that the Kansas constitutional amendment was an attempt to regulate purely personal conduct not subject to a compelling state interest. Counsel quoted Mill and the common law principles of *sic utere* as the basic founding principles of the English and American legal tradition. As counsel for the plaintiff argued: "If a state convention or legislature can punish a citizen for manufacturing beer . . . for his own use, then instead of civil liberty, we are living under the most unlimited and brutal despotism known in history. . . . Broad and comprehensive as this [police] power is, it cannot extend to the individual tastes and habits of the citizen, which are confined entirely to himself and have no effect upon others."

The Supreme Court ruled against the plaintiff and held for the state of Kansas. Justice Harlan, writing for the majority, had this to say:

> There is no justification for holding that the State under the guise merely of police regulations, is aiming to deprive the citizen of his constitutional rights: for we cannot shut out of view the fact, within the knowledge of all, that the public health, the public morals, and the public safety, may be endangered by the general use of intoxicating drinks. . . . So far from such a regulation having no relation to the general end sought to be accomplished, the entire scheme of prohibition, as embodied in the [state] constitution and laws of Kansas, might fail, if the right of each citizen to manufacture intoxicating liquors for his own use as a beverage were recognized. . . . Such a right does not inhere in citizenship. Nor can it be said that government interferes with or impairs any one's constitutional rights of liberty or of property. . . . Those rights are best secured in our government, by the observance, upon the part of all, of such regulations as are established by competent authority, to promote the common good.

The Court did not, and could not, pass judgment on the *wisdom* of the state prohibition measures. This judgment, in a republican scheme of government, rests with the legislative body. But the Court did affirm the basic political principles underlying the powers of the states to control and limit the market and private property to protect the health and safety of the citizenry. During the last decades of the nineteenth century, the Supreme Court capitulated to corporate and extreme laissez-faire interests. During this period the Court sought to block the states' power to improve the working conditions for labor, and to facilitate union organization against capital. Even so, the Court continued to uphold striking powers for the states to regulate property when the health and safety of the general citizenry was at stake.

CONTEMPORARY PUBLIC HEALTH PROBLEMS

Several twentieth-century developments have obscured the philosophical roots of the regulatory power, especially as they work to protect the public health. Because the locus of action for protecting the health and safety of the public has swung to the federal government and because the justification for this federal power lies primarily with the commerce clause of the Constitution, the group principle behind public health has tended to be subordinated to the language of individual rights.

The political justification of public health has also tended to be ignored. Most contemporary legal scholars cite the 1905 Supreme Court decision, *Jacobson v. Massachusetts,* as the leading case underlying public health. *Jacobson* dealt with a Cambridge, Massachusetts ordinance requiring compulsory vaccination in a smallpox outbreak. The language of *Jacobson* contains an exemplary and classical defense of the regulatory power, but the facts of the case focus on the control of epidemics, and the overriding necessity for requiring compulsory vaccination to prevent the spread of infection. This has encouraged many scholars to interpret the regulatory power for protecting the public health on the more narrow grounds of preventing injury to others, and to overlook the use of this power to limit liberty in the market or other areas of the public realm, even if such restriction does not protect the interests of other specific individuals.

The two most recent constitutional controversies regarding public health policy and the police power are the fluoridation and the motorcycle helmet controversies. Once again these controversies show the courts willing to accept public health paternalism. However, in the case of the helmet decisions, sometimes the broad principles of the regulatory power have tended to be replaced by spurious legal reasoning.

State supreme courts have unanimously upheld the constitutionality of both measures, and the U.S. Supreme Court has refused to review fluoridation cases, presumably because they pose no threats to constitutional rights. Plaintiffs have argued that fluoridation is an attempt to employ mass medication and constitutes a violation of individual autonomy in an area that is properly private. They have argued that the use of the regulatory power to control private rights was only justified in the past by the threat of contagious diseases. . .

The courts have been less consistent on the question of helmet laws for motorcyclists. Although state supreme courts have unanimously supported the state's power to require helmet usage, the decisions have often introduced as additional justification the danger unhelmeted cyclists pose for others on the road, or the possibility that unprotected cyclists may become wards of the state. . . .

THE LANGUAGE OF PUBLIC HEALTH

What are we to make of this constitutional tradition surrounding the development of the regulatory power for health and safety? What relevance does it have for the policy disputes of today, particularly those concerning the limitation of lifestyle risks?

The constitutional tradition for public health constitutes one of those "second languages" of republicanism that Robert Bellah and his coauthors speak of in their recent book, *Habits of the Heart*. In their book, the first language (or tradition of moral discourse) of American politics is political individualism. But there are "second languages" of community rooted in the republican and biblical tradition that limit and qualify the scope and consequences of political individualism.

Public health as a second language reminds us that we are not only individuals, we are also a community and a body politic, and that we have shared commitments to one another and promises to keep. As the Preamble to the Massachusetts Constitution puts it:

> The end of the institution, maintenance and administration of government is to secure the existence of the body-politic; to protect; and to furnish the individuals who compose it, with the power of enjoying, in safety and tranquility, their natural rights, and the blessings of life. . . . The body-politic is a social compact, by which the whole people covenants with each citizen, and each citizen with the whole people, that all shall be governed by certain laws for the common good.

The danger is that we can come to discuss public health exclusively within the dominant discourse of political individualism, relying either on the harm principle or a narrow paternalism justified on grounds of self-protection alone. By ignoring the communitarian language of public health, we risk shrinking its claims. We also risk undermining the sense in which health and safety are a signal commitment of the common life—a central *practice* by which the body-politic defines itself and affirms its values.

In *Habits of the Heart,* practices are those shared activities that are not purely instrumental and that help shape and affirm the common life. Practices can be religious, aesthetic, or ethical. Public health belongs to the realm of the political and the ethical. Public health belongs to the ethical because it is concerned not only with explaining the occurrence of illness and disease in society, but also with ameliorating them. Beyond instrumental goals, public health is concerned with integrative goals—expressing the commitment of the whole people to face the threat of death and disease in solidarity.

Public health is also a practical science. Spanning the world of science and practical action, it seeks reasonable and practical means of altering property arrangements or limiting liberty to promote the health of the public generally.

These two ideas, the ideas of second languages and of social practices, shed light on why paternalism—at least public health paternalism—plays an affirmative role in the republican tradition. In the constitutional categories for protecting the public health, the regulatory power is to protect not individual citizens, but rather citizens considered as a group, the public health. In this tradition, the public, as well as the community itself, has a reality apart from the citizens who comprise it. Fundamental constituents of the community and the common life are its practices and institutions.

Practices are communal in nature, and concerned with the well-being of the community as a whole and not just the well-being of any particular person. Policy, and here public health paternalism, operates at the level of practices and not at the level of individual behavior. . . .

This suggests that public health paternalism and the language of community on which it is based fit the parent-child analogy very poorly. To Mill, all paternalism was wrong because the individual is best placed to know his own good: "He is the person most interested in his own well-being: the interest which any other person, except in cases of strong personal attachment, can have in it, is trifling. . . . "

But precisely because public health paternalism is aimed at the group and its practices, and not the specific individual, Mill's point is wrong. The good of the particular person is not the aim of health policy in a democracy which defends both the community and the individual. In fact, Mill is wrong twice, because particular individuals are often very poorly placed to judge the effects that market arrangements and practices have on the population as a whole. This is the task for legislatures, for organized groups of citizens, and for other agents of the public, including the citizen as voter.

Mill's dichotomy of either the harm principle or self-protection is too limited; the world of harms is not exhausted by self-imposed and other-imposed injuries. There is a third and very large set of problems that afflicts the community as a whole and that results primarily from inadequate safeguards over the practices of the common life. Economists and others often refer to this class of harms as "summing up problems" or "choice-in-the-small versus choice-in-the-large."

Creating, extending, or strengthening the practices of public health—and the collective goods principle that underlies it—ought to be the primary justification for our health and safety policy. Instead we usually base these regulations on the harm principle. We usually justify regulating the steel or coal industry on the grounds that workers and the general public have the risks of pollution or black lung visited on them, but consumers are not obliged to drink alcohol or smoke cigarettes. While this may be true, in the communitarian language and categories of public health, fixing blame is not the main point. We regulate the steel or coal industry because market competition undervalues collective goods like a clean environment or workers' safety. Using social organization to secure collective goods like public health, not preventing harms to others, is the proper rationale for health and safety regulations imposed on the steel or coal industry, or the alcohol or cigarette industry. . . .

Stengthening the public health includes not only the practical task of improving aggregate welfare, it also involves the task of reacquainting the American public with its republican and communitarian heritage, and encouraging citizens to share in reasonable and practical group schemes to promote a wider welfare, of which their own welfare is only a part. In political individualism, seatbelt legislation or signs on the beach restricting swimming when a lifeguard is not present restrict the individual's liberty for his or her own good. In this circumstance the appropriate slogan is: "The life you save may be your own." But in the second language of public health these restrictions define a common practice which shapes our life together, for the general or the common good. In the language of public health, the motto for such "paternalistic" legislation might be: "The lives we save together might include your own."

Security and Welfare

MICHAEL WALZER

MEMBERSHIP AND NEED

Membership is important because of what the members of a political community owe to one another and to no one else, or to no one else in the same degree. And the first thing they owe is the communal provision of security and welfare. This claim might be reversed: communal provision is important because it teaches us the value of membership. If we did not provide for one another, if we recognized no distinction between members and strangers, we would have no reason to form and maintain political communities. 'How shall men love their country', Rousseau asked, 'if it is nothing more for them than for strangers, and bestows on them only that which it can refuse to none?' Rousseau believed that citizens ought to love their country and therefore that their country ought to give them particular reasons to do so. Membership (like kinship) is a special relation. It's not enough to say, as Edmund Burke did, that 'to make us love our country, our country ought to be lovely.' The crucial thing is that it be lovely for us—though we always hope that it will be lovely for others (we also love its reflected loveliness).

Political community for the sake of provision, provision for the sake of community: the process works both ways, and that is perhaps its crucial feature. Philosophers and political theorists have been too quick to turn it into a simple calculation. Indeed, we are rationalists of everyday life; we come together, we sign the social contract or reiterate the signing of it, in order to provide for our needs. And we value the contract insofar as those needs are met. But one of our needs is community itself: culture, religion, and politics. It is only under the aegis of these three that all the other things we need become *socially recognized needs,* take on historical and determinate form. The social contract is an agreement to reach decisions together about what goods are necessary to our common life, and then to provide those goods for one another. The signers owe

From Chapter 3 (partial) in *Spheres of Justice: A Defense of Pluralism and Equality* by Michael Walzer. Copyright © 1983 by Basic Books, Inc. Reprinted by permission of BasicBooks, a subsidiary of Perseus Books Group, LLC, and also Blackwell Publishers.

one another more than mutual aid, for that they owe or can owe to anyone. They owe mutual provision of all those things for the sake of which they have separated themselves from mankind as a whole and joined forces in a particular community. *Amour social* is one of those things; but though it is a distributed good—often unevenly distributed—it arises only in the course of other distributions (and of the political choices that the other distributions require). Mutual provision breeds mutuality. So the common life is simultaneously the prerequisite of provision and one of its products.

Men and women come together because they literally cannot live apart. But they can live together in many different ways. Their survival and then their well-being require a common effort: against the wrath of the gods, the hostility of other people, the indifference and malevolence of nature (famine, flood, fire, and disease), the brief transit of a human life. Not army camps alone, as David Hume wrote, but temples, storehouses, irrigation works, and burial grounds are the true mothers of cities. As the list suggests, origins are not singular in character. Cities differ from one another, partly because of the natural environments in which they are built and the immediate dangers their builders encounter, partly because of the conceptions of social goods that the builders hold. They recognize but also create one another's needs and so give a particular shape to what I will call the 'sphere of security and welfare'. The sphere itself is as old as the oldest human community. Indeed, one might say that the original community is a sphere of security and welfare, a system of communal provision, distorted, no doubt, by gross inequalities of strength and cunning. But the system has, in any case, no natural form. Different experiences and different conceptions lead to different patterns of provision. Though there are some goods that are needed absolutely, there is no good such that once we see it, we know how it stands *vis-à-vis* all other goods and how much of it we owe to one another. The nature of a need is not self-evident.

Communal provision is both general and particular. It is general whenever public funds are spent so as to benefit all or most of the members without any distribution to individuals. It is particular whenever goods are actually handed over to all or any of the members.* Water, for example, is one of the bare requirements of civil life', and the building of reservoirs is a form of general provision. But the delivery of water to one rather than to another neighbour-

---

*I don't mean to reiterate here the technical distinction that economists make between public and private goods. General provision is always public, at least on the less stringent definitions of that term (which specify only that public goods are those that can't be provided to some and not to other members of the community). So are most forms of particular provision, for even goods delivered to individuals generate non-exclusive benefits for the community as a whole. Scholarships to orphans, for example, are private to the orphans, public to the community of citizens within which the orphans will one day work and vote. But public goods of this latter sort, which depend upon prior distributions to particular persons or groups, have been controversial in many societies; and I have designed my categories so as to enable me to examine them closely.

hood (where, say, the wealthier citizens live) is particular. The securing of the food supply is general; the distribution of food to widows and orphans is particular. Public health is most often general, the care of the sick, most often particular. Sometimes the criteria for general and particular provision will differ radically. The building of temples and the organization of religious services is an example of general provision designed to meet the needs of the community as a whole, but communion with the gods may be allowed only to particularly meritorious members (or it may be sought privately in secret or in noncomformist sects). The system of justice is a general good, meeting common needs; but the actual distribution of rewards and punishments may serve the particular needs of a ruling class, or it may be organized, as we commonly think it should be, to give individuals what they individually deserve. Simone Weil has argued that, with regard to justice, need operates at both the general and the particular levels, since criminals need to be punished. But that is an idiosyncratic use of the word *need*. More likely, the punishment of criminals is something only the rest of us need. But need does operate both generally and particularly for other goods: health care is an obvious example that I will later consider in some detail.

Despite the inherent forcefulness of the word, needs are elusive. People don't just have needs, they have ideas about their needs; they have priorities, they have degrees of need; and these priorities and degrees are related not only to their human nature but also to their history and culture. Since resources are always scarce, hard choices have to be made. I suspect that these can only be political choices. They are subject to a certain philosophical elucidation, but the idea of need and the commitment to communal provision do not by themselves yield any clear determination of priorities or degrees. Clearly we can't meet, and we don't have to meet, every need to the same degree or any need to the ultimate degree. The ancient Athenians, for example, provided public baths and gymnasiums for the citizens but never provided anything remotely resembling unemployment insurance or social security. They made a choice about how to spend public funds, a choice shaped presumably by their understanding of what the common life required. It would be hard to argue that they made a mistake. I suppose there are notions of need that would yield such a conclusion, but these would not be notions acceptable to—they might not even be comprehensible to—the Athenians themselves.

The question of degree suggests even more clearly the importance of political choice and the irrelevance of any merely philosophical stipulation. Needs are not only elusive; they are also expansive. In the phrase of the contemporary philosopher Charles Fried, needs are voracious; they eat up resources. But it would be wrong to suggest that therefore need cannot be a distributive principle. It is, rather, a principle subject to political limitation; and the limits (within limits) can be arbitrary, fixed by some temporary coalition of interests or majority of voters. Consider the case of physical security in a modern American city. We could provide absolute security, eliminate every source of violence except domestic violence, if we put a street light every ten yards and stationed a policeman every thirty yards throughout the city. But that would be very expensive, and so we settle for something less. How much less can only be decided politically.* One can imagine the sorts of things that would figure in the debates. Above all, I think, there would be a certain understanding—more or less widely shared, controversial only at the margins—of what constitutes 'enough' security or of what level of insecurity is simply intolerable. The decision would also be affected by other factors: alternative needs, the state of the economy, the agitation of the policemen's union, and so on. But whatever decision is ultimately reached, for whatever reasons, security is provided because the citizens need it. And because, at some level, they all need it, the criterion of need remains a critical standard (as we shall see) even though it cannot determine priority and degree. . . .

THE EXTENT OF PROVISION

Distributive justice in the sphere of welfare and security has a twofold meaning: it refers, first to the recognition of need and, second, to the recognition of membership. Goods must be provided to needy members because of their neediness, but they must also be provided in such a way as to sustain their membership. It's not the case, however, that members have a claim on any specific set of goods. Welfare rights are fixed only when a community adopts some programme of mutual provision. There are strong arguments to be made that, under given historical conditions, such-and-such a programme should be adopted. But these are not arguments about individual rights; they are arguments about the character of a particular political community. No one's rights were violated because the Athenians did not allocate public funds for the education of children. Perhaps they believed, and perhaps they were right, that the public life of the city was education enough.

The right that members can legitimately claim is of a more general sort. It undoubtedly includes some version of the Hobbesian right to life, some claim on communal resources for bare subsistence. No community can allow its members to starve to death when there is food available to feed them; no government can stand passively by at such a time—not if it claims to be a government of or by or for the community. The indifference of Britain's rulers during the Irish potato famine in the 1840s is a sure sign that Ireland was a colony, a

---

*And should be decided politically: that is what democratic political arrangements are for. Any philosophical effort to stipulate in detail the rights or the entitlements of individuals would radically constrain the scope of democratic decision making. I have argued this point elsewhere.

conquered land, no real part of Great Britain. This is not to justify the indifference—one has obligations to colonies and to conquered peoples—but only to suggest that the Irish would have been better served by a government, virtually any government, of their own. Perhaps Burke came closest to describing the fundamental right that is at stake here when he wrote: 'Government is a contrivance of human wisdom to provide for human wants. Men have a right that these wants should be provided for by this wisdom.' It only has to be said that the wisdom in question is the wisdom not of a ruling class, as Burke seems to have thought, but of the community as a whole. Only its culture, its character, its common understandings can define the 'wants' that are to be provided for. But culture, character, and common understandings are not givens; they don't operate automatically; at any particular moment, the citizens must argue about the extent of mutual provision.

They argue about the meaning of the social contract, the original and reiterated conception of the sphere of security and welfare. This is not a hypothetical or an ideal contract of the sort John Rawls has described. Rational men and women in the original position, deprived of all particular knowledge of their social standing and cultural understanding, would probably opt, as Rawls has argued, for an equal distribution of whatever goods they were told they needed. But this formula doesn't help very much in determining what choices people will make, or what choices they should make, once they know who and where they are. In a world of particular cultures, competing conceptions of the good, scarce resources, elusive and expansive needs, there isn't going to be a single formula, universally applicable. There isn't going to be a single universally approved path that carries us from a notion like, say, 'fair shares' to a comprehensive list of the goods to which that notion applies. Fair shares of what?

Justice, tranquillity, defence, welfare, and liberty: that is the list provided by the United States Constitution. One could construe it as an exhaustive list, but the terms are vague; they provide at best a starting point for public debate. The standard appeal in that debate is to a larger idea: the Burkeian general right, which takes on determinate force only under determinate conditions and requires different sorts of provision in different times and places. The idea is simply that we have come together, shaped a community, in order to cope with difficulties and dangers that we could not cope with alone. And so whenever we find ourselves confronted with difficulties and dangers of that sort, we look for communal assistance. As the balance of individual and collective capacity changes, so the kinds of assistance that are looked for change, too.

The history of public health in the West might usefully be told in these terms. Some minimal provision is very old, as the Greek and Jewish examples suggest; the measures adopted were a function of the community's sense of danger and the extent of its medical knowledge. Over the years, living arrangements on a larger scale bred new dangers, and scientific advance generated a new sense of danger and a new awareness of the possibilities of coping. And then groups of citizens pressed for a wider programme of communal provision, exploiting the new science to reduce the risks of urban life. That, they might rightly say, is what the community is for. A similar argument can be made in the case of social security. The very success of general provision in the field of public health has greatly extended the span of a normal human life and then also the span of years during which men and women are unable to support themselves, during which they are physically but most often not socially, politically, or morally incapacitated. Once again, support for the disabled is one of the oldest and most common forms of particular provision. But now it is required on a much larger scale than ever before. Families are overwhelmed by the costs of old age and look for help to the political community. Exactly what ought to be done will be a matter of dispute. Words like *health, danger, science,* even *old age,* have very different meanings in different cultures; no external specification is possible. But this is not to say that it won't be clear enough to the people involved that something—some particular set of things—ought to be done.

Perhaps these examples are too easy. Disease is a general threat; old age, a general prospect. Not so unemployment and poverty, which probably lie beyond the ken of many well-to-do people. The poor can always be isolated, locked into ghettos, blamed and punished for their own misfortune. At this point, it might be said, provision can no longer be defended by invoking anything like the 'meaning' of the social contract. But let us look more closely at the easy cases; for, in fact, they involve all the difficulties of the difficult ones. Public health and social security invite us to think of the political community, in T. H. Marshall's phrase, as a 'mutual benefit club'. All provision is reciprocal; the members take turns providing and being provided for, much as Aristotle's citizens take turns ruling and being ruled. This is a happy picture, and one that is really understandable in contractualist terms. It is not only the case that rational agents, knowing nothing of their specific situation, would agree to these two forms of provision; the real agents, the ordinary citizens, of every modern democracy have in fact agreed to them. The two are, or so it appears, equally in the interests of hypothetical and of actual people. Coercion is only necessary in practice because some minority of actual people don't understand, or don't consistently understand, their real interests. Only the reckless and the improvident need to be forced to contribute—and it can always be said of them that they joined in the social contract precisely in order to protect themselves against their own recklessness and improvidence. In fact, however, the reasons for coercion go much deeper than this; the political community is something more than a mutual benefit club; and the extent of communal provision in any given case—what it is and what it should be—is determined by conceptions of need that are more problematic than the argument thus far suggests.

Consider again the case of public health. No communal provision is possible here without the constraint of a wide range of activities profitable to individual members of the community but threatening to some larger number. Even something so simple, for example, as the provision of uncontaminated milk to large urban populations requires extensive public control; and control is a political achievement, the result (in the United States) of bitter struggles, over many years, in one city after another. When the farmers or the middlemen of the dairy industry defended free enterprise, they were certainly acting rationally in their own interests. The same thing can be said of other entrepreneurs who defend themselves against the constraints of inspection, regulation, and enforcement. Public activities of these sorts may be of the highest value to the rest of us; they are not of the highest value to all of us. Though I have taken public health as an example of general provision, it is provided only at the expense of some members of the community. Moreover, it benefits most the most vulnerable of the others: thus, the special importance of the building code for those who live in crowded tenements, and of anti-pollution laws for those who live in the immediate vicinity of factory smokestacks or water drains. Social security, too, benefits the most vulnerable members, even if, for reasons I have already suggested, the actual payments are the same for everyone. For the well-to-do can, or many of them think they can, help themselves even in time of trouble and would much prefer not to be forced to help anyone else. The truth is that every serious effort at communal provision (insofar as the income of the community derives from the wealth of its members) is redistributive in character. The benefits it provides are not, strictly speaking, mutual.

Once again, rational agents ignorant of their own social standing would agree to such a redistribution. But they would agree too easily, and their agreement doesn't help us understand what sort of a redistribution is required: How much? For what purposes? In practice, redistribution is a political matter, and the coercion it involves is foreshadowed by the conflicts that rage over its character and extent. Every particular measure is pushed through by some coalition of particular interests. But the ultimate appeal in these conflicts is not to the particular interests, not even to a public interest conceived as their sum, but to collective values, shared understandings of membership, health, food and shelter, work and leisure. The conflicts themselves are often focused, at least overtly, on questions of fact; the understandings are assumed. Thus the entrepreneurs of the dairy industry denied as long as they could the connection between contaminated milk and tuberculosis. But once that connection was established, it was difficult for them to deny that milk should be inspected: *caveat emptor* was not, in such a case, a plausible doctrine. Similarly, in the debates over old-age pensions in Great Britain, politicians mostly agreed on the traditional British value of self-help but disagreed sharply about whether self-help was still possible through the established working-class friendly societies. These were real mutual-benefit clubs organized on a strictly voluntary basis, but they seemed about to be overwhelmed by the growing numbers of the aged. It became increasingly apparent that the members simply did not have the resources to protect themselves and one another from poverty in old age. And few British politicians were prepared to say that they should be left unprotected.

Here, then, is a more precise account of the social contract: it is an agreement to redistribute the resources of the members in accordance with some shared understanding of their needs, subject to ongoing political determination in detail. The contract is a moral bond. It connects the strong and the weak, the lucky and the unlucky, the rich and the poor, creating a union that transcends all differences of interest, drawing its strength from history, culture, religion, language, and so on. Arguments about communal provision are, at the deepest level, interpretations of that union. The closer and more inclusive it is, the wider the recognition of needs, the greater the number of social goods that are drawn into the sphere of security and welfare. I don't doubt that many political communities have redistributed resources on very different principles, not in accordance with the needs of the members generally but in accordance with the power of the wellborn or the wealthy. But that, as Rousseau suggested in his *Discourse on Inequality,* makes a fraud of the social contract. In any community, where resources are taken away from the poor and given to the rich, the rights of the poor are being violated. The wisdom of the community is not engaged in providing for their wants. Political debate about the nature of those wants will have to be repressed, else the fraud will quickly be exposed. When all the members share in the business of interpreting the social contract, the result will be a more or less extensive system of communal provision. If all states are in principle welfare states, democracies are most likely to be welfare states in practice. Even the imitation of democracy breeds welfarism, as in the 'people's democracies', where the state protects the people against every disaster except those that it inflicts on them itself.

So democratic citizens argue among themselves and opt for many different sorts of security and welfare, extending far beyond my 'easy' examples of public health and old-age pensions. The category of socially recognized needs is open-ended. For the people's sense of what they need encompasses not only life itself but also the good life, and the appropriate balance between these two is itself a matter of dispute. The Athenian drama and the Jewish academies were both financed with money that could have been spent on housing, say, or on medicine. But drama and education were taken by Greeks and Jews to be not merely enhancements of the common life but vital aspects of communal welfare. I want to stress again that these are not judgements that can easily be called incorrect.

AN AMERICAN WELFARE STATE

What sort of communal provision is appropriate in a society like our own? It's not my purpose here to anticipate the outcomes of democratic debate or to stipulate in detail the extent or the forms of provision. But it can be argued, I think, that the citizens of a modern industrial democracy owe a great deal to one another, and the argument will provide a useful opportunity to test the critical force of the principles I have defended up until now: that every political community must attend to the needs of its members as they collectively understand those needs; that the goods that are distributed must be distributed in proportion to need; and that the distribution must recognize and uphold the underlying equality of membership. These are very general principles; they are meant to apply to a wide range of communities—to any community, in fact, where the members are each other's equals (before God or the law), or where it can plausibly be said that, however they are treated in fact, they ought to be each other's equals. The principles probably don't apply to a community organized hierarchically, as in traditional India, where the fruits of the harvest are distributed not according to need but according to caste—or rather, as Louis Dumont has written, where 'the needs of each are conceived to be different, depending on [his] caste.' Everyone is guaranteed a share, so Dumont's Indian village is still a welfare state, 'a sort of co-operative where the main aim is to ensure the subsistence of everyone in accordance with his social function', but not a welfare state or a co-operative whose principles we can readily understand. (But Dumont does not tell us how food is supposed to be distributed in time of scarcity. If the subsistence standard is the same for everyone, then we are back in a familiar world.)

Clearly, the three principles apply to the citizens of the United States; and they have considerable force here because of the affluence of the community and the expansive understanding of individual need. On the other hand the United States currently maintains one of the shabbier systems of communal provision in the Western world. This is so for a variety of reasons: the community of citizens is loosely organized; various ethnic and religious groups run welfare programmes of their own; the ideology of self-reliance and entrepreneurial opportunity is widely accepted; and the movements of the left, particularly the labour movement, are relatively weak. Democratic decision-making reflects these realities, and there is nothing in principle wrong with that. Nevertheless, the established pattern of provision doesn't measure up to the internal requirements of the sphere of security and welfare, and the common understandings of the citizens point toward a more elaborate pattern. One might also argue that American citizens should work to build a stronger and more intensely experienced political community. But this argument, though it would have distributive consequences, is not, properly speaking, an argument about distributive justice. The question is, What do the citizens owe one another, given the community they actually inhabit?

Consider the example of criminal justice. The actual distribution of punishments is an issue I will take up in a later chapter. But the autonomy of punishment, the certainty that people are being punished for the right reasons (whatever those are), depends upon the distribution of resources within the legal system. If accused men and women are to receive their rightful share of justice, they must first have a rightful share of legal aid. Hence the institution of the public defender and the assigned counsel: just as the hungry must be fed, so the accused must be defended; and they must be defended in proportion to their needs. But no impartial observer of the American legal system today can doubt that the resources necessary to meet this standard are not generally available. The rich and the poor are treated differently in American courts, though it is the public commitment of the courts to treat them the same. The argument for a more generous provision follows from that commitment. If justice is to be provided at all, it must be provided equally for all accused citizens without regard to their wealth (or their race, religion, political partisanship, and so on). I don't mean to underestimate the practical difficulties here; but this, again, is the inner logic of provision, and it makes for an illuminating example of complex equality. For the inner logic of reward and punishment is different, requiring, as I shall argue later, that distributions be proportional to desert and not to need. Punishment is a negative good that ought to be monopolized by those who have acted badly—and who have been found guilty of acting badly (after a resourceful defence).

Legal aid raises no theoretical problems because the institutional structures for providing it already exist, and what is at stake is only the readiness of the community to live up to the logic of its own institutions. I want to turn now to an area where American institutions are relatively underdeveloped, and where communal commitment is problematic, the subject of continuing political debate: the area of medical care. But here the argument for a more extensive provision must move more slowly. It isn't enough to summon up a 'right to treatment.' I shall have to recount something of the history of medical care as a social good.

THE CASE OF MEDICAL CARE

Until recent times, the practice of medicine was mostly a matter of free enterprise. Doctors made their diagnosis, gave their advice, healed or didn't heal their patients, for a fee. Perhaps the private character of the economic relationship was connected to the intimate character of the professional relationship. More likely, I think, it had to do with the relative marginality of medicine itself. Doctors could, in fact, do very little for their patients; and the common attitude in the face of disease (as in the face of poverty) was a stoical fatalism. Or, popular remedies were developed that were not much less effective, sometimes more effective, than those prescribed by established physicians. Folk medicine sometimes produced a kind of communal provision at the local level, but it was equally likely to generate new practitioners, charging fees in their turn. Faith healing followed a similar pattern.

Leaving these two aside, we can say that the distribution of medical care has historically rested in the hands of the medical profession, a guild of physicians that dates at least from the time of Hippocrates in the fifth century BC. The guild has functioned to exclude unconventional practitioners and to regulate the number of physicians in any given community. A genuinely free market has never been in the interest of its members. But it is in the interest of the members to sell their services to individual patients; and thus, by and large, the well-to-do have been well cared for (in accordance with the current understanding of good care) and the poor hardly cared for at all. In a few urban communities—in the medieval Jewish communities, for example—medical services were more widely available. But they were virtually unknown for most people most of the time. Doctors were the servants of the rich, often attached to noble houses and royal courts. With regard to this practical outcome, however, the profession has always had a collective bad conscience. For the distributive logic of the practice of medicine seems to be this: that care should be proportionate to illness and not to wealth. Hence, there have always been doctors, like those honoured in ancient Greece, who served the poor on the side, as it were, even while they earned their living from paying patients. Most doctors, present in an emergency, still feel bound to help the victim without regard to his material status. It is a matter of professional Good Samaritanism that the call 'Is there a doctor in the house?' should not go unanswered if there is a doctor to answer it. In ordinary times, however, there was little call for medical help, largely because there was little faith in its actual helpfulness. And so the bad conscience of the profession was not echoed by any political demand for the replacement of free enterprise by communal provision.

In Europe during the Middle Ages, the cure of souls was public, the cure of bodies private. Today, in most European countries, the situation is reversed. The reversal is best explained in terms of a major shift in the common understanding of souls and bodies: we have lost confidence in the cure of souls, and we have come increasingly to believe, even to be obsessed with, the cure of bodies. Descartes's famous declaration that the 'preservation of health' was the 'chief of all goods' may be taken to symbolize the shift—or to herald it, for in the history of popular attitudes, Descartes's *Discourse on Method* came very early. Then, as eternity receded in the popular consciousness, longevity moved to the fore. Among medieval Christians, eternity was a socially recognized need; and every effort was made to see that it was widely and equally distributed, that every Christian had an equal chance at salvation and eternal life: hence, a church in every parish, regular services, catechism for the young, compulsory communion, and so on. Among modern citizens, longevity is a socially recognized need; and increasingly every effort is made to see that it is widely and equally distributed, that every citizen has an equal chance at a long and healthy life: hence doctors and hospitals in every district, regular check-ups, health education for the young, compulsory vaccination, and so on.

Parallel to the shift in attitudes, and following naturally from it, was a shift in institutions: from the church to the clinic and the hospital. But the shift has been gradual: a slow development of communal interest in medical care, a slow erosion of interest in religious care. The first major form of medical provision came in the area of prevention, not of treatment, probably because the former involved no interference with the prerogatives of the guild of physicians. But the beginnings of provision in the area of treatment were roughly simultaneous with the great public health campaigns of the late nineteenth century, and the two undoubtedly reflect the same sensitivity to questions of physical survival. The licensing of physicians, the establishment of state medical schools and urban clinics, the filtering of tax money into the great voluntary hospitals: these measures involved, perhaps, only marginal interference with the profession— some of them, in fact, reinforced its guildlike character; but they already represent an important public commitment. Indeed, they represent a commitment that ultimately can be fulfilled only by turning physicians, or some substantial number of them, into public physicians (as a smaller number once turned themselves into court physicians) and by abolishing or constraining the market in medical care. But before I defend that transformation, I want to stress the unavoidability of the commitment from which it follows.

What has happened in the modern world is simply that disease itself, even when it is endemic rather than epidemic, has come to be seen as a plague. And since the plague can be dealt with, it *must* be dealt with. People will not endure what they no longer believe they have to endure. Dealing with tuberculosis, cancer, or heart failure, however, requires a common effort. Medical research is expensive, and the treatment of many particular diseases lies far beyond the resources of ordinary citizens. So the community must step in, and any democratic community will in fact step in, more or less vigorously, more or less effectively, depending on the outcome of particular political battles. Thus, the role of the American Government (or governments, for much of the activity is at the state and local levels): subsidizing research, training doctors, providing hospitals and equipment, regulating voluntary insurance schemes, underwriting the treatment of the very old. All this represents 'the contrivance of human wisdom to provide for human wants.' And all that is required to make it morally necessary is the development of a 'want' so widely and deeply felt that it can plausibly be said that it is the want not of this or that person alone but of the community generally—a 'human want' even though culturally shaped and stressed.*

But once communal provision begins, it is subject to further moral constraints: it must provide what is 'wanted' equally to all the members of the community; and it must do so in ways that respect their membership. Now, even the pattern of medical provision in the United States, though it stops far short of a national health service, is intended to provide minimally decent care to all who need it. Once public funds are committed, public officials can hardly intend anything less. At the same time, however, no political decision has yet been made to challenge directly the system of free enterprise in medical care. And so long as that system exists, wealth will be dominant in (this part of) the sphere of security and welfare; individuals will be cared for in proportion to their ability to pay and not to their need for care. In fact, the situation is more complex than that formula suggests, for communal provision already encroaches upon the free market, and the very sick and the very old sometimes receive exactly the treatment they should receive. But it is clear that poverty remains a significant bar to adequate and consistent treatment. Perhaps the most telling statistic about contemporary American medicine is the correlation of visits to doctors and hospitals with social class rather than with degree or incidence of illness. Middle- and upper-class Americans are considerably more likely to have a private physician and to see him often, and considerably less likely to be seriously ill, than are their poorer fellow citizens. Were medical care a luxury, these discrepancies would not matter much; but as soon as medical care becomes a socially recognized need, and as soon as the community invests in its provision, they matter a great deal. For then deprivation is a double loss—to one's health and to one's social standing. Doctors and hospitals have become such massively important features of contemporary life that to be cut off from the help they provide is not only dangerous but also degrading.

But any fully developed system of medical provision will require the constraint of the guild of physicians. Indeed, this is more generally true: the provision of security and welfare requires the constraint of those men and women who had previously controlled the goods in question and sold them on the market (assuming, what is by no means always true, that the market predates

---

*Arguing against Bernard Williams's claim that the only proper criterion for the distribution of medical care is medical need, Robert Nozick asks why it doesn't then follow 'that the only proper criterion for the distribution of barbering services is barbering need'? Perhaps it does follow if one attends only to be the 'internal goal' of the activity, conceived in universal terms. But it doesn't follow if one attends to the social meaning of the activity, the place of the good it distributes in the life of a particular group of people. One can conceive of a society in which haircuts took on such central cultural significance that communal provision would be morally required, but it is something more than an interesting fact that no such society has ever existed. I have been helped in thinking about these issues by an article of Thomas Scanlon's; I adopt here his 'conventionalist' alternative.

communal provision). For what we do when we declare this or that good to be a needed good is to block or constrain its free exchange. We also block any other distributive procedure that doesn't attend to need—popular election, meritocratic competition, personal or familiar preference, and so on. But the market is, at least in the United States today, the chief rival of the sphere of security and welfare; and it is most importantly the market that is pre-empted by the welfare state. Needed goods cannot be left to the whim, or distributed in the interest, of some powerful group of owners or practitioners.

Most often, ownership is abolished, and practitioners are effectively conscripted or, at least, 'signed up' in the public service. They serve for the sake of the social need and not, or not simply, for their own sakes: thus, priests for the sake of eternal life, soldiers for the sake of national defence, public [state] school teachers for the sake of their pupils' education. Priests act wrongly if they sell salvation; soldiers, if they set up as mercenaries; teachers, if they cater to the children of the wealthy. Sometimes the conscription is only partial, as when lawyers are required to be officers of the court, serving the cause of justice even while they also serve their clients and themselves. Sometimes the conscription is occasional and temporary, as when lawyers are required to act as 'assigned counsels' for defendants unable to pay. In these cases, a special effort is made to respect the personal character of the lawyer-client relationship. I would look for a similar effort in any fully developed national health service. But I see no reason to respect the doctor's market freedom. Needed goods are not commodities. Or, more precisely, they can be bought and sold only insofar as they are available above and beyond whatever level of provision is fixed by democratic decision making (and only insofar as the buying and selling doesn't distort distributions below that level).

It might be argued, however, that the refusal thus far to finance a national health service constitutes a political decision by the American people about the level of communal care (and about the relative importance of other goods): a minimal standard for everyone—namely, the standard of the urban clinics; and free enterprise beyond that. That would seem to me an inadequate standard, but it would not necessarily be an unjust decision. It is not, however, the decision the American people have made. The common appreciation of the importance of medical care has carried them well beyond that. In fact, federal, state, and local governments now subsidize different levels of care for different classes of citizens. This might be all right, too, if the classification were connected to the purposes of the care—if, for example, soldiers and defence workers were given special treatment in time of war. But the poor, the middle class, and the rich make an indefensible triage. So long as communal funds are spent, as they currently are, to finance research, build hospitals, and pay the fees of doctors in private practice, the services that these expenditures underwrite must be equally available to all citizens.

This, then, is the argument for an expanded American welfare state. It follows from the three principles with which I began, and it suggests that the tendency of those principles is to free security and welfare from the prevailing patterns of dominance. Though a variety of institutional arrangements is possible, the three principles would seem to favour provision in kind; they suggest an important argument against current proposals to distribute money instead of education, legal aid, or medical care. The negative income tax, for example, is a plan to increase the purchasing power of the poor—a modified version of simply equality. This plan would not, however, abolish the dominance of wealth in the sphere of need. Short of a radical equalization, men and women with greater purchasing power could still, and surely would, bid up the price of needed services. So the community would be investing, though now only indirectly, in individual welfare but without fitting provision to the shape of need. Even with equal incomes, health care delivered through the market would not be responsive to need; nor would the market provide adequately for medical research. This is not an argument against the negative income tax, however, for it may be the case that money itself, in a market economy, is one of the things that people need. And then it too, perhaps, should be provided in kind.

I want to stress again that no *a priori* stipulation of what needs ought to be recognized is possible; nor is there any *a priori* way of determining appropriate levels of provision. Our attitudes toward medical care have a history; they have been different; they will be different again. The forms of communal provision have changed in the past and will continue to change. But they don't change automatically as attitudes change. The old order has its clients; there is a lethargy in institutions as in individuals. Moreover, popular attitudes are rarely so clear as they are in the case of medical care. So change is always a matter of political argument, organization, and struggle. All that the philosopher can do is to describe the basic structure of the arguments and the constraints they entail. Hence the three principles, which can be summed up in a revised version of Marx's famous maxim: From each according to his ability (or his resources); to each according to his socially recognized needs. This, I think, is the deepest meaning of the social contract. It only remains to work out the details—but in everyday life, the details are everything.

Medicine and Public Health, Ethics and Human Rights

JONATHAN M. MANN

The relationships among medicine, public health, ethics, and human rights are now evolving rapidly, in response to a series of events, experiences, and struggles. These include the shock of the worldwide epidemic of human immunodeficiency virus and AIDS, continuing work on diverse aspects of women's health, and challenges exemplified by the complex humanitarian emergencies of Somalia, Iraq, Bosnia, Rwanda, and now, Zaire.

From among the many impacts of these experiences, three seem particularly salient. First, human rights thinking and action have become much more closely allied to, and even integrated with, public health work. Second, the long-standing absence of an ethics of public health has been highlighted. Third, the human rights-related roles and responsibilities of physicians and other medical workers are receiving increased attention.

PUBLIC HEALTH AND MEDICINE

To explore the first of these issues—the connections between human rights and public health—it is essential to review several central elements of modern public health.

Medicine and public health are two complementary and interacting approaches for promoting and protecting health—defined by the World Health Organization (WHO) as a state of physical, mental, and social well-being. Yet medicine and public health can, and also must be differentiated, because in several important ways they are not the same. The fundamental difference involves the population emphasis of public health, which contrasts with the essentially individual focus of medical care. Public health identifies and measures threats to the health of populations, develops governmental policies in response

From *The Hastings Center Report*, May–June 1997, 6-13. Copyright © The Hastings Center. Reproduced by permission.

to these concerns, and seeks to assure certain health and related services. In contrast, medical care focuses upon individuals—diagnosis, treatment, relief of suffering, and rehabilitation.

Several specific points follow from this essential difference. For example, different instruments are called for: while public health measures population health status through epidemiological, survey, and other statistically based methods, medicine examines biophysical and psychological status using a combination of techniques, including dialogue, physical examination, and laboratory study of the individual. Public health generally values most highly (or at least is supposed to) primary prevention, that is, preventing the adverse health event in the first place, such as helping to prevent the automobile accident or the lead poisoning from happening at all. In contrast, medicine generally responds to existing health conditions, in the context of either secondary or tertiary prevention. Secondary prevention involves avoiding or delaying the adverse impact of a health condition like hypertension or diabetes. Thus, while the hypertension or insulin deficiency exists, its effects, such as heart disease, kidney failure, or blindness, can be avoided or delayed. So-called tertiary prevention involves those efforts to help sustain maximal functional and psychological capacity despite the presence of both the disease, such as hypertension, and its outcomes, heart disease, stroke, or kidney failure.

Accordingly, the skills and expertise needed in public health include epidemiology, biostatistics, policy analysis, economics, sociology, and other behavioral sciences. In contrast, medical skills and expertise center on the exploration, analysis, and response to the biophysical status of individuals, based principally on an understanding of biology, biochemistry, immunology, pharmacology, pathology, pathophysiology, anatomy, and psychology.

Naturally, the settings in which public health and medicine operate also differ: governmental organizations, large-scale public programs, and various fora associated with developing and implementing public policy are inherently part of public health, while private medical offices, clinics, and medical care facilities of varying complexity and sophistication are the settings in which medical care is generally provided.

Finally, the relationship between the profession and the people with whom it deals differs: in a sense, public health comes to you, while you go to the doctor. And expectations associated with each domain differ: from medicine, individual care and treatment are sought; from public health, protection against broad health threats like epidemic disease, unsafe water, or chemical pollution is expected.

Therefore, public health and medicine are principally distinguished by their focus on collectivities or on individuals, respectively, with a series of subsidiary differences involving methods of work, systems of analysis and measurement, emphasis on primary versus secondary or tertiary prevention, types of expertise and relevant skill, settings in which work is conducted, and client/public relationships and expectations.

Yet obviously, there is substantial overlap. Public health requires a sound biomedical basis, and involves many medical practitioners, whose services are organized in settings such as maternal and child health clinics, or immunization programs. Also, medical practice operates within a context highly influenced and governed by law and public policy. The potentially fluid relationship between public health and medicine is further suggested by recent proposals in this country that certain traditional public health functions be delegated to the private medical sector.

Despite these many differences, people equate medical care with health. Certainly, this basic confusion has informed the recent discussions of health care in the United States; and coverage of health issues in the popular press around the world reflects this perspective, in which access to medical care and the quality of that care are seen as the principal health needs of individuals and populations.

MEDICINE AND HEALTH

Yet the contribution of medicine to health, while undeniably important (and vital in certain situations), is actually quite limited. For example, it is estimated that only about one-sixth of the years of life expectancy gained in this country during this century can be attributed to the beneficial impact of medicine, medical care, and medical research. And it has been estimated that only about 10 percent of preventable premature deaths are associated with a lack of medical care. . . .

The vast majority of research into the health of populations identifies so-called "societal factors" as the major determinants of health status. Most of the work in this area has focused on socioeconomic status as the key variable, for it is clear, throughout history and in all societies, that the rich live generally longer and healthier lives than the poor. Thus, in the United Kingdom in 1911, the age-adjusted standardized mortality rate among members of the lowest social class was 1.6 times higher than for the highest social class. Interestingly, following creation of the National Health Services to ensure full access to medical care, and despite a dramatic change in major causes of death (from mainly infectious to mainly chronic diseases), in 1981 this societal gradient not only persisted, but increased, to a 2.1-fold higher standardized mortality rate among the lowest compared with the highest social class.

A major question arising from the socioeconomic status-health gradient is why there is a gradient. For example, among over 10,000 British civil servants followed for many years, health status and longevity were better for each successive category of civil servants, from lowest to highest. This raises two issues: first, while we believe we can—at least intuitively—explain poor health among the destitute when compared with the rich, associated with a lack of good food, housing, and with poor sanitary conditions, even the lowest class of British civil servants cannot be considered poor. Secondly, why should the civil servants in the next-to-highest group, living in quite comfortable circumstances, experience poorer health than the highest group?

Beyond these unanswered issues, many recent studies have pointed to the limited explanatory power of socioeconomic status, generally measured in terms of current income, years of education, and job classification. Other measures, such as the extent of socioeconomic inequality within a community, the nature, level, and temporal pattern of unemployment, societal connectedness and the extent of involvement in social networks, marital status, early childhood experiences, and exposure to dignity-denying situations have all been suggested as powerful potential components of a "black box" of societal factors whose dominant role in determining levels of preventable disease, disability, and premature death is beyond dispute.

AN ETHICS FOR PUBLIC HEALTH

Public health, although it began as a social movement, has—at least in recent years—responded relatively little to this most profound and vital knowledge about the dominant impact of society on health. To illustrate: we all know that certain behaviors have an enormous impact on health, such as cigarette smoking, excess alcohol intake, dietary choices, or levels of exercise and physical fitness. How these behaviors are conceptualized determines how they will be addressed by public health. The basic question is whether and to what extent these behaviors can be considered, and therefore responded to, as isolated individual choices.

Public health practitioners share a strong belief that important health-related behaviors are substantially influenced by societal factors and context. Yet examining public health programs designed to address the health problems associated with these same behaviors reveals that they generally consist of activities which assume that individuals have essentially complete control over their health-related behaviors. Traditional public health seeks to provide individuals with information and education about risks associated with diet or lack of exercise, along with various clinic-based services such as counseling, or distribution of condoms and other contraceptives. However, while public health may cite, or blame, or otherwise identify the societal-level or contextual issues—which it acknowledges to be of dominant importance, both in influencing individual behavior and for determining health status more broadly—it does not deal directly with these societal factors.

At least three reasons for this paradoxical inaction may be proposed. First, public health has lacked a conceptual framework for identifying and analyzing the essential societal factors that represent the "conditions in which people can be healthy." Second, a related problem: public health lacks a vocabulary with which to speak about and identify commonalities among health problems experienced by very different populations. Third, there is no consensus about the nature or direction of societal change that would be necessary to address the societal conditions involved. Lacking a coherent conceptual framework, a consistent vocabulary, and consensus about societal change, public health assembles and then tries valiantly to assimilate a wide variety of disciplinary perspectives, from economists, political scientists, social and behavioral scientists, health systems analysts, and a range of medical practitioners. Yet, while each of these perspectives provides some useful insight, public health becomes thereby a little bit of everything and thus not enough of anything.

With this background in mind, it would be expected that in the domains of public health and medicine, different, yet complementary languages for describing and incorporating values would be developed. For even when values are shared at a higher level of abstraction, the forms in which they are expressed, the settings in which they are evoked, and their practical application may differ widely.

Not surprisingly, medicine has chosen the language of ethics, as ethics has been developed in a context of individual relationships, and is well adapted to the nature, practice, settings, and expectations of medical care. The language of medical ethics has also been applied when medicine seeks to deal with issues such as the organization of medical care or the allocation of societal resources. However, the contribution of medical ethics to these societal issues has been less powerful when compared, for example, with its engagement in the behavior of individual medical practitioners.

Public health, at least in its contemporary form, is struggling to define and articulate its core values. In this context, the usefulness of the language and structure of ethics as we know it today has been questioned. Given its population focus, and its interest in the underlying conditions upon which health is predicated (and that these major determinants of health status are societal in nature), it seems evident that a framework which expresses fundamental values in societal terms, and a vocabulary of values which links directly with societal structure and function, may be better adapted to the work of public health than a more individually oriented ethical framework.

For this reason, modern human rights, precisely because they were initially developed entirely outside the health domain and seek to articulate the societal preconditions for human well-being, seem a far more useful framework, vocabulary, and form of guidance for public health efforts to analyze and respond directly to the societal determinants of health than any inherited from the past biomedical or public health tradition.

PUBLIC HEALTH AND HUMAN RIGHTS

The linkage between public health and human rights can be explored further by considering three relationships. The first focuses on the potential burden on human rights created by public health policies, programs, and practices. As public health generally involves direct or indirect state action, public health officials represent the state power toward which classical human rights concerns are traditionally addressed. Thus, in the modern world, public health officials have, for the first time, two fundamental responsibilities to the public: to protect and promote public health, and to protect and promote human rights. While public health officials may be unlikely to seek deliberately to violate human rights, there is great unawareness of human rights concepts and norms among public health practitioners. In stark contrast to the large number of bioethics courses available in medical educational settings, a recent survey of all twenty-eight accredited schools of public health in the United States and schools of public health in thirty-four other countries identified only seven formal courses in human rights for the presumed future leaders of public health.

Public health practice is heavily burdened by the problem of inadvertent discrimination. For example, outreach activities may "assume" that all populations are reached equally by a single, dominant-language message on television; or analysis "forgets" to include health problems uniquely relevant to certain groups, like breast cancer or sickle cell disease; or a program "ignores" the actual response capability of different population groups, as when lead poisoning warnings are given without concern for financial ability to ensure lead abatement. Indeed, inadvertent discrimination is so prevalent that all public health policies and programs should be considered discriminatory until proven otherwise, placing the burden on public health to affirm and ensure its respect for human rights.

In addition, in public health circles there is often an unspoken sense that public health and human rights concerns are inherently confrontational. At times, this has been true. In the early years of the HIV epidemic, the knee-jerk response of various public health officials to invoke mandatory testing, quarantine, and isolation did create a major clash with protectors of human rights. Even quite recently, an opinion piece in the *British Medical Journal* purports that excessive respect for human rights crippled public health efforts and is therefore responsible for the intensifying and expanding AIDS epidemic.

However, while modern human rights explicitly acknowledges that public health is a legitimate reason for limiting rights, more recently the underlying complementarity rather than inherent confrontation between public health and human rights has been emphasized. Again in the context of AIDS, public health has learned that discrimination toward HIV-infected people and people with AIDS is counterproductive. Specifically, when people found to be infected were deprived of employment, education, or ability to marry and travel, participation in prevention programs diminished. Thus, recent attention has been directed to a negotiation process for optimizing both the achievement of complementary public health goals and respect for human rights norms.

A second relationship between public health and human rights derives from the observation that human rights violations have health impacts, that is, adverse effects on physical, mental, and social well-being. For some rights, such as the right not to be tortured or imprisoned under inhumane conditions, the health damage seems evident, indeed inherent in the rights violation. However, even for torture, only more recently has the extensive, life-long, family and communitywide, and transgenerational impact of torture been recognized.

For many other rights, such as the right to information, to assembly, or to association, health impacts resulting from violation may not be initially so apparent. The violation of any right has measurable impacts on physical, mental, and social well-being; yet these health effects still remain, in large part, to be discovered and documented. Yet gradually, the connection is being established.

The right to association provides a useful example of this relationship. Public health benefits substantially—even requires—involvement of people in addressing problems that affect them. Because the ability of people concerned about a health problem to get together, talk, and search for effective solutions is so essential to public health, wherever the right to association is restricted, public health suffers. Taking a positive example from the history of HIV/AIDS: needle exchange—the trading-in of needles used for drug injection for clean needles, so as to avoid needle-sharing with consequent risk of HIV transmission—was invented by a union of drug users in Amsterdam. Needle exchange was a classic example of an innovative, local response to a pressing local problem. Needle exchange was not and would have been highly unlikely to have been developed by academics, government officials, or hired consultants! Yet the creative solution of needle exchange and respect for the right of association are closely linked. Thus, in societies in which people generally, or specific population groups, cannot associate around health, or other issues, such as injection drug users in the United States, or sex workers, or gay and lesbian people in many countries, local solutions are less able to emerge or be applied and public health is correspondingly compromised.

A third relationship between health and human rights has already been suggested; namely, that promoting and protecting human rights is inextricably linked with promoting and protecting health. Once again, this is because human rights offers a societal-level framework for identifying and responding to the underlying—societal—determinants of health. It is important to emphasize that human rights are respected not only for their instrumental value in contributing to public health goals, but for themselves, as societal goods of pre-eminent importance.

For example, a cluster of rights, including the rights to health, bodily integrity, privacy, information, education, and equal rights in marriage and divorce, have been called "reproductive rights," insofar as their realization (or violation) is now understood to play a major role in determining reproductive health. From an early focus on demographic targets for population control, to an emphasis on ensuring "informed consent" of women to various contraceptive methods, a new paradigm for population policies *and* reproductive health has recently emerged. Articulated most forcefully at the United Nations Conference on Population and Development in 1994 in Cairo, the focus has shifted to ensuring that women can make and effectuate real and informed choices about reproduction. And in turn, this is widely acknowledged to depend on realization of human rights.

Similarly, in the context of HIV/AIDS, vulnerability to the epidemic has now been associated with the extent of realization of human rights. For as the HIV epidemic matures and evolves within each community and country, it focuses inexorably on those groups who, before HIV/AIDS arrived, were already discriminated against, marginalized, and stigmatized within each society. Thus, in the United States the brunt of the epidemic today is among racial and ethnic minority populations, inner city poor, injection drug users, and, especially women in these communities. In Brazil, an epidemic that started among the jet set of Rio and São Paulo with time has become a major epidemic among the slum-dwellers in the *favelas* of Brazil's cities. The French, with characteristic linguistic precision, identify the major burden of HIV/AIDS to exist among "*les exclus*," those living at the margins of society. Now that a lack of respect for human rights has been identified as a societal level risk factor for HIV/AIDS vulnerability, HIV prevention efforts—for example, for women—are starting to go beyond traditional educational and service-based efforts to address the rights issues that will be a precondition for greater progress against the epidemic.

Ultimately, ethics and human rights derive from a set of quite similar, if not identical, core values. As with medicine and public health, rather than seeing human rights and ethics as conflicting domains, it seems more appropriate to consider a continuum, in which human rights is a language most useful for guiding societal level analysis and work, while ethics is a language most useful for guiding individual behavior. From this perspective, and precisely because public health must be centrally concerned with the structure and function of society, the language of human rights is extremely useful for expressing, considering, and incorporating values into public health analysis and response.

Thus, public health work requires both ethics applicable to the individual public health practitioner and a human rights framework to guide public health in its societal analysis and response. . . .

At the hypothetical extreme of individual medical care, ethics would be the most useful language. However, to the extent that the individual practitioner is cognizant of the societal forces acting upon the individual patient, societal level considerations may also be articulated in human rights terms. At the other extreme of public health, human rights is the most useful language, speaking as it does directly to the societal level determinants of well-being. Nevertheless, the ethical framework remains critical, for public health is carried out by individuals within specific professional roles and competencies. In practice, of course, positions between the hypothetical extremes of medicine and public health are more common, calling for mixtures of human rights and ethical concepts and language.

PROFESSIONAL ROLES AND RESPONSIBILITIES

The placement of both human rights and ethics and public health and medicine at ends of a continuum suggests also that the interest domains of individuals and organizations can be "mapped" and areas calling for additional attention can be highlighted.

According to this mapping approach, the "French Doctors" movement can be seen as primarily medical, primarily ethics-based, yet with growing involvement in the public health dimensions of health emergencies and in human rights issues raised by these complex humanitarian crises. Similarly, many traditional, medical ethics-based institutes and centers can be placed on this map. At the Harvard School of Public Health, the François-Xavier Bagnoud Center for Health and Human Rights, along with several others, is now focusing on the health-human rights territory. This map also suggests two major gaps in current work: on the ethics of public health, and on the relationships between medicine and human rights.

Where are the ethics of public health? In contrast to the important declarations of medical ethics such as the International Code of Medical Ethics of the World Medical Association and the Nuremberg Principles, the world of public health does not have a reasonably explicit set of ethical guidelines. In part, this deficiency may stem from the broad diversity of professional identities within public health. Yet, curiously, many of the occupational groups central to public health (epidemiologists, policy analysts, social scientists, biostatisticians, nutritionists, health system managers) have not yet developed, or are only now developing, widely accepted ethical guidelines or statements of principle for their work in the public health context. Thus, while a public health physician may draw upon medical ethics for guidance, the ethics of a public health physician have yet to be clearly articulated.

The central problem is one of coherence and identity: public health cannot develop an ethics until it has achieved clarity about its own identity; technical expertise and methodology are not substitutes for conceptual coherence. Or, as one student remarked a few years ago, public health spends too much time on the "p" values of biostatistics and not enough time on values.

To have an ethic, a profession needs clarity about central issues, including its major role and responsibilities. Two steps will be essential for public health to reach toward this analytic and definitional clarity.

First, public health must divest itself of its biomedical conceptual foundation. The language of disease, disability, and death is not the language of well-being; the vocabulary of diseases may detract from analysis and response to underlying societal conditions, of which traditional morbidity and mortality are expressions. It is clear that we do not yet know all about the universe of human suffering. Just as in the microbial world, in which new discoveries have become the norm—Ebola virus, hantavirus, toxic shock syndrome, Legionnaires' disease, AIDS—we are explorers in the larger world of human suffering and well-being. And our current maps of this universe, like world maps from sixteenth century Europe, have some very well-defined, familiar coastlines and territories and also contain large blank spaces, which beckon the explorer.

The language of biomedicine is cumbersome and ultimately perhaps of little usefulness in exploring the impacts of violations of dignity on physical, mental, and social well-being. The definition of dignity itself is complex and thus far elusive and unsatisfying. While the Universal Declaration of Human Rights starts by placing dignity first, "all people are born equal in dignity and rights," we do not yet have a vocabulary, or taxonomy, let alone an epidemiology of dignity violations.

Yet it seems we all know when our dignity is violated or impugned. Perform the following experiment: recall, in detail, an incident from your own life in which your dignity was violated, for whatever reason. If you will immerse yourself in the memory, powerful feelings will likely arise—of anger, shame, powerlessness, despair. When you connect with the power of these feelings, it seems intuitively obvious that such feelings, particularly if evoked repetitively, could have deleterious impacts on health. Yet most of us are relatively privileged, we live in a generally dignity-affirming environment, and suffer only the occasional lapse of indignity. However, many people live constantly in a dignity-impugning environment, in which affirmations of dignity may be the exceptional occurrence. An exploration of the meanings of dignity and the forms of its violation—and the impact on physical, mental, and social well-being—may help uncover a new universe of human suffering, for which the biomedical language may he inapt and even inept. After all, the power of naming, describing, and then measuring is truly enormous—child abuse did not exist in meaningful societal terms until it was named and then measured; nor did domestic violence.

A second precondition for developing an ethics of public health is the adoption and application of a human rights framework for analyzing and responding to the societal determinants of health. The human rights framework can provide the coherence and clarity required for public health to identify and work with conscious attention to its roles and responsibilities. At that point, an ethics of public health, rather than the ethics of individual constituent disciplines within public health, can emerge.

Issues of respect for autonomy, beneficence, nonmaleficence, and justice can then be articulated from within the set of goals and responsibilities called for by seeking to improve public health through the combination of traditional approaches and those that strive concretely to promote realization of human rights. This is not to replace health education, information, and clinical service-based activities of public health with an exclusive focus on human rights and dignity. Both are necessary.

For example, the challenges for public health officials in balancing the goals of promoting and protecting public health and ensuring that human rights and dignity are not violated call urgently for ethical analysis. The official nature of much public health work places public health practitioners in a complex environment, in which work to promote rights inevitably challenges the state system within which the official is employed. Ethical dimensions are highly relevant to collecting, disseminating, and acting on information about the health impacts of the entire range of human rights violations. And as public health seeks to "ensure the conditions in which people can be healthy," and as those conditions are societal, to be engaged in public health necessarily involves a commitment to societal transformation. The difficulties in assessing human rights status and in developing useful and appropriate ways to promote human rights and dignity necessarily engage ethical considerations. For example, beyond accurate diagnosis, beyond efforts to cure, and even beyond the ever-present responsibility for relief of pain, the physician agrees to accompany the patient, to stand by the patient through her suffering, even to the edge of life itself, even when the only thing the physician can offer is the fact of his or her presence. Is this not as relevant to public health? For public health must engage difficult issues even when no cure or effective instruments are yet available, and public health also must accompany, remain with, and not abandon vulnerable populations.

That this work—added to, not substituted for, the current approach of public health—will require major changes in public health reflection, analysis, action, and education, is clear. That it is urgently required, in order to confront the major health challenges of the modern world, is equally clear. . . .

3

PREVENTION AND ITS LIMITS

Public health is known for its stress on preventing disease before it occurs, and doing so through "primary, secondary, and tertiary" prevention.[1] Prevention is the hallmark of public health. Yet the word can quickly become a cliche. We sometimes speak of prevention as if it were a simple and obvious remedy to all social ills, when it is anything but simple or obvious. Readers should be alert to three critical questions in prevention: (1) What is to be prevented? (2) Who is responsible for prevention and who must pay the cost? (3) What level of safety should be the standard for prevention measures?

Preventive measures in public health aim to reduce the exposure of communities to the major hazards of our time. Some of these hazards are diseases: The HIV virus and other viral threats; the recurrence of plague, cholera, and malaria; and gastrointestinal disease caused by deadly parasites and other pathogens are examples. Others are environmental hazards such as air pollution and chemical exposures. Still other hazards have both environmental and behavioral elements, like tobacco and alcohol, and highway crashes. When preventing exposure is not possible, other strategies can be used to protect populations, such as immunization against infectious disease or the use of air bags or seat belts in automobiles.

Reducing exposure to dangers usually necessitates overcoming established conceptions of why epidemics or highway crashes or gunshot injuries occur. These established conceptions focus on the role of particular agents in bringing about the unfortunate result: hence, the term *agent-causality*. In agent-causality the stress is placed upon what the individual did wrong to invite or to accept exposure to dangerous conditions. Someone gets AIDS because he or she had unprotected sex or shared needles. The cause of a workplace accident is the worker's failure to wear safety goggles. The accident was caused by the driver's speeding.

Public health does not deny individual contributions to injury and disease; that would be absurd. However, it is more interested in how hazards might be reduced or mitigated than in blaming individuals. It finds explanations that

95

focus on exposure to risk within populations more helpful than explanations that focus on agent-causality. In exposure (as opposed to agent) causality, the emphasis is less on what individuals do and more on measures to reduce the exposure of whole communities or groups to hazards.

In prevention, the focus is upon the predictable and stable occurrence of disease conditions in society. William Ryan spoke of this perspective a number of years ago: "Adherents of this [public health] approach tended to search for defects in the community and the environment rather than in the individual; to emphasize predictability and usualness rather than random deviance."[2]

Sometimes a measure which seems sensible from an individual standpoint does not reduce risk in the aggregate. One of the more interesting examples comes from the field of injury control. Research indicates that driver education for young people actually results in higher crash rates in this age group.[3] This is surprising because driver education should improve the safety records of young drivers (which is why insurance companies offer a discount on the insurance of teenagers who have taken driver education). However, the incentive for young people to take driver education is the ability to drive at a younger age, say 16 or 17 rather than 18. The mere fact that a greater number of younger, licensed drivers are consequently on the road and exposed to risks, accounts for the increase in the crash rate. The research suggests that states might eliminate the programs in the name of safety.

An emphasis on aggregate harm and exposure to risks suggests an answer to our second question: Who is responsible for taking action to protect the public's health? Responsibility for protecting the public's health is best seen as a collective function, a task of government, because making preventive responsibility an individual matter seldom reduces rates of disease and injury sharply. Cigarette smoking seems the exception, as smoking levels have fallen over the past three decades without massive government regulation. But cigarette advertising was banished from television, there were widely publicized reports from the Office of the U.S. Surgeon General, and the national news media has saturated the public with the dangers of smoking. This, coupled with legal restrictions on smoking in public and increases in tobacco taxes, has sharply cut smoking levels.

The third critical issue in prevention is, How safe should we seek to make the public from the hazards in the workplace, in transportation, or in the environment? This question is difficult, if not impossible, to answer in the abstract, as the answer depends on multiple factors, including the seriousness of the hazard, its prevalence, and the cost of prevention. We cannot give a formula for determining the right level of prevention here but can argue against one way of deciding what risks are acceptable, namely, in terms of individuals' voluntary acceptance of risk. It is sometimes argued that we often voluntarily accept risks that are much more dangerous than other risks that are imposed on us, and from which we, as members of the public, expect government to protect us. For example, we drive automobiles when trains are forced to be much safer. We fly in private planes which are far more dangerous than commercial aircraft. This leads some to suggest that the level of risk individuals are willing to accept in their voluntary choices constitutes a general acceptable level of safety. The implications of such a view are startling. It would mean that airline safety could be allowed to decrease far below the current level, perhaps to the level of automobile traffic. It would allow consumer product safety to decrease in a comparable way, perhaps to the level of risk individuals take when they smoke cigarettes. Because this approach to risk sets the level of safety so low, it is inconsistent with a public health perspective.

The first selection in this chapter, "Public Health as Social Justice," by Dan Beauchamp, was written in the mid-1970s as the Great Society programs were being challenged by a business backlash. The business community resented being forced to carry the burden of making the public safer. Beauchamp analyzes preventive measures such as regulations to control air and water pollution, or to make automobiles and other consumer products safer, in terms of exposure causality and the norms of social justice, showing how this differs markedly from liberal and market models of justice.

This is today an enduring theme in public health—the attempt to persuade democratic bodies to legislate rules for economic production and distribution that are safer. Community public health interests are ranged against powerful, well-organized entities such as corporations and interest groups (like the National Rifle Association). The struggle for the common health and safety is further complicated by the fact that the redistribution of the burdens of health and safety legislation is on behalf of "statistical lives." This resembles a struggle for social justice because the effort is on behalf of the less well-organized and less powerful against the power of the market and its masters.

The second article in this chapter, "Analysis of Cause—Long-cut to Prevention?" by J. H. Renwick, suggests that too much emphasis on the causation of social problems or health problems can be misleading and may distract us from effective measures of prevention. Often we know how to abate (prevent) problems long before we know the causes of problems.

Finally, we turn to the limits to prevention and to the whole idea of community. This is the issue of paternalism. Is it the case that public health, in its zeal to promote the health of the public, goes too far and neglects the rights and interests of the individual?

Paternalism has been a major theme in bioethics. A principal problem facing philosophers who began work in bioethics about three decades ago was the paternalism of American medicine. This gave rise to an entire literature on paternalism in the health field.[4] In the third selection for this chapter, paternalism is defined by Gerald Dworkin as "the interference with a person's liberty of action for reasons referring exclusively to the welfare, good, happiness, needs, interests, or values of the person being coerced." Physicians who seek to promote the individual patient's own good by withholding information (which the physician may think the patient is not qualified to evaluate) or by withholding facts (which the physician may feel might be too painful for the patient), act paternalistically, and indefensibly in the eyes of most bioethicists. The struggle to define a defensible notion of patient autonomy, and to rethink the responsibilities of physicians and other health professionals in honoring that autonomy, has been a major part of the development of biomedical ethics over the past 30 years. This struggle, while not over, has won a respected place for the idea of patient autonomy in American medicine. When philosophers turn to public health and find that its proponents advocate legislation requiring the wearing of motorcycle helmets or seat belts or buying cars with air bags installed, this looks to them like paternalism because the individual's liberty is being restricted to promote his or her own well-being. Influenced by John Stuart Mill's famous essay, "On Liberty,"[5] which is a powerful attack on paternal government, philosophers tend to regard public health as objectionably paternalistic. Indeed, for many in bioethics, public health is synonymous with paternalism.

The term *paternal government* has an interesting history. (The actual term *paternalism* was never used by Mill and seems to be a term of the 20th century.) The idea of paternal government likely first arose in England and dealt with the responsibilities of landed gentry for the welfare of persons who lived on their estates. In this case, the owners and minor nobility were responsible for the well-being and safety of persons who lived on their lands and who were known to them, personally. Thus, paternalism today reminds us of a government which, knowing its citizenry to be unlikely to take care of themselves, passes legislation to require seat belts, to wear motorcycle helmets, and so on. To most people, this idea is anachronistic, condescending, and vaguely insulting because it second-guesses people's own evaluations about what is best for them, treating them like children in need of protection. Most people resent this. They want to be able to make up their own minds and shape their own destiny, even when they make choices that others regard as foolish or unwise.

Mill argued that coercing individuals for their own good was never justified. The sole justification for interfering with a person's liberty was to prevent harm to others. The "harm principle," as it has become known, has been used by some to justify certain public health measures that may seem at first glance paternalistic. On this view, some choices made by individuals impose harms on society even if they do not directly impose harms on specific others. We may call this the *burdens-to-society thesis*. It holds, for example, that individuals who eat fatty foods may think they are harming only themselves, but in truth (or so this argument goes) they are creating future medical bills and higher insurance costs, burdens which all of society has to bear. One article went so far as to argue that the obese impose burdens on society through higher fuel costs, in the form of food and fossil fuels for transportation![6]

A different justification of paternalism focuses on the fact that people sometimes act against their *own* considered judgments about how they ought to act. They overeat when they want to lose weight. They continue to smoke, even though they do not want to get cancer or emphysema. Philosophers call this kind of acting against one's own best judgment "weakness of will." Are coercive measures aimed at getting people to do what they agree they should do, and would do, if only they were not weak-willed, paternalistic? Some argue that they are not, that paternalism inherently involves forcing people to act against their own values, for their own good. Others regard paternalism to counteract weakness of will as a *kind* of paternalism, which may be called "weak" or "soft" paternalism. It seems likely that many public health measures, such as seatbelt legislation, come under the heading of weak paternalism. The legislation forces people to do what they really know they should do but are too lazy or weak-willed to do without the added incentive of a law.

A third approach to the problem of paternalism is to argue that public health measures are not, in fact, paternalistic because the proposed interventions are not aimed at promoting the individual's *own* good. This is the argument suggested by Dan Beauchamp in his article on community and public health in the last chapter. While he termed this form of regulation *public health paternalism,* he means that these limits are not, strictly speaking, classical paternalism. Rather, the legislation in question is aimed at a population and is intended to reduce the rates of premature death and serious injury among that population. Put another way, what is being promoted is the good of the group, not the good of specific individuals.

Because of its emphasis on the good of the group, we can call this the *communitarian perspective.* The communitarian perspective is not vulnerable to the objection that it is condescending or patronizing because the rationale for the coercive measures is *not* that the government knows better than the individual what is in his or her own best interest. It is rather that minor infringements on the liberty of individuals (like buckling up in the car) are justified by the great good that can be accomplished (saving thousands of lives a year). Unlike the burdens-on-society thesis, the communitarian perspective does not blame individuals for imposing costs on society. However, both views justify preventive measures on harm-principle grounds and therefore do not threaten the autonomy of individuals any more than any other harm-preventing measures. The communitarian perspective argues that public health has devised, if not very self-consciously, a theory of individual autonomy that is distinctive and different from the one proposed by Mill in "On Liberty," different from the burdens-on-society thesis, and one that is not a form of soft paternalism, or *paternalism lite.*

NOTES

1. Primary prevention is preventing damaging events from ever occurring. Secondary prevention is reducing the damage or harm from damaging events after they occur (for example, with air bags or seat belts in automobiles). Tertiary prevention is arranging clinical treatment to reduce the level of damage among a population.

2. William Ryan, *Blaming the Victim* (New York: Vintage, 1971 p. 17).

3. Leon S. Robertson, "Crash Involvement of Teenaged Drivers When Driver Education Is Eliminated From High School," *American Journal of Public Health* 70 (1980), pp. 599–603.

4. See Daniel Wikler, "Lifestyles and Public Health," *Encyclopedia of Bioethics, Revised Edition* (New York: Macmillan Library Reference, 1995, v. 3, pp. 1366–69), and Dennis Thompson, *Paternalism in Medicine, Law, and Public Policy,*" in Daniel Callahan and Sissela Bok, eds. *Ethics Teaching in Higher Education.* (New York: Plenum, 1980, pp. 245–272). For a defense of paternalism that somewhat resembles the public health position, see Richard Bonnie, "Discouraging Unhealthy Personal Choices: Reflections on New Directions in Substance Abuse Policy," *Journal of Drug Issues* 8 (1978), pp. 199–219. See also Robert M. Veatch, "Voluntary Risks to Health, the Ethical Issues," *Journal of the American Medical Association* 243 (1980), pp. 50–55. See Dan Beauchamp, "Life-Style, Public Health and Paternalism," in S. Doxiadis, ed. *Ethical Dilemmas in Health Promotion.* (London: John Wiley, 1987).

5. J. S. Mill, "On Liberty," in Marshall Cohen, ed. *Philosophy of John Staurt Mill: Ethical, Political, Religious* (New York: Modern Library, 1961, 185–319).

6. B. M. Hannon and T. G. Lohman, "The Energy Cost of Overweight in the United States," *American Journal of Public Health* 68 (1978), 765–767. Others point out that people with poor health habits probably *save* society money in the long run. By dying prematurely, they avoid large medical costs that typically occur at the end of life, as well as Social Security and pension payments. If cost is the issue, perhaps we ought to give smokers a tax break!

Public Health As Social Justice

DAN E. BEAUCHAMP

Anthony Downs has observed that our most intractable public problems have two significant characteristics. First, they occur to a relative minority of our population (even though that minority may number millions of people). Second, they result in significant part from arrangements that are providing substantial benefits or advantages to a majority or to a powerful minority of citizens. Thus solving or minimizing these problems requires painful losses, the restructuring of society and the acceptance of new burdens by the most powerful and the most numerous on behalf of the least powerful or the least numerous. As Downs notes, this bleak reality has resulted in recent years in cycles of public attention to such problems as poverty, racial discrimination, poor housing, unemployment or the abandonment of the aged; however, this attention and interest rapidly wane when it becomes clear that solving these problems requires painful costs that the dominant interests in society are unwilling to pay. Our public ethics do not seem to fit our public problems.

It is not sufficiently appreciated that these same bleak realities plague attempts to protect the public's health. Automobile-related injury and death; tobacco, alcohol and other drug damage; the perils of the workplace; environmental pollution; the inequitable and ineffective distribution of medical care services; the hazards of biomedicine—all of these threats inflict death and disability on a minority of our society at any given time. Further, minimizing or even significantly reducing the death and disability from these perils entails that the majority or powerful minorities accept new burdens or relinquish existing privileges that they presently enjoy. Typically, these new burdens or restrictions involve more stringent controls over these and other hazards of the world.

This somber reality suggests that our fundamental attention in public health policy and prevention should not be directed toward a search for new technology, but rather toward breaking existing ethical and political barriers to minimizing death and disability. This is not to say that technology will never again help avoid painful social and political adjustments. Nonetheless, only the technological Pollyannas will ignore the mounting evidence that the critical barriers to protecting the public against death and disability are not the barriers to technological progress—indeed the evidence is that it is often technology itself that is our own worst enemy. The critical barrier to dramatic reductions in death and disability is a social ethic that unfairly protects the most numerous or the most powerful from the burdens of prevention.

This is the issue of justice. In the broadest sense, justice means that each person in society ought to receive his due and that the burdens and benefits of society should be fairly and equitably distributed. But what criteria should be followed in allocating burdens and benefits: Merit, equality or need? What end or goal in life should receive our highest priority: Life, liberty or the pursuit of happiness? The answer to these questions can be found in our prevailing theories or models of justice. These models of justice, roughly speaking, form the foundation of our politics and public policy in general, and our health policy (including our prevention policy) specifically. Here I am speaking of politics not as partisan politics but rather the more ancient and venerable meaning of the political as the search for the common good and the just society.

These models of justice furnish a symbolic framework or blueprint with which to think about and react to the problems of the public, providing the basic rules to classify and categorize problems of society as to whether they necessitate public and collective protection, or whether individual responsibility should prevail. These models function as a sort of map or guide to the common world of members of society, making visible some conditions in society as public issues and concerns, and hiding, obscuring or concealing other conditions that might otherwise emerge as public issues or problems were a different map or model of justice in hand.

In the case of health, these models of justice form the basis for thinking about and reacting to the problems of disability and premature death in society. Thus, if public health policy requires that the majority or a powerful minority accept their fair share of the burdens of protecting a relative minority threatened with death or disability, we need to ask if our prevailing model of justice contemplates and legitimates such sacrifices.

MARKET-JUSTICE

The dominant model of justice in the American experience has been market-justice. Under the norms of market-justice people are entitled only to those valued ends such as status, income, happiness, etc., that they have acquired by fair rules of entitlement, e.g., by their own individual efforts, actions or abilities. Market-justice emphasizes individual responsibility, minimal collective action and freedom from collective obligations except to respect other persons' fundamental rights.

While we have as a society compromised pure market-justice in many ways to protect the public's health, we are far from recognizing the principle that death and disability are collective problems and that all persons are entitled to health protection. Society does not recognize a general obligation to protect the individual against disease and injury. While society does prohibit individuals from causing direct harm to others, and has in many instances regulated clear public health hazards, the norm of market-justice is still dominant and the primary duty to avert disease and injury still rests with the individual. The individual is ultimately alone in his or her struggle against death.

Barriers to Protection

This individual isolation creates a powerful barrier to the goal of protecting all human life by magnifying the power of death, granting to death an almost supernatural reality. Death has throughout history presented a basic problem to humankind, but even in an advanced society with enormous biomedical technology, the individualism of market-justice tends to retain and exaggerate pessimistic and fatalistic attitudes toward death and injury. This fatalism leads to a sense of powerlessness, to the acceptance of risk as an essential element of life, to resignation in the face of calamity, and to a weakening of collective impulses to confront the problems of premature death and disability.

Perhaps the most direct way in which market-justice undermines our resolve to preserve and protect human life lies in the primary freedom this ethic extends to all individuals and groups to act with minimal obligations to protect the common good. Despite the fact that this rule of self-interest predictably fails to protect adequately the safety of our workplaces, our modes of transportation, the physical environment, the commodities we consume, or the equitable and effective distribution of medical care, these failures have resulted so far in only half-hearted attempts at regulation and control. This response is explained in large part by the powerful sway market-justice holds over our imagination, granting fundamental freedom to all individuals to be left alone—even if the "individuals" in question are giant producer groups with enormous capacities to create great public harm through sheer inadvertence. Efforts for truly effective controls over these perils must constantly struggle against a prevailing ethical paradigm that defines as threats to fundamental freedoms attempts to assure that all groups—even powerful producer groups—accept their fair share of the burdens of prevention.

Market-justice is also the source of another major barrier to public health measures to minimize death and disability—the category of voluntary behavior. Market-justice forces a basic distinction between the harm caused by a factory

polluting the atmosphere and the harm caused by the cigarette or alcohol industries, because in the latter case those that are harmed are perceived as engaged
in "voluntary" behavior. It is the radical individualism inherent in the market
model that encourages attention to the individual's behavior and inattention to
the social preconditions of that behavior. In the case of smoking, these preconditions include a powerful cigarette industry and accompanying social and cultural forces encouraging the practice of smoking. These social forces include
norms sanctioning smoking as well as all forms of media, advertising, literature, movies, folklore, etc. Since the smoker is free in some ultimate sense to
not smoke, the norms of market-justice force the conclusion that the individual
voluntarily "chooses" to smoke; and we are prevented from taking strong collective action against the powerful structures encouraging this so-called voluntary behavior.

Yet another way in which the market ethic obstructs the possibilities for
minimizing death and disability, and alibis the need for structural change, is
through explanations for death and disability that "blame the victim." Victim-
blaming misdefines structural and collective problems of the entire society as
individual problems, seeing these problems as caused by the behavioral failures
or deficiencies of the victims. These behavioral explanations for public problems tend to protect the larger society and powerful interests from the burdens
of collective action, and instead encourage attempts to change the "faulty" behavior of victims.

Market-justice is perhaps the major cause for our over-investment and over-
confidence in curative medical services. It is not obvious that the rise of medical science and the physician, taken alone, should become fundamental obstacles to collective action to prevent death and injury. But the prejudice found in
market-justice against collective action perverts these scientific advances into
an unrealistic hope for "technological shortcuts" to painful social change.
Moreover, the great emphasis placed on individual achievement in market-justice has further diverted attention and interest away from primary prevention
and collective action by dramatizing the role of the solitary physician-scientist,
picturing him as our primary weapon and first line of defense against the threat
of death and injury. . . .

Public Health Measures

I have saved for last an important class of health policies—public health measures to protect the environment, the workplace, or the commodities we purchase and consume. Are these not signs that the American society is willing to
accept collective action in the face of clear public health hazards?

I do not wish to minimize the importance of these advances to protect the
public in many domains. But these separate reforms, taken alone, should be

cautiously received. This is because each reform effort is perceived as an iso-lated exception to the norm of market-justice; the norm itself still stands. Con-sequently, the predictable career of such measures is to see enthusiasm for enforcement peak and wane. These public health measures are clear signs of hope. But as long as these actions are seen as merely minor exceptions to the rule of individual responsibility, the goals of public health will remain beyond our reach. What is required is for the public to see that protecting the public's health takes us beyond the norms of market-justice categorically, and necessi-tates a completely new health ethic. . . .

SOCIAL JUSTICE

The fundamental critique of market-justice found in the Western liberal tradition is social justice. Under social justice all persons are entitled equally to key ends such as health protection or minimum standards of income. Further, unless col-lective burdens are accepted, powerful forces of environment, heredity or social structure will preclude a fair distribution of these ends. While many forces influenced the development of public health, the historic dream of public health that preventable death and disability ought to be minimized is a dream of social justice. Yet these egalitarian and social justice implications of the public health vision are either still not widely recognized or are conveniently ignored. . . .

Ideally, then, the public health ethic is not simply an alternative to the market ethic for health—it is a fundamental critique of that ethic as it unjustly protects powerful interests from the burdens of prevention and as that ethic serves to legitimate a mindless and extravagant faith in the efficacy of medical care. In other words, the public health ethic is a *counter-ethic* to market-justice and the ethics of individualism as these are applied to the health problems of the public. . . .

This new ethic has several key implications which are referred to here as "principles": 1) Controlling the hazards of this world, 2) to prevent death and disability, 3) through organized collective action, 4) shared equally by all ex-cept where unequal burdens result in increased protection of everyone's health and especially potential victims of death and disability.

These ethical principles are not new to public health. To the contrary, making the ethical foundations of public health visible only serves to highlight the social justice influences at work behind pre-existing principles.

Controlling the Hazards

A key principle of the public health ethic is the focus on the identification and control of the hazards of this world rather than a focus on the behavioral defects of those individuals damaged by these hazards. Against this principle it is often argued that today the causes of death and disability are multiple and frequently behavioral in origin. Further, since it is usually only a minority of the public that fails to protect itself against most known hazards, additional controls over these perilous sources would not seem to be effective or just. We should look instead for the behavioral origins of most public health problems, asking why some people expose themselves to known hazards or perils, or act in an unsafe or careless manner.

Public health should—at least ideally—be suspicious of behavioral paradigms for viewing public health problems since they tend to "blame the victim" and unfairly protect majorities and powerful interests from the burdens of prevention. It is clear that behavioral models of public health problems are rooted in the tradition of market-justice, where the emphasis is upon individual ability and capacity, and individual success and failure.

Public health, ideally, should not be concerned with explaining the successes and failures of differing individuals (dispositional explanations) in controlling the hazards of this world. . . .

Prevention

Like the other principles of public health, prevention is a logical consequence of the ethical goal of minimizing the numbers of persons suffering death and disability. The only known way to minimize these adverse events is to prevent the occurrence of damaging exchanges or exposures in the first place, or to seek to minimize damage when exposures cannot be controlled.

Prevention, then, is that set of priority rules for restructuring existing market rules in order to maximally protect the public. These rules seek to create policies and obligations to replace the norm of market-justice, where the latter permits specific conditions, commodities, services, products, activities or practices to pose a direct threat or hazard to the health and safety of members of the public, or where the market norm fails to allocate effectively and equitably those services (such as medical care) that are necessary to attend to disease at hand.

Thus, the familiar public health options:

1. Creating rules to minimize exposure of the public to hazards (kinetic, chemical, ionizing, biological, etc.) so as to reduce the rates of hazardous exchanges.
2. Creating rules to strengthen the public against damage in the event damaging exchanges occur anyway, where such techniques (fluoridation, seatbelts, immunization) are feasible.

3. Creating rules to organize treatment resources in the community so as to minimize damage that does occur since we can rarely prevent all damage.

Collective Action

Another principle of the public health ethic is that the control of hazards cannot be achieved through voluntary mechanisms but must be undertaken by governmental or non-governmental agencies through planned, organized and collective action that is obligatory or non-voluntary in nature. This is for two reasons.

The first is because market or voluntary action is typically inadequate for providing what are called public goods. Public goods are those public policies (national defense, police and fire protection, or the protection of all persons against preventable death and disability) that are universal in their impacts and effects, affecting everyone equally. These kinds of goods cannot easily be withheld from those individuals in the community who choose not to support these services (this is typically called the "free rider" problem). Also, individual holdouts might plausibly reason that their small contribution might not prevent the public good from being offered.

The second reason why self-regarding individuals might refuse to voluntarily pay the costs of such public goods as public health policies is because these policies frequently require burdens that self-interest or self-protection might see as too stringent. For example, the minimization of rates of alcoholism in a community clearly seems to require norms or controls over the substance of alcohol that limit the use of this substance to levels that are far below what would be safe for individual drinkers.

With these temptations for individual noncompliance, justice demands assurance that all persons share equally the costs of collective action through obligatory and sanctioned social and public policy.

Fair-Sharing of the Burdens

A final principle of the public health ethic is that all persons are equally responsible for sharing the burdens—as well as the benefits—of protection against death and disability, except where unequal burdens result in greater protection for every person and especially potential victims of death and disability. In practice this means that policies to control the hazards of a given substance, service or commodity fall unequally (but still fairly) on those involved in the production, provision or consumption of service, commodity or substance. The clear implication of this principle is that the automotive industry, the tobacco industry, the coal industry and the medical care industry—to mention only a few key groups—have an unequal responsibility to bear the costs of reducing death and disability since their actions have far greater impact than those of individual citizens.

DOING JUSTICE: BUILDING A NEW PUBLIC HEALTH

I have attempted to show the broad implications of a public health commitment to protect and preserve human life, setting out tentatively the logical consequences of that commitment in the form of some general principles. We need, however, to go beyond these broad principles and ask more specifically: What implications does this model have for doing public health and the public health profession?

The central implication of the view set out here is that doing public health should not be narrowly conceived as an instrumental or technical activity. Public health should be a way of doing justice, a way of asserting the value and priority of all human life. The primary aim of all public health activity should be the elaboration and adoption of a new ethical model or paradigm for protecting the public's health. This new ethical paradigm will necessitate a heightened consciousness of the manifold forces threatening human life, and will require thinking about and reacting to the problems of disability and premature death as primarily collective problems of the entire society. . . .

CONCLUSION

The central thesis of this article is that public health is ultimately and essentially an ethical enterprise committed to the notion that all persons are entitled to protection against the hazards of this world and to the minimization of death and disability in society. I have tried to make the implications of this ethical vision manifest, especially as the public health ethic challenges and confronts the norms of market-justice.

I do not see these goals of public health as hopelessly unrealistic nor destructive of fundamental liberties. Public health may be an "alien ethic in a strange land." Yet, if anything, the public health ethic is more faithful to the traditions of Judeo-Christian ethics than is market-justice.

The image of public health that I have drawn here does raise legitimate questions about what it is to be a professional, and legitimate questions about reasonable limits to restrictions on human liberty. These questions must be addressed more thoroughly than I have done here. Nonetheless, we must never pass over the chaos of preventable disease and disability in our society by simply celebrating the benefits of our prosperity and abundance, or our technological advances. What are these benefits worth if they have been purchased at the price of human lives?

Nothing written here should be construed as a per se attack on the market system. I have, rather, surfaced the moral and ethical norms of that system and argued that, whatever other benefits might accrue from those norms, they are woefully inadequate to assure full and equal protection of all human life.

The adoption of a new public health ethic and a new public health policy must and should occur within the context of a democratic polity. I agree with Terris that the central task of the public health movement is to persuade society to accept these measures.

Finally, it is a peculiarity of the word freedom that its meaning has become so distorted and stretched as to lend itself as a defense against nearly every attempt to extend equal health protection to all persons. This is the ultimate irony. The idea of liberty should mean, above all else, the liberation of society from the injustice of preventable disability and early death. Instead, the concept of freedom has become a defense and protection of powerful vested interests, and the central issue is viewed as a choice between freedom on the one hand, and health and safety on the other. I am confident that ultimately the public will come to see that extending life and health to all persons will require some diminution of personal choices, but that such restrictions are not only fair and do not constitute abridgement of fundamental liberties, they are a basic sign and imprint of a just society and a guarantee of that most basic of all freedom—protection against man's most ancient foe.

Analysis of Cause—Long Cut to Prevention?

J. H. RENWICK

Although in biomedical research prevention of a disease is customarily considered complementary to its cause, most of the scientific working hypotheses are framed around testing the supposed cause directly. In some circumstances, however, there are advantages in framing hypotheses around prevention.

I shall consider first the circumstances in which the classical causal hypothesis is more or less adequate. These arise either when a disease situation occurs naturally that superficially resembles a laboratory experiment or when a true experiment is possible in an animal that is acceptable as a valid analogue of man.

The thalidomide incident is an example of the natural or at least unplanned experiment. When thalidomide was taken by pregnant women and a defined range of otherwise rare malformations was observed in many of their offspring but not in the offspring of other women, the hypothesis was proposed that thalidomide was at least a contributory cause of these malformations in humans. Indeed, for any new ailment (disease, malformation or injury), it is simple and effective to state a proposition in the causal mode. As in a classical experiment, a known background situation is modified and an effect produced.

An animal experiment with thalidomide would be an example of the other situation (of adequacy of a causal hypothesis) but only when the test animal is trusted as a valid analogue of man. Rhesus monkeys and certain marmosets are so trusted; the malformations produced in them by this drug are almost identical with those in man. A causal hypothesis even for man, being therefore indirectly testable, can usefully be proposed.

NEED FOR ABATIVE HYPOTHESES

The position is different for ailments to which man has been subject for a long time and for which no convincing animal analogue is available. Unfortunately, we are in the habit of constructing causal claims about even these ailments although the relevant experiments to test the claims directly would usually be unethical. The causal experiments are therefore impracticable except in imagination. In a 'thought experiment' of this sort, an artificial base-line for the population has to be created. In one example, it could involve the (imaginary) absence of refined sucrose. This basal situation would then be modified (in imagination) by the addition of sucrose and various alimentary disorders would ensue. Such at least is the experiment that seems to be suggested by a causal claim that sucrose is an important factor in the cause of colonic diverticulosis, for example. The hypothesis cannot be tested directly because it is nearly always unethical to increase the risk of ailment in a real experiment.

If we can overcome the habit of allowing cause to dominate our thinking, we have a very simple way of bypassing such a problem. This is to perform a real intervention experiment on a part of the population with its present, known burden of disease. This basal situation is then modified—by some procedure such as reduction of intake of refined sucrose. The degree of abatement of the disease is then the outcome of the experiment. With such an experiment in mind, a preventative hypothesis can be formed that is in principle testable, and there are usually no major ethical objections to an experiment of this sort. Further, the statement can be framed briefly yet accurately in terms of deviation from the present state because the 'present state' is known widely enough for it to require, in many cases, no detailed description. Many intervention experiments of exactly this type are done. The change that I am suggesting is that they should be acknowledged as testing preventative statements and not causal ones.

Preventative statements, when confirmed, will sometimes summon up practical measures to control disease. Any such measure—it may be preventative or therapeutic or both—will be called 'abative' as its purpose is to produce some abatement of the ailment and of its burden to the individual and to society.

NON-RECIPROCAL RELATIONSHIP BETWEEN CAUSE AND ABATIVE

Wherever a necessary-and-sufficient abative measure exists there must, in principle, be a corresponding necessary-and-sufficient cause and *vice versa*. The search for cause or abative then comes to much the same task. But the relationship between cause and abative is not always so exactly reciprocal. For instance, a sufficient abative is one that removes a necessary cause. A somewhat oversimplified example of a 'sufficient abative' would be the banning of rye cultivation to prevent poisoning by the ergot fungus, for which rye is the preferred host. The corresponding causal statement is that rye is the 'necessary cause' of ergot poisoning. As in this example, so in general—an abative measure that has the property of sufficiency but not of necessity is the counterpart of a cause that is necessary but not sufficient.

The degree of reciprocity is also limited in a more subjective way. Even though abatives, like causes, do interact, the percentage abatement of a disease incidence by a single manipulation is an unambiguous and complete concept. By contrast, the concept of the percentage effect of a single cause is more likely to be misleading unless the interactions with other causes are fully specified. Specifying these interactions by the disclaimer—other things being equal—is rarely adequate.

Few such difficulties apply to statements or hypotheses on abatement. The effects of single causes or abatives are best expressed as percentage change from the initial situation. The effects (causal or abative) may sum to several times the incidence of the disease. This is not awkward if it is abative effects that are being summed since each is operative only potentially and mainly in the future. We are not surprised at the existence of alternative means of prevention nor at the possibility of their interacting, so when the sum exceeds 100% effectiveness, we are not disturbed. But there is a seeming absurdity in the statement, say, that 50% of the present incidence of a disease is caused by each of three factors, x, y, z. For the claim to be explicit, interactions or options must be invoked because, obviously, the realised effect of the three factors combined does not exceed the present overall incidence.

As already noted, intervention studies of abative measure are already an established part of epidemiological practice. For example, there have been nonsmoking studies, breathalyser studies, and, on the positive side, fluoridation studies. But the conceptual framework has not been adequately spelled out to my knowledge. In some intervention studies, by a curious inversion, the investigators even imply that causes are being studied rather than abatives. The distinction is worth making as it reflects a difference. Abatement is the aim of medicine; the study of causation of an ailment, say, in experimental animals, is frequently a useful intermediate but may not be an essential one in all cases. Even the very concept of causation can, on occasion, be dispensed with in considering abatement strategies.

REMAINING PROBLEM DISEASES ARE A SELECTED SAMPLE

I suggest that if neither causes nor abatives are yet known—and I shall call such an ailment a problem ailment—causation is probably complex. The more complex the causation, the more likely it is to be currently unknown. In tackling such a problem ailment, then, we would be wise to turn at least some of our attention from causes to abatives. For example, the causal mechanism of carcinoma of the colon is unknown and probably complex. From its geographical distribution the simple and testable abative measure of a high residue diet has been proposed. From past neglect, simple abatives like this have not always been adequately excluded.

ADVANTAGES OF ABATIVE STATEMENTS

For old-established conditions, three major advantages of abative compared with causal statements have so far been mentioned—direct testability on the human species itself; expressibility in simpler terms; and the opportunity to include a quantitative component that expresses the percentage of prevention anticipated.

This last advantage is well illustrated in the case of road accidents. We should like to make statements such as "20% of accidents in the United Kingdom are caused by alcohol", but such statements are intrinsically misleading because of the interactions: practically no cause operates in isolation. An abative statement that the introduction of the breathalyser laws in the United Kingdom reduced the accident rate by a certain percentage is simpler and open to a smaller range of interpretations.

This example introduces another important advantage of abative propositions. They are directly relevant to the achievement of human goals such as the partial prevention of accidents, and so are directly relevant to decision making in public and private life. The quantitative aspect is the most important in this context, as the predicted advantage has to be balanced against the cost of introducing the abative measure.

It is at least arguable that if the observed association between smoking and lung cancer had led to an abative rather than a causal claim, society's 20 year delay in taking action would have been shorter. The claim would have been directly confirmed by the results now available of non-smoking intervention studies and the question of the identification of the presumed carcinogen(s) could have been deferred. Further, the genetic red herring would have been more clearly recognised for what it is—a matter of intellectual interest but with little practical relevance, in this instance, in decision making.

PERSPECTIVES ON CAUSATION AND ABATEMENT

The properties of abative statements are so attractive that we need to ask why they are rarely made. After all, if prevention of disease is an aim of medicine, why have we departed so completely from the folklore mode of expression exemplified by 'an apple a day keeps the doctor away'? The historian might well find an influence of the philosophy of non-medical science—the dominance of how (does it happen) over how not. Waddington in *The Scientific Attitude* roughly defined science as "the organised attempt of mankind to discover how things work as causal systems". Perhaps the absence of specific mention of abatement in such definitions has been taken to imply that abative statements are less scientific than causal ones, despite the fact that, for both types, the "criterion of truth is experimental" and objective.

Alternatively, did the current emphasis on causation spring from the need of the legal system to apportion blame? Or, equally plausibly, was the need to study epidemics more pressing than the need to study the less dramatic non-epidemic state? The manifest success of laboratory methodology in so many non-human fields undoubtedly played a large part in establishing the habit of thinking in the causal mode. We correctly believe that we have not understood anything at a fundamental level unless we have understood the mechanism of causation. And we often think (incorrectly) that such understanding is a prerequisite of wise action. Kant knew better—that "it is often necessary to make a decision on the basis of knowledge sufficient for action but insufficient to satisfy the intellect".

It is true, even today, that wise action can occasionally be based at least temporarily on empirical knowledge alone and there are many examples of this from the past. From the time of Admiral Wager, scurvy was controlled in the Navy by the provision of citrus fruits before ascorbic acid was known to be a vitamin. Penicillin was used effectively, even before its mode of action was understood; and tobacco avoidance dramatically reduces bronchocarcinoma incidences although we still do not know how.

Decision-making in medicine is more directly concerned with prevention and treatment rather than causation, so we should often express claims in terms of abatement rather than causation as at present. A few scientists disagree. They argue that causation and abatement are simply converse concepts and, at the same time, that one is scientific, the other empirical. Both arguments are rather shallow assessments. Abatement is not always the simple converse of causation. Further, an abative statement can be as scientific and testable experimentally as any other. It may even be just as possible to discover general laws concerning abatement as laws concerning causation.

Abative and causal hypotheses are not mutually exclusive. Indeed, there is a one-to-one relationship between them. The abative statement is usually simpler in practice. This is particularly true for complex problems. And most real-life problems are complex.

Paternalism

GERALD DWORKIN

. . . I take as my starting point the "one very simple principle" proclaimed by Mill in *On Liberty* . . . "That principle is, that the sole end for which mankind are warranted, individually or collectively, in interfering with the liberty of action of any of their number, is self-protection. That the only purpose for which power can be rightfully exercised over any member of a civilized community, against his will, is to prevent harm to others. He cannot rightfully be compelled to do or forbear because it will be better for him to do so, because it will make him happier, because, in the opinion of others, to do so would be wise, or even right."

This principle is neither "one" nor "very simple." It is at least two principles; one asserting that self-protection or the prevention of harm to others is sometimes a sufficient warrant and the other claiming that the individual's own good is *never* a sufficient warrant for the exercise of compulsion either by the society as a whole or by its individual members. I assume that no one with the possible exception of extreme pacifists or anarchists questions the correctness of the first half of the principle. This essay is an examination of the negative claim embodied in Mill's principle—the objection to paternalistic interferences with a man's liberty.

I

By paternalism I shall understand roughly the interference with a person's liberty of action justified by reasons referring exclusively to the welfare, good, happiness, needs, interests or values of the person being coerced. One is always well-advised to illustrate one's definitions by examples but it is not easy to find "pure" examples of paternalistic interferences. For almost any piece of legislation is justified by several different kinds of reasons and even if historically a piece of legislation can be shown to have been introduced for purely paternalistic motives, it may be that advocates of the legislation with an anti-paternalistic outlook can find sufficient reasons justifying the legislation without appealing to the reasons which were originally adduced to support it. Thus, for example, it may be that the original legislation requiring motorcyclists to wear safety helmets was introduced for purely paternalistic reasons. But the Rhode Island Supreme Court recently upheld such legislation on the grounds that it was "not persuaded that the legislature is powerless to prohibit individuals from pursuing a course of conduct which could conceivably result in their becoming public charges," thus clearly introducing reasons of a quite different kind. Now I regard this decision as being based on reasoning of a very dubious nature but it illustrates the kind of problem one has in finding examples. The following is a list of the kinds of interferences I have in mind as being paternalistic.

II

1. Laws requiring motorcyclists to wear safety helmets when operating their machines.
2. Laws forbidding persons from swimming at a public beach when lifeguards are not on duty.
3. Laws making suicide a criminal offense.
4. Laws making it illegal for women and children to work at certain types of jobs.
5. Laws regulating certain kinds of sexual conduct, e.g. homosexuality among consenting adults in private.
6. Laws regulating the use of certain drugs which may have harmful consequences to the user but do not lead to anti-social conduct.
7. Laws requiring a license to engage in certain professions with those not receiving a license subject to fine or jail sentence if they do engage in the practice.
8. Laws compelling people to spend a specified fraction of their income on the purchase of retirement annuities. (Social Security)
9. Laws forbidding various forms of gambling (often justified on the grounds that the poor are more likely to throw away their money on such activities than the rich who can afford to).
10. Laws regulating the maximum rate of interest for loans.
11. Laws against duelling.

In addition to laws which attach criminal or civil penalties to certain kinds of action there are laws, rules, regulations, decrees, which make it either difficult or impossible for people to carry out their plans and which are also justified on paternalistic grounds. Examples of this are:

1. Laws regulating the types of contracts which will be upheld as valid by the courts, e.g. (an example of Mill's to which I shall return) no man may make a valid contract for perpetual involuntary servitude.

2. Not allowing as a defense to a charge of murder or assault the consent of the victim.

3. Requiring members of certain religious sects to have compulsory blood transfusions. This is made possible by not allowing the patient to have recourse to civil suits for assault and battery and by means of injunctions.

4. Civil commitment procedures when these are specifically justified on the basis of preventing the person being committed from harming himself. (The D.C. Hospitalization of the Mentally Ill Act provides for involuntary hospitalization of a person who "is mentally ill, and because of that illness, is likely to injure *himself* or others if allowed to remain at liberty." The term injure in this context applies to unintentional as well as intentional injuries.)

5. Putting fluorides in the community water supply.

All of my examples are of existing restrictions on the liberty of individuals. Obviously one can think of interferences which have not yet been imposed. Thus one might ban the sale of cigarettes, or require that people wear safety-belts in automobiles (as opposed to merely having them installed) enforcing this by not allowing motorists to sue for injuries even when caused by other drivers if the motorist was not wearing a seat-belt at the time of the accident.

I shall not be concerned with activities which though defended on paternalistic grounds are not interferences with the liberty of persons, e.g. the giving of subsidies in kind rather than in cash on the grounds that the recipients would not spend the money on the goods which they really need, or not including a $1000 deductible provision in a basic protection automobile insurance plan on the ground that the people who would elect it could least afford it. Nor shall I be concerned with measures such as "truth-in-advertising" acts and the Pure Food and Drug legislation which are often attacked as paternalistic but which should not be considered so. In these cases all that is provided—it is true by the use of compulsion—is information which it is presumed that rational persons are interested in having in order to make wise decisions. There is no interference with the liberty of the consumer unless one wants to stretch a point beyond good sense and say that his liberty to apply for a loan without knowing the true rate of interest is diminished. It is true that sometimes there is sentiment for going further than providing information, for example when laws against usurious interest are passed preventing those who might wish to contract loans at high rates of interest from doing so, and these measures may correctly be considered paternalistic.

III

Bearing these examples in mind let me return to a characterization of paternalism. I said earlier that I meant by the term, roughly, interference with a person's liberty for his own good. But as some of the examples show, the class of persons whose good is involved is not always identical with the class of persons whose freedom is restricted. Thus in the case of professional licensing it is the practitioner who is directly interfered with and it is the would-be patient whose interests are presumably being served. Not allowing the consent of the victim to be a defense to certain types of crime primarily affects the would-be aggressor but it is the interests of the willing victim that we are trying to protect. Sometimes a person may fall into both classes as would be the case if we banned the manufacture and sale of cigarettes and a given manufacturer happened to be a smoker as well.

Thus we may first divide paternalistic interferences into "pure" and "impure" cases. In "pure" paternalism the class of persons whose freedom is restricted is identical with the class of persons whose benefit is intended to be promoted by such restrictions. Examples: the making of suicide a crime, requiring passengers in automobiles to wear seat-belts, requiring a Christian Scientist to receive a blood transfusion. In the case of "impure" paternalism in trying to protect the welfare of a class of persons we find that the only way to do so will involve restricting the freedom of other persons besides those who are benefitted. Now it might be thought that there are no cases of "impure" paternalism since any such case could always be justified on non-paternalistic grounds, i.e. in terms of preventing harms to others. Thus we might ban cigarette manufacturers from continuing to manufacture their product on the grounds that we are preventing them from causing illness to others in the same way that we prevent other manufacturers from releasing pollutants into the atmosphere, thereby causing danger to the members of the community. The difference is, however, that in the former but not the latter case the harm is of such a nature that it could be avoided by those individuals affected if they so chose. The incurring of the harm requires, so to speak, the active co-operation of the victim. It would be mistaken theoretically and hypocritical in practice to assert that our interference in such cases is just like our interference in standard cases of protecting others from harm. At the very least someone interfered with in this way can reply that no one is complaining about his activities. It may be that impure paternalism requires arguments or reasons of a stronger kind in order to be justified since there are persons who are losing a portion of their liberty and they do not even have the solace of having it be done "in their own interest." Of course in some sense, if paternalistic justifications are ever correct, then we are protecting others, we are preventing some from injuring others, but it is important to see the differences between this and the standard case.

Paternalism then will always involve limitations on the liberty of some individuals in their own interest but it may also extend to interferences with the liberty of parties whose interests are not in question.

IV

Finally, by way of some more preliminary analysis, I want to distinguish paternalistic interferences with liberty from a related type with which it is often confused. Consider, for example, legislation which forbids employees to work more than, say, 40 hours per week. It is sometimes argued that such legislation is paternalistic for if employees desired such a restriction on their hours of work they could agree among themselves to impose it voluntarily. But because they do not the society imposes its own conception of their best interests upon them by the use of coercion. Hence this is paternalism.

Now it may be that some legislation of this nature is, in fact, paternalistically motivated. I am not denying that. All I want to point out is that there is another possible way of justifying such measures which is not paternalistic in nature. It is not paternalistic because as Mill puts it in a similar context such measures are "required not to overrule the judgment of individuals respecting their own interest, but to give effect to that judgment: they being unable to give effect to it except by concert, which concert again cannot be effectual unless it receives validity and sanction from the law."

The line of reasoning here is a familiar one first found in Hobbes and developed with great sophistication by contemporary economists in the last decade or so. There are restrictions which are in the interests of a class of persons taken collectively but are such that the immediate interest of each individual is furthered by his violating the rule when others adhere to it. In such cases the individuals involved may need the use of compulsion to give effect to their collective judgment of their own interest by guaranteeing each individual compliance by the others. In these cases compulsion is not used to achieve some benefit which is not recognized to be a benefit by those concerned, but rather because it is the only feasible means of achieving some benefit which *is* recognized as such by all concerned. This way of viewing matters provides us with another characterization of paternalism in general. Paternalism might be thought of as the use of coercion to achieve a good which is not recognized as such by those persons for whom the good is intended. Again while this formulation captures the heart of the matter—it is surely what Mill is objecting to in *On Liberty*—the matter is not always quite like that. For example, when we force motorcyclists to wear helmets we are trying to promote a good—the protection of the person from injury—which is surely recognized by most of the individuals concerned. It is not that a cyclist doesn't value his bodily integrity; rather, as a supporter of such legislation would put it, he either places, perhaps irrationally, another value or good (freedom from wearing a helmet) above that of physical well-being or, perhaps, while recognizing the danger in the abstract, he either does not fully appreciate it or he underestimates the likelihood of its occurring. But now we are approaching the question of possible justifications of paternalistic measures and the rest of this essay will be devoted to that question.

V

I shall begin for dialectical purposes by discussing Mill's objections to paternalism and then go on to discuss more positive proposals.

An initial feature that strikes one is the absolute nature of Mill's prohibitions against paternalism. It is so unlike the carefully qualified admonitions of Mill and his fellow Utilitarians on other moral issues. He speaks of self-protection as the *sole* end warranting coercion, of the individual's own goals as *never* being a sufficient warrant. Contrast this with his discussion of the prohibition against lying in *Util[itarianism]*.

> Yet that even this rule, sacred as it is, admits of possible exception, is acknowledged by all moralists, the chief of which is where the with-holding of some fact . . . would save an individual . . . from great and unmerited evil.

The same tentativeness is present when he deals with justice.

> It is confessedly unjust to break faith with any one: to violate an engagement, either express or implied, or disappoint expectations raised by our own conduct, at least if we have raised these expectations knowingly and voluntarily. Like all the other obligations of justice already spoken of, this one is not regarded as absolute, but as capable of being overruled by a stronger obligation of justice on the other side.

This anomaly calls for some explanation. The structure of Mill's argument is a follows:

1. Since restraint is an evil, the burden of proof is on those who propose such restraint.
2. Since the conduct which is being considered is purely self-regarding, the normal appeal to the protection of the interests of others is not available.
3. Therefore we have to consider whether reasons involving reference to the individual's own good, happiness, welfare, or interests are sufficient to overcome the burden of justification.

4. We either cannot advance the interests of the individual by compulsion, or the attempt to do so involves evil which outweighs the good done.
5. Hence the promotion of the individual's own interests does not provide a sufficient warrant for the use of compulsion.

Clearly the operative premise here is 4 and it is bolstered by claims about the status of the individual as judge and appraiser of his welfare, interests, needs, etc.

> With respect to his own feelings and circumstances, the most ordinary man or woman has means of knowledge immeasurably surpassing those that can be possessed by any one else. . . .
> He is the man most interested in his own well-being: the interest which any other person, except in cases of strong personal attachment, can have in it, is trifling, compared to that which he himself has.

These claims are used to support the following generalizations concerning the utility of compulsion for paternalistic purposes.

> The interferences of society to overrule his judgment and purposes in what only regards himself must be grounded on general presumptions, which may be altogether wrong, and even if right, are as likely as not to be misapplied to individual cases. . . .
> But the strongest of all the arguments against the interference of the public with purely personal conduct is that when it does interfere, the odds are that it interferes wrongly and in the wrong place. . . .
> All errors which the individual is likely to commit against advice and warning are far outweighed by the evil of allowing others to constrain him to what they deem his good.

Performing the utilitarian calculation by balancing the advantages and disadvantages we find that:

> Mankind are greater gainers by suffering each other to live as seems good to themselves, than by compelling each other to live as seems good to the rest.

From which follows the operative premise 4.

This classical case of a utilitarian argument with all the premises spelled out is not the only line of reasoning present in Mill's discussion. There are asides, and more than asides, which look quite different and I shall deal with them later. But this is clearly the main channel of Mill's thought and it is one which has been subjected to vigorous attack from the moment it appeared—most often by fellow Utilitarians. The link that they have usually seized on is, as Fitzjames Stephen put it, the absence of proof that the "mass of adults are so well acquainted with their own interests and so much disposed to pursue them that no compulsion or restraint put upon them by any others for the purpose of promoting their interest can really promote them." Even so sympathetic a critic as Hart is forced to the conclusion that:

> In Chapter 5 of his essay Mill carried his protests against paternalism to lengths that may now appear to us as fantastic . . . No doubt if we no longer sympathise with this criticism this is due, in part, to a general decline in the belief that individuals know their own interest best.
>
> Mill endows the average individual with "too much of the psychology of a middle-aged man whose desires are relatively fixed, not liable to be artificially stimulated by external influences; who knows what he wants and what gives him satisfaction of happiness; and who pursues these things when he can."

Now it is interesting to note that Mill himself was aware of some of the limitations on the doctrine that the individual is the best judge of his own interests. In his discussion of government intervention in general (even where the intervention does not interfere with liberty but provides alternative institutions to those of the market), after making claims which are parallel to those just discussed, e.g.,

> People understand their own business and their own interests better, and care for them more, than the government does, or can be expected to do,

he goes on to an intelligent discussion of the "very large and conspicuous exceptions" to the maxim that:

> Most persons take a juster and more intelligent view of their own interest, and of the means of promoting it than can either be prescribed to them by a general enactment of the legislature, or pointed out in the particular case by a public functionary.

Thus there are things

> of which the utility does not consist in ministering to inclinations, nor in serving the daily uses of life, and the want of which is least felt where the need is greatest. This is peculiarly true of those things which are chiefly useful as tending to raise the character of human beings. The uncultivated cannot be competent judges of cultivation. Those who most need to be made wiser and better, usually desire it least, and, if they desired it, would be incapable of finding the way to it by their own lights.
>
> . . . A second exception to the doctrine that individuals are the best judges of their own interest, is when an individual attempts to decide irrevocably now what will be best for his interest at some future and distant time. The presumption in favor of individual judgment is only legitimate, where the judgment is grounded on actual, and especially on present, personal experience; not where it is formed antecedently to experience, and not suffered to be reversed even after experience has condemned it.

The upshot of these exceptions is that Mill does not declare that there should never be government interference with the economy but rather that

> . . . in every instance, the burden of making out a strong case should be thrown not on those who resist but on those who recommend government interference. Letting alone, in short, should be the general practice: every departure from it, unless required by some great good, is a certain evil.

In short, we get a presumption not an absolute prohibition. The question is, why doesn't the argument against paternalism go the same way?

I suggest that the answer lies in seeing that in addition to a purely utilitarian argument Mill uses another as well. As a Utilitarian Mill has to show, in Fitz-james Stephen's words, that:

> Self-protection apart, no good object can be attained by any compulsion which is not in itself a greater evil than the absence of the object which the compulsion obtains.

To show this is impossible; one reason being that it isn't true. Preventing a man from selling himself into slavery (a paternalistic measure which Mill himself accepts as legitimate), or from taking heroin, or from driving a car without wearing seat-belts may constitute a lesser evil than allowing him to do any of these things. A consistent Utilitarian can only argue against paternalism on the grounds that it (as a matter of fact) does not maximize the good. It is always a contingent question that may be refuted by the evidence. But there is also a non-contingent argument which runs through *On Liberty*. When Mill states that "there is a part of the life of every person who has come to years of discretion, within which the individuality of that person ought to reign uncontrolled either by any other person or by the public collectively," he is saying something about what it means to be a person, an autonomous agent. It is because coercing a person for his own good denies this status as an independent entity that Mill objects to it so strongly and in such absolute terms. To be able to choose is a good that is independent of the wisdom of what is chosen. A man's "mode of laying out his existence is the best, not because it is the best in itself, but because it is his own mode."

> It is the privilege and proper condition of a human being, arrived at the maturity of his faculties, to use and interpret experience in his own way.

As further evidence of this line of reasoning in Mill consider the one exception to his prohibition against paternalism.

> In this and most civilised countries, for example, an engagement by which a person should sell himself, or allow himself to be sold, as a slave, would be null and void;

neither enforced by law nor by opinion. The ground for thus limiting his power of voluntarily disposing of his own lot in life, is apparent, and is very clearly seen in this extreme case. The reason for not interfering, unless for the sake of others, with a person's voluntary acts, is consideration for his liberty. His voluntary choice is evidence that what he so chooses is desirable, or at least endurable, to him, and his good is on the whole best provided for by allowing him to take his own means of pursuing it. But by selling himself for a slave, he abdicates his liberty; he foregoes any future use of it beyond that single act.

He therefore defeats, in his own case, the very purpose which is the justification of allowing him to dispose of himself. He is no longer free; but is thenceforth in a position which has no longer the presumption in its favour, that would be afforded by his voluntarily remaining in it. The principle of freedom cannot require that he should be free not to be free. It is not freedom to be allowed to alienate his freedom.

Now leaving aside the fudging on the meaning of freedom in the last line, it is clear that part of this argument is incorrect. While it is true that *future* choices of the slave are not reasons for thinking that what he chooses then is desirable for him, what is at issue is limiting his immediate choice; and since this choice is made freely, the individual may be correct in thinking that his interests are best provided for by entering such a contract. But the main consideration for not allowing such a contract is the need to preserve the liberty of the person to make future choices. This gives us a principle—a very narrow one—by which to justify some paternalistic interferences. Paternalism is justified only to preserve a wider range of freedom for the individual in question. How far this principle could be extended, whether it can justify all the cases in which we are inclined upon reflection to think paternalistic measures justified remains to be discussed. What I have tried to show so far is that there are two strains of argument in Mill—one a straight-forward Utilitarian mode of reasoning and one which relies not on the goods which free choice leads to but on the absolute value of the choice itself. The first cannot establish any absolute prohibition but at most a presumption and indeed a fairly weak one, given some fairly plausible assumptions about human psychology; the second, while a stronger line of argument, seems to me to allow on its own grounds a wider range of paternalism than might be suspected. I turn now to a consideration of these matters.

VI

. . . Let me suggest types of situations in which it seems plausible to suppose that fully rational individuals would agree to having paternalistic restrictions imposed upon them. It is reasonable to suppose that there are "goods" such as health which any person would want to have in order to pursue his own good— no matter how that good is conceived. This is an argument that is used in connection with compulsory education for children but it seems to me that it can be extended to other goods which have this character. Then one could agree that the attainment of such goods should be promoted even when not recognized to be such, at the moment, by the individuals concerned.

An immediate difficulty that arises stems from the fact that men are always faced with competing goods and that there may be reasons why even a value such as health—or indeed life—may be overridden by competing values. Thus the problem with the Christian Scientist and blood transfusions. It may be more important for him to reject "impure substances" than to go on living. The difficult problem that must be faced is whether one can give sense to the notion of a person irrationally attaching weights to competing values.

Consider a person who knows the statistical data on the probability of being injured when not wearing seat-belts in an automobile and knows the types and gravity of the various injuries. He also insists that the inconvenience attached to fastening the belt every time he gets in and out of the car outweighs for him the possible risks to himself. I am inclined in this case to think that such a weighing is irrational. Given his life plans which we are assuming are those of the average person, his interests and commitments already undertaken, I think it is safe to predict that we can find inconsistencies in his calculations at some point. I am assuming that this is not a man who for some conscious or unconscious reasons is trying to injure himself nor is he a man who just likes to "live dangerously." I am assuming that he is like us in all the relevant respects but just puts an enormously high negative value on inconvenience—one which does not seem comprehensible or reasonable.

It is always possible, of course to assimilate this person to creatures like myself. I, also, neglect to fasten my seat-belt and I concede such behavior is not rational but not because I weigh the inconvenience differently from those who fasten the belts. It is just that having made (roughly) the same calculation as everybody else, I ignore it in my actions. [Note: a much better case of weakness of the will than those usually given in ethics texts.] A plausible explanation for this deplorable habit is that although I know in some intellectual sense what the probabilities and risks are, I do not fully appreciate them in an emotionally genuine manner.

We have two distinct types of situation in which a man acts in a non-rational fashion. In one case he attaches incorrect weights to some of his values; in the other he neglects to act in accordance with his actual preferences and desires. Clearly there is a stronger and more persuasive argument for paternalism in the latter situation. Here we are really not—by assumption—imposing a good on another person. But why may we not extend our interference to what we might call evaluative delusions? After all, in the case of cognitive delusions we are prepared, often, to act against the expressed will of the person involved. If a man believes that when he jumps out the window he will float upwards—

Robert Nozick's example—would not we detain him, forcibly if necessary? The reply will be that this man doesn't wish to be injured and if we could convince him that he is mistaken as to the consequences of his action he would not wish to perform the action. But part of what is involved in claiming that a man who doesn't fasten his seat-belts is attaching an irrational weight to the inconvenience of fastening them is that if he were to be involved in an accident and severely injured he would look back and admit that the inconvenience wasn't as bad as all that. So there is a sense in which if I could convince him of the consequences of his action he also would not wish to continue his present course of action. Now the notion of consequences being used here is covering a lot of ground. In one case it's being used to indicate what will or can happen as a result of a course of action and in the other it's making a prediction about the future evaluation of the consequences—in the first sense—of a course of action. And whatever the difference between facts and values—whether it be hard and fast or soft and slow—we are genuinely more reluctant to consent to interferences where evaluative differences are the issue. Let me now consider another factor which comes into play in some of these situations which may make an important difference in our willingness to consent to paternalistic restrictions.

Some of the decisions we make are of such a character that they produce changes which are in one or another way irreversible. Situations are created in which it is difficult or impossible to return to anything like the initial stage at which the decision was made. In particular, some of these changes will make it impossible to continue to make reasoned choices in the future. I am thinking specifically of decisions which involve taking drugs that are physically or psychologically addictive and those which are destructive of one's mental and physical capacities.

I suggest we think of the imposition of paternalistic interferences in situations of this kind as being a kind of insurance policy which we take out against making decisions which are far-reaching, potentially dangerous and irreversible. Each of these factors is important. Clearly there are many decisions we make that are relatively irreversible. In deciding to learn to play chess I could predict in view of my general interest in games that some portion of my free-time was going to be preempted and that it would not be easy to give up the game once I acquired a certain competence. But my whole life-style was not going to be jeopardized in an extreme manner. Further it might be argued that even with addictive drugs such as heroin one's normal life plans would not be seriously interfered with if an inexpensive and adequate supply were readily available. So this type of argument might have a much narrower scope than appears to be the case at first.

A second class of cases concerns decisions which are made under extreme psychological and sociological pressures. I am not thinking here of the making of the decision as being something one is pressured into—e.g., a good reason for making duelling illegal is that unless this is done many people might have to manifest their courage and integrity in ways in which they would rather not do so—but rather of decisions such as that to commit suicide which are usually made at a point where the individual is not thinking clearly and calmly about the nature of his decision. In addition, of course, this comes under the previous heading of all-too-irrevocable decision. Now there are practical steps which a society could take if it wanted to decrease the possibility of suicide—for example not paying social security benefits to the survivors or as religious institutions do, not allowing such persons to be buried with the same status as natural deaths. I think we may count these as interferences with the liberty of persons to attempt suicide and the question is whether they are justifiable.

Using my argument schema the question is whether rational individuals would consent to such limitations. I see no reason for them to consent to an absolute prohibition but I do think it is reasonable for them to agree to some kind of enforced waiting period. Since we are all aware of the possibility of temporary states, such as great fear or depression, that are inimical to the making of well-informed and rational decisions, it would be prudent for all of us if there were some kind of institutional arrangement whereby we were restrained from making a decision which is (all too) irreversible. What this would be like in practice is difficult to envisage and it may be that if no practical arrangements were feasible, then we would have to conclude that there should be no restriction at all on this kind of action. But we might have a "cooling off" period, in much the same way that we now require couples who file for divorce to go through a waiting period. Or, more far-fetched, we might imagine a Suicide Board composed of a psychologist and another member picked by the applicant. The Board would be required to meet and talk with the person proposing to take his life, though its approval would not be required.

A third class of decisions—these classes are not supposed to be disjoint—involves dangers which are either not sufficiently understood or appreciated correctly by the persons involved. Let me illustrate, using the example of cigarette smoking, a number of possible cases.

1. A man may not know the facts—e.g., smoking between 1 and 2 packs a day shortens life expectancy 6.2 years, the costs and pain of the illness caused by smoking, etc.
2. A man may know the facts, wish to stop smoking, but not have the requisite willpower.
3. A man may know the facts but not have them play the correct role in his calculation because, say, he discounts the danger psychologically because it is remote in time and/or inflates the attractiveness of other consequences of his decision which he regards as beneficial.

In case 1 what is called for is education, the posting of warnings, etc. In case 2 there is no theoretical problem. We are not imposing a good on someone who rejects it. We are simply using coercion to enable people to carry out their own goals. (Note: There obviously is a difficulty in that only a subclass of the individuals affected wish to be prevented from doing what they are doing.) In case 3 there is a sense in which we are imposing a good on someone since given his current appraisal of the facts he doesn't wish to be restricted. But in another sense we are not imposing a good since what is being claimed—and what must be shown or at least argued for—is that an accurate accounting on his part would lead him to reject his current course of action. Now we all know that such cases exist, that we are prone to disregard dangers that are only possibilities, that immediate pleasures are often magnified and distorted.

If in addition the dangers are severe and far-reaching, we could agree to allowing the state a certain degree of power to intervene in such situations. The difficulty is in specifying in advance, even vaguely, the class of cases in which intervention will be legitimate. . . .

I have suggested in this essay a number of types of situations in which it seems plausible that rational men would agree to granting the legislative powers of a society the right to impose restrictions on what Mill calls "self-regarding" conduct. However, rational men knowing something about the resources of ignorance, ill-will and stupidity available to the law-makers of a society—a good case in point is the history of drug legislation in the United States—will be concerned to limit such intervention to a minimum. I suggest in closing two principles designed to achieve this end.

In all cases of paternalistic legislation there must be a heavy and clear burden of proof placed on the authorities to demonstrate the exact nature of the harmful effects (or beneficial consequences) to be avoided (or achieved) and the probability of their occurrence. The burden of proof here is twofold—what lawyers distinguish as the burden of going forward and the burden of persuasion. That the authorities have the burden of going forward means that it is up to them to raise the question and bring forward evidence of the evils to be avoided. Unlike the case of new drugs where the manufacturer must produce some evidence that the drug has been tested and found not harmful, no citizen has to show with respect to self-regarding conduct that it is not harmful or promotes his best interests. In addition the nature and cogency of the evidence for the harmfulness of the course of action must be set at a high level. To paraphrase a formulation of the burden of proof for criminal proceedings—better 10 men ruin themselves than one man be unjustly deprived of liberty.

Finally I suggest a principle of the least restrictive alternative. If there is an alternative way of accomplishing the desired end without restricting liberty, then although it may involve great expense, inconvenience, etc., the society must adopt it.

III

MODERN CHALLENGES TO THE PUBLIC'S HEALTH

4

ALCOHOL, TOBACCO, AND OTHER DRUGS

Public health approaches have worked a fundamental change in perspective on the causes and prevention of alcoholism and alcohol abuse. Something similar is taking place with regard to other drugs, including tobacco and the illegal drugs.

There has been a remarkable transformation in this century of our policy toward alcohol, from laissez-faire to national Prohibition to a disease concept of addiction and a more public-health-oriented policy. Today our alcohol policies are an amalgam of these successive eras of prevention; older attitudes persist, unintegrated. A prohibitionist approach is reflected in laws prohibiting the sale of alcohol in some counties, while a more public health approach is seen in imposing state age limits on drinking in order to reduce teenage deaths related to drunk driving. Higher taxes on alcohol to discourage heavy drinking is another example of a public health approach.

Up until the American revolution, there was relatively little interest in officially regulating drinking. The Puritans accepted alcohol, while controlling its use through informal social sanctions, such as those of the local tavernkeepers, the local communities, and the church. Yet the Revolutionary period was a time when drunkenness came to be seen as a rising problem in the towns and cities of the new country. This was intensified by the rise of a new industry: the distilled spirits or whiskey industry among farmers further to the west and inland.

For the next century and a half, Temperance and later Prohibition dominated the American political agenda. The coming of Prohibition in 1917 as a World War I wartime measure, and the institutionalizing of Prohibition with the passage of the Volstead Amendment, are major landmarks in American social and political history. As an experiment in a moralistic approach to alcohol, Prohibition was a serious failure, despite the fact that Prohibition caused drinking to fall precipitously in the United States and to remain low for several decades after repeal. It was a failure because a less restrictive set of measures, like heavy taxation or shorter hours for sale, could have produced the same results in falling drinking levels and declining cirrhosis rates. It was also a failure because its chief aim was less to improve the public's health and instead improve the public morality, to produce the Sober Republic, which would increase well-being in all realms.

Alcoholism, or the concept that heavy drinking is a disease, is one of the legacies of Prohibition. Alcoholism as an idea is based on the "two types of people" theory: There are drinkers who can control their drinking, and alcoholics who can not, and these two groups are fairly fixed in their distribution across the population, with alcoholics constituting a small minority. The idea that drinking behavior is distributed across a population and is constantly changing was not fully appreciated until the late 1960s and early 70s, when researchers began to study the patterning of drinking in the United States.

In the first selection, James Mosher and David Jernigan detail the fundamental shift in thinking about alcohol problems that has occurred in the past three decades, beginning with epidemiological analysis of the relationship between levels of per capita consumption of alcohol and rates of alcohol-related problems like cirrhosis. They describe the growth of a public health perspective inside and outside government circles and how this new conception has changed our stance toward alcohol problems. The public health perspective for alcohol problems is similar to that for other public health problems: The focus is on the distribution of risk and hazard (alcohol) in the whole population and the need for policies that limit and control this hazard. The whole community, including all who drink, bears responsibility for preventing alcohol problems. This new focus shifts attention from drinkers who have a disease and puts far more attention on regulating the sale and price and advertising of alcohol products for the whole community. This new perspective makes limits to consumption of alcohol for everyone a central policy issue. Of course the new perspective is staunchly resisted by the alcohol industry, which prefers to see the problem defined as "treating alcoholism" rather than reducing alcohol consumption (and the profits of the liquor industry) in the whole population.

What about illegal drugs? Is our experience with the prohibition of alcohol such that we should consider legalizing other drugs, like marijuana, heroin, or cocaine? Most public health experts would likely say no, but with considerable hesitance. On one hand, the lesson of the recent decades has been that increasing access to a substance will almost surely increase its consumption. On the other hand, the prohibition of drugs is a very costly and divisive policy in itself. The drug trade takes a terrible social and environmental toll, and the courts and police have been ineffective in combating it, despite the fact that our prisons are filled with people there for drug-related offenses.

Whether we should dismantle part of our national policy against illegal drugs is deeply controversial. Bonnie Steinbock provides a public health perspective on the whole debate over legalizing drugs.[1] As we note in Chapter 6, a public health perspective rejects policies based on moralism. It also demands that any policy be based on empirical evidence. The public health perspective also focuses less on the debate over legalization versus prohibition and more on ways of reducing the harm of using dangerous drugs to individuals and to groups. Steinbock presents a long, sad litany of failures in our current drug policy, including the use of criminal sanctions to discourage even minor drug use and the huge infrastructure we have erected to suppress the trade in drugs. Jails have become overcrowded as long jail sentences have been given for both users and minor drug traffickers. The war on drugs has had a chilling effect on civil liberties, resulting in illicit police searches of vehicles and homes. Based on tips from informants, armed police have burst into apartments in search of drugs, terrifying the inhabitants, who sometimes have nothing to do with drugs. Our drug policy demands cannabis (the active substance in marijuana) not be used to counteract pain and nausea in AIDS and cancer patients. Moreover, we have been ineffective in persuading other nations to reduce the production of drugs, given our inability to curb our domestic consumption.

As Steinbock notes, there are other options to legalization, such as decriminalization or the decision to not arrest and prosecute use of drugs like marijuana, even if laws forbidding their use remain on the books. Several European nations have a more forgiving stance toward those who use drugs; they offer users low-cost drugs or therapy but are strict about the sale or provision of illegal drugs.

The moralistic approach has admittedly had certain benefits. Millions of Americans use little or no alcohol as the result of moral and religious disapproval. Social disapproval is also having an impact on smoking. The decline in smoking in recent decades is not only due to the scare put into the public by a series of Surgeon General reports, but also to the stigmatizing of smokers in our society. Social disapproval is a form of moralism, seeing the smoker as someone who is persisting in a socially condemned practice, a kind of deviancy. While this can go too far, it is nonetheless effective in discouraging people from smoking. The cigarette's long fall from the celluloid lips of Humphrey Bogart and Lauren Bacall to the chilled lips of office workers huddled outside buildings in the winter is a remarkable social transformation ushered in by more than the fear of lung cancer.

In the third selection, Leonard Glantz reviews the debate over regulating advertising for tobacco. This is an important public health issue since tobacco, a legal product, causes far more harm than do illegal drugs. It is important for another reason. The percentage of those smoking tobacco, especially cigarettes, have fallen precipitously since the 1960s, resulting in major declines in heart disease and more recently lung cancer. These declines occurred as a result of aggressive reports by U.S. Surgeons General, as a result of counteradvertising on television and the eventual omission of cigarette advertising on television, and as a result of a constant barrage of public discussion regarding the lethality of smoking.

For these reasons, the battle to control tobacco and smoking has centered on advertising and the media, with some arguing that all advertising for tobacco products should be banned, especially when these advertisements seem targeted at people who are not yet old enough to smoke. (The same issues arise for the promotion of beer by the alcohol industry.) Thus, the question arises: Can the state can legitimately ban advertising for a legal product, one sold in the stream of commerce? Many argue that this would be unconstitutional. As Glantz points out, it may be that the doctrine of "commercial speech," developed by liberal justices on the Supreme Court beginning in the 1970s, may accord advertising, even for dangerous products like alcohol and tobacco, a measure of the protections now granted to ordinary speech in newspapers, television, and elsewhere.

NOTES

1. See also James Mosher and Karen Yanagisako, "Public Health, Not Social Warfare: A Public Health Approach to Illegal Drug Policy," *Journal of Public Health Policy,* 12 (1991), pp. 278–321.

New Directions in Alcohol Policy

JAMES F. MOSHER AND DAVID H. JERNIGAN

INTRODUCTION

An exciting drama is unfolding in the public health field today. As previous
reviews have indicated, a new consensus is emerging regarding the prevention
of alcohol-related problems, one of our most serious health issues. Built on
public health theory and experience, this new alcohol policy movement offers
the entire public health field the opportunity to reach new constituencies. In
keeping with the nature of the problems it is designed to prevent, the approach
cuts across ideological, racial, ethnic, and socioeconomic divisions in our society and provides the means to build a coalition for broad social change in
regard to health policy.

As was the case with the antismoking and other public health movements
that preceded it, this new alcohol policy movement is opposed by powerful
economic and political interests. Classic tactics to divert and blunt health policy
reform are now a familiar part of the alcohol field—industry denials of health
risks associated with their product; industry-financed research designed to cast
doubt on studies documenting adverse consequences of its use; strong-arm
lobbying at local, state, and federal levels, including massive contributions to
legislators; industry "donations" to a variety of social groups to deter their
participation in the reform movement; massive advertising budgets that are used
to silence and shape media attention to alcohol problems; and much more. That
the tactics have a familiar ring is no coincidence: many alcohol companies are
owned by tobacco conglomerates, and draw on that industry's experience in
conducting a sophisticated and heavily financed campaign to blunt efforts to
prevent tobacco-related disease.

As indicated in previous reviews, implementing the new approaches to alcohol-related problem prevention is not an easy task. The theoretical soundness of
the new approaches has been thoroughly documented, and thus this review
focuses on both the barriers and promising routes to implementation. Drawing

on concrete experiences in researching and implementing policy approaches, we argue that the alcohol field is moving into a new implementation stage, requiring new kinds of knowledge and skills. Although much remains to be learned regarding the nature of alcohol problems and the impact of different strategies for their treatment and prevention, and research and programmatic agendas concerning these issues should remain high priorities, it is time for public health advocates to address the challenge of becoming effective in the process of policy change.

Changing policy requires learning to organize new constituencies, becoming effective in the political and economic arena, developing new funding sources, and offsetting the barriers to effective public health reform. It demands as well a coordinated, concerted effort from diverse professionals—researchers and evaluators, program personnel, citizen activists, government administrators, educators, health care providers, health planners, and others. The potential benefits are enormous. Not only do we have a chance to reduce dramatically the tragic toll of alcohol-related problems on society. The approach envisioned here also holds the potential of broadening citizen support and activism on behalf of public health goals and agendas across the board.

The review is divided into four sections: the first section outlines the public health approach to the prevention of alcohol-related problems and documents the consensus that has developed over the last five years regarding this approach. The second section analyzes the barriers to implementation of effective prevention policies. The third section describes current research and activities that address the barriers to change, and the concluding section discusses both lessons learned and future agendas.

THE PUBLIC HEALTH MODEL: ALCOHOL POLICY AND THE NEW CONSENSUS

The public health field has experienced a revolution in the last 20 years regarding its understanding of alcohol problems. As documented by Room in the 1984 edition of the *Annual Review of Public Health*, this has involved at least three basic conceptual shifts:

1. Change in focus from "alcoholism" to "alcohol-related problems" or "alcohol problems": In the wake of the repeal of Prohibition, researchers and community workers alike increasingly viewed alcohol problems as exclusively due to "alcoholics," whose presumed inherent defect caused their disease. This view divided society into two groups: social drinkers, who suffer no adverse consequences from alcohol consumption; and alcoholics, who had no choice but to abstain to avoid alcohol problems. In this model, prevention activities were limited primarily to early case finding to locate the second group as early as possible. Empirical findings from research studies during the late 1960s and early 1970s undermined these assumptions. Epidemiologic studies found that all parts of the drinking population reported a variety of alcohol problems, and that individuals may drastically change their problematic drinking patterns over time.

2. Renewed emphasis on the diverse health consequences of alcohol use: The focus on the individual alcoholic tended to blind the field to the diverse problems associated with alcohol use—particularly trauma, cirrhosis of the liver, and other long-term health effects such as cancer. Research on alcohol has become increasingly sensitive to alcohol's role as a risk factor in a wide variety of health consequences that include and reach beyond the issue of alcoholism.

3. New attention placed on "alcohol control policy" as an integral prevention strategy: The dominant paradigm that emerged following repeal considered the control of alcohol availability (including the price and physical availability of alcohol, as well as the marketing strategies of the alcohol industry) irrelevant to the incidence and severity of alcohol problems. Alcoholics were assumed to be unaffected by availability, whereas social drinkers, whose consumption might be affected by controls on availability, were assumed to be free of alcohol problems. Indeed, some proponents of this model viewed alcohol controls as potentially counterproductive, stigmatizing alcoholics and creating barriers to the learning of "responsible drinking" norms. As Room has documented, the ferocious and vitriolic condemnation of those propounding even the most mild dissent documents the dominance of this model. Even in the public health field, advocates of control policy faced ostracism and charges that they sought a return to moralistic and prohibitionary alcohol policies.

Again, research findings undercut and eventually discredited this widely held view. As reviewed by Ashley & Rankin, a wide variety of studies have documented the impact of alcohol control variables on health consequences. Contrary to expectations, many control policies affect heavy drinkers more than light and moderate drinkers. The studies do not show uniform results, and differing control strategies have differing impacts. Researchers have found it difficult to measure the impact of relatively modest changes in alcohol availability, and societal and cultural variables must be taken into account. Nevertheless, "taken all together, there is substantial evidence that controls on physical availability can reduce rates of alcohol-related problems, and that the consumption of heavy, as well as moderate drinkers can be reduced".

The Public Health Model

In recent years, alcohol and public health researchers have placed these alcohol control strategies solidly in the public health tradition through the application of the familiar epidemiologic triad of environment-agent-host to alcohol-related problems. In addition to strategies already in place targeting the host—i.e. the individual drinker—with education, deterrence, treatment, and so on, this "public health model" of alcohol-related problems calls attention to the role of environmental factors (the social and physical structures within which alcohol problems occur) and agent factors (the presentation of alcohol, including alcohol packaging, labeling, and price) in the spread of alcohol problems.[1]

The alcohol field has increasingly focused on the interaction of the individual with his or her environment. "Environment" is defined broadly to include not only the physical availability of the agent alcohol, but also the cultural, social, political, and economic arena within which alcohol consumption and alcohol problems take place. According to Wallack,

> In effect, alcohol problems are seen as properties of systems rather than individuals. Individuals are viewed only as they exist in this larger system. Because alcohol problems exist across many different levels of the broader system (i.e. individual, family, peer group, school, community group, societal), prevention efforts must ultimately address all of these levels.

Messages about alcohol consumption abound in every part of the environment. Wallack stresses the importance of making those messages consistent at all levels.

This application of the public health model to alcohol-related problems builds on the research findings discussed above. It recognizes that alcohol problems reach beyond alcoholism. It focuses on populations as well as individuals, and stresses the importance of alcohol availability policies. It also acknowledges the importance of cultural and social norms and their interaction with control policies.

The new approach also creates two important bridges in the field. First, it acknowledges that prevention strategies aimed at individuals are appropriate and needed, provided they take into account and are consistent with strategies for changing problematic environmental factors. Conversely, those working to change environmental factors must be attentive to the impact of and reaction to those changes by individuals. This has helped to defuse some of the unease felt between "control" advocates and health educators. Second, it places treatment/recovery strategies as complementary, rather than opposed, to prevention. Alcoholism recovery, which occurs at the individual level, will be enhanced in a social and physical environment consistent with recovery goals. Concerns re-

---

[1]Alcohol is not always in the agent role in what we term alcohol-related problems. In the case of alcohol-related illnesses, ethanol is the agent, carried by beverage alcohol. In the case of alcohol-related injuries, however, the agent (that which is necessary and sufficient to cause harm to the host) is energy; alcohol is a significant environmental factor increasing the likelihood that an injurious energy exchange will occur.

garding recovery thus must be taken into account as prevention strategies targeting environmental factors are designed. This recognition, which is central to the "social model" recovery movement in California, has helped to overcome the suspicions that historically have separated those involved in recovery and those working for environmental change.

Alcohol Policy and the Public Health Model

Influencing the interaction between the individual and his or her environment involves addressing policy issues—those laws, regulations, formal and informal rules, and understandings that are adopted on a collective basis to guide individual and collective behavior. For the purposes here, the term is not limited to public policy or formal law. Rather it incorporates rules and procedures used by private organizations—commercial and noncommercial—to affect the organizations' members.

Policies at a variety of levels may influence a given situation. For example, a party given at a university dormitory may be subject to state law (no service to underaged persons), university regulation (e.g. a proctor must be present), dormitory regulation (e.g. no guests allowed), and party organizer party planning rules (e.g. no drinking contests). If policies in these overlapping settings are inconsistent, the chances for successful prevention drop significantly. It will be difficult or impossible to establish a moderate drinking norm in a university fraternity that encourages drinking contests and hazing. Such an environment will cause alcohol problems to increase and will undermine the effectiveness of university efforts to educate students about alcohol use.

The public health model, then, involves attention to alcohol policies and their impact on both individuals and their environments. Because the field has historically focused on individual-based strategies, a major contribution of the model is to provide a means for analyzing and addressing environmental factors. Alcohol control policies—the formal laws affecting alcohol availability and price—are an important, but not exclusive, part of this analysis. Numerous new priorities regarding environmental factors have emerged, based primarily on research conducted in the last 20 years:

TAX POLICIES State and federal government policies have resulted in steadily decreasing tax rates. Alcohol prices have fallen 28% relative to inflation since 1967, and the differential pricing between alcohol and other nonalcoholic beverages has practically disappeared. Research relating price and consumption shows this trend to be contrary to public health goals. Other tax policies serve to promote drinking as well, for example, the deduction given to corporations for alcohol purchases, which are assumed to be "ordinary and necessary to the conduct of business".

ADVERTISING AND OTHER PROMOTIONAL PRACTICES OF THE ALCOHOL INDUSTRY The dominant source of information on alcohol in our society comes from the multibillion dollar promotional efforts of the alcohol industry. Research has shown these messages to be deliberately distorted and deceptive, excluding health information, promoting denial of problems, and targeting groups at high risk for alcohol problems. Huge promotional campaigns overwhelm and contradict the accurate health information available from other sources and inhibit media coverage of alcohol issues. A variety of reforms in advertising practice have been proposed to counteract the impact of the alcohol industry's promotional campaigns. These include bans on alcohol advertisements on radio and television; regulation of advertising content; equal time for health messages on airwaves; and health warning labels on public health containers, on advertisements, and in retail establishments.

Research is equivocal regarding the direct impact of advertising on drinking practices and drinking problems. The industry has used the lack of clear evidence of such an impact as an argument against advertising reforms. The purpose of advertising is to "educate" consumers—affect their beliefs and attitudes—regarding the rewards and benefits of the product. Advertising is not designed to impact consumption directly except on a very long-term basis and in conjunction with other marketing and societal variables. Proving a direct impact is probably impossible given the confounding variables and the long-term strategy involved. From the viewpoint provided by the public health model, however, the degree to which aggressive and deceptive advertising practices cause an inconsistency of messages about alcohol in the environment is a serious problem, which has an adverse impact on other prevention strategies. Proving the direct impact of advertising on drinking practices and problems is thus tangential from the standpoint of a public health model that stresses the need for consistency throughout the environment.

PHYSICAL AVAILABILITY OF ALCOHOL Research has shown a direct link between the physical availability of alcohol and the level of alcohol problems in a society. The regulation of alcohol availability involves a complex set of governmental and private rules and regulations affecting who may serve and sell, where, in what kinds of establishments, in what manner, and at what time. As discussed by Makela et al, the impact of particular reforms is difficult to assess, although research suggests caution in loosening current availability regulations. A recent focus in the field has been to encourage local communities to develop availability regulations that meet the needs and concerns of community members, thus ensuring that regulations have community support. Server intervention, which focuses on the serving practices of both commercial and noncommercial servers, has also been a major focus among alcohol policy advocates (see below for discussion).

SPECIAL PROTECTIONS FOR YOUNG PEOPLE Restricting availability to young people is a major subcategory of control efforts. Research has demonstrated that minimum age drinking laws affect drinking and alcohol-related vehicle crashes among young people. Efforts have been made to regulate industry promotional campaigns on college campuses.

OTHER INSTITUTIONAL TARGETS FOR PREVENTION Social institutions do much to shape the alcohol environment. Beyond the institutions listed above, the agenda for policy change includes the actions of corporations, the military, educational and medical institutions, professional sports, the insurance industry, private foundations, and so on. Corporations have made important strides in developing Employee Assistance Programs to help employees identified as having alcohol problems. Practices in the corporate environment that may foster heavy drinking have come under increasing scrutiny. Alcohol policies on military reservations—notably price promotions—have been targeted. In each institution an agenda for change has been developed, as we have written elsewhere.

These policy agendas, flowing from the public health model, augment and help to shape other activities and priorities found in the alcohol field—adequate recovery services, educational and mass media compaigns, strict drinking-driving laws, and victim assistance programs. Under the model, the comprehensiveness and coordination of the agendas is central. Omitting these environmental influences will severely limit the viability of individual-based strategies. . . .

BARRIERS TO CHANGE: THE CURRENT ALCOHOL ENVIRONMENT

Many agencies and organizations responding to alcohol problems have not adopted the public health model and express fears that the focus on alcohol policy will restigmatize alcoholics and serve as an excuse to abandon treatment priorities. Yet a clear shift in perspective has occurred in this decade, and vocal opposition to this shift has become muted. . . .

The shift in perspective has not, however, been matched by success in achieving alcohol policy reforms. Environmental change requires reform of collective rules and understandings. These rules may be found on an informal or private level or may exist in formal laws and regulations. As discussed below, policy reform has succeeded most often at the local level. Furthermore, these successes tend to be modest and are frequently rolled back by state legislatures overruling local decision-makers. Action at the federal level, except for the legislation encouraging 21-year-old drinking age laws at the state level and the 1988 legislation requiring a health warning on all alcoholic beverage containers, has been notably unsuccessful.

Given a high level of public support and the emergence of a core leadership group, why have efforts to reform alcohol taxes, advertising practices, and availability policies been so unsuccessful? One obvious problem, noted by Room, is that public support is very shallow. The dominant public understanding of alcohol problems remains at the individual level. As Room suggests, a top priority with any alcohol policy reform effort is to focus on public awareness and understanding of the new perspective, which may be more important than whether the reform is actually implemented. Mosher has labeled this public apathy or misunderstanding "societal denial"—a countervailing tendency to deny that alcohol problems are collective problems requiring collective attention and solutions. Rather, the problems are viewed as the "fault" of the individual—as a crime, moral failing, or disease. Thus, although public opinion polls evidence support for alcohol policy reform, that support is easily diverted in the public policy arena.

As Ashley & Rankin point out, the second, more powerful and more profound barrier to implementation involves the alcohol industry and its allies. In part because of the public health field's historical lack of attention to environmental factors, the shape of the alcohol environment since the repeal of Prohibition has largely been determined by the marketing practices of a very powerful and sophisticated industry. As with the tobacco industry, the alcohol industry strongly opposes any attempt to limit marketing practices. Yet these practices are inevitable targets of an environmental approach to prevention. The industry's opposition can be felt not only in the legislatures, but throughout society, fostering continuing societal denial and apathy. Alcohol policy reform, if it is to succeed, must build on a knowledge of the industry, its structure, tactics, strengths, and weaknesses, and how these combine to define and control the current alcohol environment. We now turn to these topics.

Industry Marketing Strategy

The first step in addressing industry tactics is understanding the industry's interest in the alcohol policy debate. Cowan & Mosher have documented the industry's reliance on "total marketing" to maintain and expand its sales and profitability. Total marketing involves first defining the competition. During the last ten years, the industry has defined itself as being part of the "beverage market," competing for "stomach share" with other beverages—soft drinks, tap water, coffee, milk, etc. The beverage industry estimates that Americans drink approximately two quarts of liquid a day, and there is fierce competition among the beverage types (except of course from the "tap water" segment) to maintain and expand market share.

The alcohol industry operates in this "beverage market" by defining the target groups to be reached and developing a marketing plan tailored to each group. The population is broken down by demographic variables: age, sex, race, ethnicity, drinking patterns, etc. Each group so defined receives a distinct marketing effort. The most important group to the industry is the heaviest drinking 10% of the population (a plurality of whom are young men), who consume approximately 57% of all alcohol sold.

The marketing plan for each targeted group has four key components. First, a product is developed suited to the group's tastes, mores, and attitudes. Malt liquor, for example, is a product designed for young black men; fortified wine targets public inebriates; imported scotch is intended to reach upper class men. Wine coolers, one of the newest products on the market, clearly targets young people and women. The industry strongly denies it targets teenagers deliberately; recent polls demonstrate that, whatever the intent, the product has indeed penetrated this market.

The second component involves the promotion of the product that has been developed or identified to its target audience. Sophisticated advertising campaigns are designed to give the product a mythos—a message that ties it to the targeted group's desires, fears, and fantasies. Alcohol promotions are notably lacking in any factual information, particularly regarding potential health consequences. In this context, alcohol advertising is in reality a form of education, one that is dominated by deceptive and irrelevant material. Instead of providing health information, advertising seeks to promote "societal denial," saturating the environment with positive messages. The industry's response in recent years to growing concerns about health and fitness has been to focus promotional campaigns on images of young, physically fit people being active while drinking.

Third, each product in the product line is given a price. The price is set to meet the targeted group's ability and willingness to pay. For upper class and sophisticated drinkers, relatively high prices are expected; for those with limited income or entering the market, such as students, the lowest possible prices are established. Thus, alcohol products have a wide range of prices, but it is of critical importance that the range begin at the lowest price possible. This is particularly important because of the competition with other beverages. A major development in the last 20 years has been the ability of the beer and wine industries to compete in price with soft drinks and other types of nonalcoholic beverages.

Finally, the product needs to be in a place that is easily and widely available to the targeted group. This involves developing new packaging that is suited to the target group and the ability to place the packaging in the appropriate outlets where the group is likely to purchase. Women, for example, do not like to shop in liquor stores, preferring super markets. Thus, for example, in New York the wine industry moved aggressively to change state laws to allow wine coolers, a product targeted to the women's market, to be sold in grocery stores. Again, the competition with other nonalcoholic beverages has led the alcohol industry to become increasingly aggressive in seeking new outlets. From the point of view of the industry, alcohol products need to be as accessible to the target groups as soft drinks if they are to compete effectively.

These four marketing components—product, promotion, price, and place— are carefully coordinated with each other to reach each targeted audience. Thus the marketing plan to reach public inebriates is quite different from the plan for reaching young women. For the former, a very cheap product (fortified wine) is made available primarily in skid row liquor stores. Promotions are done primarily on billboards and in the stores themselves, since the target group is relatively small and does not watch television. Young women, on the other hand, are reached with a sweet, light wine (wine coolers) that avoids an "alcohol" taste, is promoted as a fun, light, healthful beverage, and is sold in grocery and convenience stores.

An understanding of the alcohol industry's marketing strategy helps explain recent trends in alcohol sales. The distilled spirits industry, which has suffered decreased sales over the last ten years, is at a distinct disadvantage. It does not have access to television and radio advertising, and is taxed at a much higher rate than beer and wine, resulting in higher prices relative to the rest of the "beverage market." Both beer and wine producers have suffered stagnated sales in recent years, which the industry attributes to societal concerns for health and fitness and drinking–driving. The industry has avoided an erosion of their markets by developing new "healthful" products—lower calorie beer and wine coolers—that have been very heavily promoted on television and radio and are widely available at low prices.

The ideal social environment from the industry's perspective, then, is one that is saturated with low-cost alcohol and positive alcohol messages, where alcohol is available in a wide and ever expanding array of beverage types, containers, and places of sale. The industry has been remarkably successful in creating this environment since Prohibition. Yet these are precisely the variables that have come under scrutiny in recent years by the public health movement as critical to the prevention of alcohol problems. It is not surprising, then, that reform efforts have met severe resistance from the industry, which feels under siege and views its ability to compete effectively in the beverage market as under attack. . . .

Organizing Local Constituencies

Successful application of environmental approaches to prevention requires the development of organized, educated, and active constituencies at the local level. Public health advocates need to counter industry lobbying with the mobilization of large numbers of people for policy change. Beginning at the local level, this mobilization provides an experiential base for learning about the alcohol environment and about industry tactics. Although many people are concerned over the impact of alcohol on their lives, public consciousness-raising and organizing are usually necessary to channel their interest into action on policy issues. Campaigns at the local level provide a sense of community power and ownership of the alcohol environment. Concerted collective action combats the sense of helplessness that often pervades community discussions of environmental issues. Campaigns build on each other: to a certain degree, whether a particular campaign succeeds matters less than that it sows seeds of awareness and recognition of the utility of community control over the alcohol environment that can be transferred to other policy issues.

Little research as yet documents process or outcomes from community organizing projects. Recent initiatives by major research centers to convene a conference on the implementation of community-based prevention signals a research direction that the field needs to pursue. As mentioned above, most policy successes have been achieved at the local level. Examples from community organizing campaigns already underway indicate the promise this approach holds for policy change. In Mill Valley, California, community organizing efforts recently produced a city ordinance controlling the service of alcohol on city property. At all events serving alcoholic beverages, the ordinance outlaws "no-host" bars; requires nonalcoholic beverage alternatives, low-alcohol beer and wine, and free food be visible and available; and mandates the prominent display of signs about drinking and driving. In Santa Cruz, a decision by law enforcement officials to enforce an ordinance banning drinking on the public beach has contributed to a reduction in police reports and emergency room admissions. San Diego County has instituted a wide variety of environmental policies that are in the process of being evaluated. A comprehensive community organizing project in Castro Valley, California has resulted in a citizen's task force that uses local zoning ordinances to combat proliferation of alcohol outlets. Numerous communities throughout California have successfully organized to mandate point-of-sale warnings about alcohol and birth defects.

Local organizing has intrinsic value in the contributions made toward improvement of the local environment. Local efforts also feed larger organizing agendas. Much about the nature of the alcoholic beverage industry and the policy process can be learned only through the experience of organizing for an apparently simple objective, which then turns out to be connected to a much wider agenda for change. The industry's opposition to birth defect-related warning posters, for example, illustrates a level of callousness to the health impact of alcoholic beverages that often must be witnessed to be believed. Through the experience of confronting the industry on a policy issue, communities can begin to analyze and understand the alcohol environment, and comprehend the contributions of such environmental factors as low excise taxes and widespread availability to alcohol-related problems.

Coalition-Building at the State and Federal Levels

Finally, local organizing provides the basis for the development of much broader coalitions to take on policy issues at the state and federal levels. The warning label issue provides a good example of building on local efforts to mount broad-based statewide and federal campaigns. This issue also exemplifies the potential for health-policy coalition-building that alcohol issues hold. Through the warning label efforts, groups with broad health agendas have become active on alcohol issues, while alcohol-focused organizations have recognized their stake in broader public health issues. Local successes in California have fed into a statewide coalition backing a warning label bill in the state legislature. Led by Consumers Union, the coalition includes entities as diverse as right-to-lifers and Planned Parenthood, as well as the PTA, the California Medical and Nurses Associations, and a host of public and private health and alcohol service delivery organizations.

State and local campaigns both feed into and draw from efforts at the federal level. CSPI and NCA have led the way in organizing two major national coalitions, the National Alcohol Tax Coalition (NATC) and Project SMART. NATC brought the American Association of Retired Persons, the Association of Junior Leagues, the Children's Defense Fund, the National Women's Health Fund, and over 25 other major national organizations together on behalf of excise tax increases. Project SMART, a petition drive that collected over a million signatures in support of equal time for health-oriented counteradvertising on the nation's broadcast media, won the support of the United Methodist Church, Action for Children's Television, Americans for Democratic Action, National PTA, Remove Intoxicated Drivers, and over 20 other national organizations. The recent successful effort to pass warning label legislation at the federal level, again spearheaded by NCA and CSPI, garnered support from over 100 health, consumer action, educational, treatment, and religious organizations. The existence of statewide warning label efforts supported the drive for a federal mandate, while membership in a federal coalition often leads to activism by state-level chapters.

As Room points out, beyond the concrete gains of the coalitions lies the significant contribution that such efforts make to public discourse on alcohol policy. Creating this consciousness-raising about sources and contributors to alcohol-related problems can be as important in the long run as winning a particular alcohol policy reform. This suggests a building block approach, choosing issues on the basis of their ability to raise consciousness and broaden coalitions rather than their ability to ameliorate the problem quickly. Warning labels will have less impact on public education than changes in advertising regulations, but they are politically more accessible and may lay the groundwork for an effective coalition to change advertising practices.

CONCLUSION: LESSONS LEARNED AND FUTURE AGENDAS

The past decade has witnessed a groundswell of support for alcohol policy change. Although major campaigns to raise excise taxes, require health warning labels, and restrict advertising have not yet found success at state or federal levels, much has been learned in the past decade about what a successful movement for alcohol policy change requires. These efforts have done much to raise the consciousness and clarify the goals of the alcohol policy reform movement. The last ten years have produced an efflorescence of research and consensus documents supporting those goals. They are relatively modest and specific. Industry allegations notwithstanding, the movement does not seek the prohibition of alcohol use. As Wallack and others point out, the overall goal is to reduce the risk associated with alcohol use, by altering the environments in which alcohol is available to make abstinence acceptable in all situations, discourage heavy use, and eliminate all use in situations where there is high risk for alcohol-related problems. Because prohibition is not a goal, it is assumed that alcohol-related problems will continue, albeit at significantly lower levels, even if the implementation of this approach to prevention is successful beyond the highest hopes of its proponents. Thus there will continue to be other research activities, lying outside of the realm of primary prevention and adding to our knowledge about treatment and recovery, which will remain important.

In this article we have attempted to outline some of the new knowledge needed to achieve policy reform. A cursory review of the environment permitting harmful actions between host and agent reveals that this environment has been largely determined, not by public health advocates, but by the alcohol industry. Internationally, as in the case of tobacco, the growing concentration of the alcoholic beverage industry and the stagnation of the domestic market are pushing alcohol multinationals to develop markets in the developing countries, exporting their total marketing approach to create the kinds of alcohol environments causing problems in the developed nations. This growing internationalization of alcohol problems only increases the need for effective action on the domestic front.

Familiarity with the industry's definition of the alcohol environment and the tactics used by the industry and its allies to maintain that environment are necessary prerequisites to successful alcohol policy change. The policy agenda articulated in the Alcohol Policy Bill of Rights and elsewhere responds to each of the industry's four P's with prevention strategies designed to create a healthy environment. Successful implementation of that agenda requires a response to the seven areas of industry tactics articulated above that is at least as comprehensive and coordinated as the industry's efforts. Industry attempts to influence legislators must be met by broad-based coalitions dedicated to safeguarding the health of the public. Linkages within the industry and with other industries can be weakened through server intervention, dram shop liability, and research and dissemination on the impact of alcohol problems on industry. The role of industry money in rewarding and punishing allies and opponents, and in improving the industry's image, can be exposed through case studies and through providing organizations and coalitions with experiences and training that demonstrate the function of donations in furthering industry agendas. The tactic of organizing drinkers must be countered by organizing those affected by and concerned about alcohol problems, including recovering people. Finally, sources of funding for research and training on environmental factors must be identified, encouraged, and developed to counter industry-sponsored research.

Prevention research has begun to focus on some of these crucial implementation issues. Research needs to be responsive to and supportive of emerging community agendas for change, and to inform community-based efforts in implementation. Process evaluations and case study analyses of community-based organizing and policy change projects are needed to provide direction to community action. These should be supplemented by outcome studies that document the impact of various policy changes on alcohol-related problems over time. Studies of various institutions and institutional environments, including the alcohol industry but also corporations, professional sports, higher education, the military, and other institutions that may be targets for change or barriers to or promoters of it, are also needed.

Research dissemination needs to take on a new form as well. Most organizations and individuals understand alcohol issues, and are moved to action about them, through a single issue: drinking-driving, alcoholism, injury prevention, domestic violence, etc. The task of implementing the public health approach is to build on these individualized understandings of the problem, shifting people's consciousness of alcohol problems to include an understanding of the importance of environmental forces. Researchers have an important role to play in accomplishing this shift in consciousness by providing a broad range of training and technical assistance activities. These include the development and dissemination of action-oriented informational resources—newsletter articles, action guides, slide and video presentations, information sheets summarizing recent research for the lay public—that introduce environmental issues and provide clear routes for community action. Seminars, conferences, and workshops tailored to the interests of specific groups but introducing broader prevention agendas as well are a high priority. Identification and training of leaders at the local level and the provision of technical expertise to emergent issue-oriented coalitions are also vital roles potentially filled by those with the research expertise to teach others to move with confidence in the face of industry opposition and obfuscation. Finally, researchers need to become active in the funding world, encouraging support of projects that will add to the knowledge base regarding implementation of the new approach.

Several leading alcohol researchers have argued that the current wave of temperance sentiment is merely another in a series of temperance "waves," which inevitably come and go with the tides of history. Although there is undoubtedly some truth to this, the differences between this period in alcohol policy and prevention and previous ones are sufficient to support the argument that we are in a new stage. Never before has the industry been so concentrated in the hands of a few corporations, and so sophisticated in its tactics of opposition to reform. On the public health side, alcohol policy advocates are working from a new understanding of the problem, one that is more comprehensive than earlier formulations, that is based in public health theory and research, and that both seeks more modest goals than past movements and provides the basis for broader coalitions.

What the current wave of temperance sentiment has done is to heighten the immediacy of individual alcohol problems. Alcohol problems grace the covers of major newsweeklies and are profiled in network specials. The challenge to the public health field is to place the problems in a public health perspective, and to organize for permanent policy reform based in that perspective. The breadth of the coalitions that have already been built suggests the potential of a public health approach for reaching new constituencies, raising popular consciousness abut new directions in alcohol policy and new ways to reduce alcohol-related problems, and swelling the ranks of the overall coalition working for a more human health policy in the US.

Drug Prohibition:
A Public-Health Perspective

BONNIE STEINBOCK

THE DRUG PROBLEM

It is estimated that over six million Americans are heavy drug users. Between 1986 and 1988, the number of cocaine addicts in New York City more than tripled, with an estimated total of 600,000 in 1988, most addicted to crack. Although middle-class cocaine use in the United States as a whole is on the decline—it has dropped 22 percent since 1988—Federal officials say that 6.4 million Americans used cocaine last year. In the poorest neighborhoods, cocaine smoking and snorting is on the rise, and a flood of potent heroin is creating new addicts. Drug abuse has caused problems for individuals, families, and society as a whole for years, but the introduction of crack cocaine has made things much worse. Let me mention just a few of the effects attributed to crack in New York City.

- Drug-related crime is far worse than it was twenty years ago. From 1987 to 1988, the number of murders in New York rose 10.4 percent. Police say that drugs, in particular, crack, played a role in at least 38 percent of the 1,867 murders in 1988, compared with a generally constant rate of 20 percent for years.
- Crack contributed to a tripling of cases in which parents under the influence of drugs abused or neglected their children. In 1987, 73 percent of the deaths in abuse and neglect cases resulted from parents abusing drugs, up from 11 percent in 1985.
- Between 1986 and 1988, the number of newborn children in New York City testing positive for drugs—mostly cocaine—almost quadrupled, going from 1,325 to 5,088. Because of crack, in some inner-city hospitals, the number of babies going directly from the hospital into foster homes has

From *Drugs, Morality, and the Law* edited by Steven Luper-Foy and Curtis Brown (Garland Publishing, Inc., 1994). Reprinted by permission.

risen from 2 percent to 15 percent. Urban child-welfare workers estimate that 70 percent of children they see are raised by grandmothers or other relatives after parents abandon them for drugs.

The impact of the crack epidemic on children is perhaps the most heartrending aspect of the drug problem. Other effects of crack, such as the tremendous increase in the prison population—up from 9,815 in New York City in 1985 to over 17,500 in 1989—can be laid to the fact that crack is *illegal.* Legalize addictive drugs, and drug arrests (1.2 million a year in the United States), which are overwhelming the criminal justice system, causing overcrowding in the prisons, and costing billions of dollars, would disappear. Moreover, according to Ira Glasser, Executive Director of the American Civil Liberties Union (ACLU) and a proponent of legalization, three-quarters of "drug-related" homicides are caused by territorial disputes and other incidents relating to the criminal trafficking system. "Only 7.5 percent of the homicides were related to the effects of the drug itself, and two-thirds of those involved alcohol, not crack."

By contrast, the effects of crack on children, both pre- and postnatally, will not be diminished by legalization. Dr. Linda A. Randolph, director of the State Office of Public Health, says that, because of drug abuse, particularly crack, "we are seeing dramatic increases in infant mortality, in congenital syphilis, and in the number of AIDS-infected women who are giving birth." Intensive hospital care for *each* crack baby costs about $90,000. That translates into $2.5 billion annually for the nation.

Crack can have devastating effects on the nervous systems of newborns. T. Berry Brazelton describes the clinical manifestations this way:

> They are either limp and unresponsive or are hyper-sensitive and behave chaotically. They have difficulty receiving and responding to the stimuli of a soothing voice or face. When they are cuddled or rocked, they react with piercing wails and jerky motions. Few people could love these babies. They are likely to suffer later from learning disabilities and to be either hyperactive or emotionally flat. They also tend to be at the mercy of their impulses. The social programs required to educate them will cost billions of dollars.

It should be noted that, although crack is ingested during pregnancy, the harmful effects are imposed on the newborn, the infant, and even the older child. The pregnant crack addict does not risk harm only to herself, but also to the baby she will bear, if she decides not to abort. The term "fetal abuse," often used to describe the use of drugs during pregnancy, is something of a misnomer, since the damage is not confined to the fetus, but is done also to the born child. However one views the fetus, born children have full legal rights, including the right not to be injured prior to live birth. That is why there is no logical contradiction in supporting the right to abortion and maintaining that

women have an obligation not to harm their not-yet-born children through in-
gestion of drugs during pregnancy.

While there is debate among the experts about how bad and long-lasting the
physical damage is to children born to crack users, there is agreement that these
babies are especially susceptible to child abuse. They suffer from neglect because, as one article put it, ". . . people who hardly bother with food for themselves can't be expected to give up precious crack to feed a baby, can they?"
And they are at risk for child abuse because their screaming and nonresponsive-
ness make them unattractive and difficult to care for. As Brazelton asks, "What
would an addicted parent in an addicted environment do to such a baby? The
ingredients for child abuse were all there."

THE LIBERTARIAN APPROACH

Even this brief recounting indicates a major social problem, something with
which society is entitled—even obligated—to concern itself. Yet a libertarian
perspective suggests otherwise. . . .

[L]ibertarian[s] . . . value individual liberty more than any other value. The
libertarian principle can be traced back to John Stuart Mill, who argued in *On
Liberty* that the only purpose for which it was permissible to restrict individual
freedom was to prevent harm to others. A person's own good was never sufficient warrant. Mill's principle has been applied in all sorts of ways: from opposition of seatbelt and helmet laws to opposition to closing gay bathhouses in an
effort to stop the spread of AIDS.

Mill attempted to defend his absolute prohibition against paternalistic intervention on utilitarian grounds, but this has been notoriously unsuccessful. There
is no reason to think that the harm of paternalistic intervention will necessarily
outweigh the benefit to be attained. Philosopher Gerald Dworkin persuasively
argues that it was not utilitarian calculation that led Mill to his absolute rejection of paternalism, but rather a non-contingent, non-utilitarian argument about
what it means to be a person, an autonomous agent. Dworkin says, "It is because coercing a person for his own good denies this status as an independent
entity that Mill objects to it so strongly and in such absolute terms. Dworkin
goes on to argue that some paternalistic intervention can be justified, even on
Millian grounds, namely, restrictions that preserve a wider range of freedom for
the individual in question.

THE PUBLIC-HEALTH APPROACH

Whereas Dworkin can be seen as attempting to justify very limited paternalistic
measures, within a Millian perspective, Dan Beauchamp, a professor of public

health, is a more outright critic of Mill. Beauchamp notes that some restrictions on individual liberty result in considerable social gain. Consider the example of seat belts. Each year roughly forty-five thousand people in the United States are killed in car crashes. Laws requiring the wearing of seat belts or making air bags compulsory would save roughly ten thousand lives a year. That's a lot of lives, a considerable social good. Libertarians object to seat-belt laws as being objectionably paternalistic. Why shouldn't I decide for myself whether to buckle up? Refusing to buckle up doesn't cause "harm to others" and so laws forcing people to use seat belts are not warranted on Millian grounds. But Beauchamp argues that, since the infringement on individual freedom is minuscule, and the social good so great, the intrusion is warranted. He supports "reasonable, minimally intrusive restrictions that yield significant gains in the health and safety of the public."

I think that Beauchamp's public-health approach is far more useful in thinking about the legalization of drugs than the libertarian approach. The libertarian insists that there isn't a drug problem, since trade is a positive sum game, and both parties gain. No one who has any experience with drug abuse and the social upheaval it has caused will agree with that conclusion. Instead of insisting, on ideological grounds, that individuals should have the right to buy whatever they want, regardless of the social costs, we should examine carefully the costs of prohibition and the costs of legalization. This means that the argument about legalization is not primarily a philosophical one. Rather, it is an empirical argument about the likely consequences of different strategies for dealing with the drug problem.

While the public-health approach rejects Mill's absolutist antipaternalism, it entirely agrees with Mill on one thing: the rejection of moralism. Mill argued that legal or social prohibitions on behavior could never be justified simply on the ground that the behavior in question was regarded by the majority as wicked or sinful. He insisted that infringements on individual liberty have to be justified by demonstrating that the conduct in question was likely to cause harm to others.

Of course it is not always easy to settle the question of whether an activity will cause harm to others: the example of violent pornography is a case in point. However, the rejection of moralism at least makes it clear what *kind* of argument is necessary to support coercive intervention. Empirical evidence of injury or the risk of injury is essential. Simply referring to moral principles, no matter how widely accepted, or moral feelings, no matter how strongly held, will not do. Someone who takes a public-health perspective may be willing to consider closing gay bathhouses *if* it is reasonable to think that this will slow the spread of a deadly disease, but will not be willing to infringe on individual liberty because the activities in such places are viewed by many as nasty or evil.

Why does the public-health perspective reject moralism? After all, if it is willing to acknowledge collective or communal values, such as health, why not acknowledge that there can be collective or communal *moral* values? Indeed, aren't free speech, equal opportunity, and the democratic process, which are essential to a democratic republic, *moral* values? Of course. The rejection of moralism does not consist in rejection of or neutrality toward all moral values. Rather, the rejection of moralism consists in opposition to coercion (as opposed to education and persuasion) to eradicate sin and vice or to make individuals morally better.

It might be objected that a public-health approach is based on a false distinction between different kinds of values. On a public-health approach, some government coercion is acceptable for the sake of certain values (for example, those connected to public health) but not others (for example, those related to private sexual behavior). A libertarian might argue that if it is permissible to infringe individual liberty for the sake of social goals, there is no principled reason for insisting that the goals to be achieved must be of a certain kind. If the majority in a society thinks that homosexuality is bad for society, then why shouldn't it pass laws against homosexuality? What justifies coercion for some social goals, but not others? The answer has to do with a certain conception of the common good. The common good should not be understood in terms of whatever the majority values or wants. Such a conception would indeed threaten individual liberty through, in Mill's phrase, "the tyranny of the majority." Rather, I suggest that we think of the common good in terms of what Rawls calls "primary goods": "things which it is supposed a rational man wants whatever else he wants." Health is an example of a primary good. By restricting our conception of the common good to primary goods, we avoid imposing goals and values on individuals that they do not happen to share. However, it may be objected that, even if it is true that everyone has reason to value his or her own health, it does not follow that everyone has reason to value the health of the community. (This was the mistake that Mill is supposed to have made in his proof of the principle of utility.) What if I am not interested in saving ten thousand lives a year? What justifies forcing me to buckle up?

I am not sure that it can be demonstrated that not caring about aggregate welfare or the good of society as a whole is *irrational*. However, the communitarian or republican morality of "We're all in this together" seems to me infinitely preferable to the extreme individualism which is concerned only with individuals' interests and rights. Republican morality balances individual virtues like self-reliance and individual responsibility against community virtues like beneficence, cooperation, and justice. As Dan Beauchamp puts it:

> Beneficence means that we wish the good and welfare of others as well as ourselves, while cooperation and justice mean that we as citizens are disposed to see

that the common welfare is extended to all alike and do not allow our private interests to frustrate achievement of the common good. While the principles of individuality and community can often pull in opposite directions, both principles are needed to assure the fullest development of the individual and his dignity both as an autonomous person and as a member of the political fellowship.

Recognition that there is a common good, as well as the separate welfares of individuals, does not preclude controversy over its nature. Moreover, even when individuals acknowledge a collective good, such as disease prevention, they may differ as to its importance relative to other collective goods. A public-health approach does not demand that we value life and health above all else. It merely supports minimally intrusive restrictions on individual liberty to promote the common good.

A related objection holds that even if it is possible to differentiate among social goods, so that infringement of individual liberty is restricted to primary collective goods, such as health, there is still a danger of imposing majoritarian moral views on individuals, because there is no morally neutral way to characterize even basic goods. All people may want to be healthy, but one's conception of health depends on one's particular moral or religious views. Whether one regards drug use, for example, as "unhealthy" depends on one's views about the body, altered consciousness, pleasure, industriousness, and, in general, the right way to live. It is this inability to characterize, in an objective fashion, basic goods that leads the libertarian to maintain that the assessment about what is worth pursuing should be left to individuals.

I think we can agree that there is an overlap between health and morality without conceding that it is impossible to distinguish the two. Individuals from widely divergent religious and moral backgrounds can agree on whether someone is sick, what disease he or she has, and whether something is a health risk. This suggests that there is a difference between health and morals, which makes it possible, in general, to distinguish arguments and reasons based on health considerations from those based on moral and religious values.

It must be admitted that much of American drug policy has been drenched in moralism. This moralistic attitude is revealed both in regarding addiction as a failure of willpower ("Just say no") and in wildly exaggerated descriptions of the effects of addiction. Here is a description of the effects of heroin from a concurring opinion by Justice Douglas in a 1962 United States Supreme Court decision:

> To be a confirmed drug addict is to be one of the walking dead. . . . The teeth have rotted out; the appetite is lost and the stomach and intestines don't function properly. The gall bladder becomes inflamed; eyes and skin turn a bilious yellow. In some cases membranes of the nose turn a flaming red; the partition separating the nostrils is eaten away—breathing is difficult. Oxygen in the blood decreases; bronchitis and tuberculosis develop. Good traits of character disappear and bad

ones emerge. Sex organs become affected. Veins collapse and livid purplish scars remain. Boils and abscesses plague the skin; gnawing pain racks the body. Nerves snap; vicious twitching develops. Imaginary and fantastic fears blight the mind and sometimes complete insanity results. Often times, too, death comes—much too early in life. . . . Such is the torment of being a drug addict; such is the plague of being one of the walking dead.

Similar lies were propagated about LSD in various newspaper stories, and about marijuana in such films as *Reefer Madness*. The effect, ironically enough, was to persuade a generation that any warnings about drug usage were likely to be completely untrustworthy.

Moralism about drugs is often coupled with hypocrisy about legal drugs. Schoolchildren are taught about the evils of illicit drugs, but the dangers of legal drugs are downplayed or ignored. A recent ad on television depicts a father confronting his child with marijuana found in his room, asking, "Who taught you to do this?" only to be told, "You did, Dad!" The announcer solemnly intones, "Parents who use drugs will have children who use drugs." Yet we don't see ads warning, "Parents who smoke and drink will have children who smoke and drink," despite the fact that far more people die from cigarettes and alcohol than from illegal drugs.

A public-health approach is pragmatic and non-ideological. It rejects moralism, and insists on sound empirical evidence for its claims. It recognizes the values of liberty and privacy, and supports the right of people to make their own choices about how they will live, free from governmental interference. At the same time, it recognizes that private acts can have social consequences. Thus, a public-health approach balances the harm to individuals of coercive laws against the social good to be achieved. It is willing to sacrifice some individual liberty in order to achieve important collective goals, such as the saving of thousands of lives or the eradication of disease.

IMPLICATIONS FOR DRUG POLICY

The Failure of the War on Drugs

There is wide consensus on one thing: the penal approach to the drug problem has been a dismal failure. The United States has poured nearly $70 billion into fighting drugs in the last twenty years, with very little to show for it. The reasons for the failure of the War on Drugs are primarily economic. Illicit drugs are big business. Seventy-nine billion dollars are generated every year by the sale of illicit drugs. Only the Exxon Corporation has higher annual revenues.

In many less-developed countries, drug trafficking, which has provided a new way to earn vast sums of hard currency, is transforming whole economies. In poor Third World countries, coca is one of the few cash crops that grows well, much better than coffee or oranges. In Colombia, Bolivia, and Peru, many farmers have turned from growing food crops to growing marijuana and coca, which make them three or four times as much money a year. In Bolivia, cocaine is estimated to generate as much as ten times the amount of Bolivia's leading official export, tin. Drug traffickers are at least as powerful as the government. They have more money than—and weapons and equipment as least as good as—the armed forces or the police. Moreover, drug traffickers are regarded by much of the populace as benefactors, not criminals. Even with the best will in the world, the government can do little to enforce laws that run counter to the vital economic interests of large numbers of its citizens. And that will is not always present. Mathea Falco, former Assistant Secretary of State for International Narcotics Matters, writes:

> It is very difficult to convince a foreign government to take the serious political and economic risks that are entailed by an all-out campaign against, say, cocaine production when the American public's predilection for cocaine is so well known. And it is virtually impossible to persuade foreign growers of marijuana to stop producing when one American in four has tried the drug—and billions of dollars in profits are being made by marijuana growers in the United States.

Occasionally, the U.S. government has been able to solicit the cooperation of foreign governments to stop production, but often with unexpected results. In 1975, the Mexican government, with American assistance, began a program to eliminate the marijuana crop by spraying it with paraquat. Mexico, then a major supplier to the U.S. market of relatively cheap, low-potency marijuana, effectively destroyed much of the crop. Jamaica and Colombia, previously only minor suppliers of marijuana, quickly stepped up production, producing a plant of much higher potency. In addition, American domestic production of marijuana began to boom. Marijuana is currently the second-largest cash crop in the United States, just after corn and ahead of soybeans.

Throughout the 1980s, the Reagan and Bush administrations acted aggressively in mobilizing the agencies of the federal government in a coordinated attack on the drug supply from abroad and the distribution of drugs within the United States. Total federal spending on the War on Drugs rose from approximately $1 billion to $9 billion during the 1980s. The crackdown yielded record numbers of drug seizures, arrests, and convictions. The Drug Enforcement Administration (DEA), the FBI, and Customs seized nearly half a billion dollars in drug-related assets in 1986. That year, the DEA arrested twice as many drug offenders as in 1982. From the end of 1980 to June 30, 1987, the prison population soared from 329,021 to 570,519. Roughly 40 percent of new prison inmates are incarcerated for drug offenses.

Should we conclude that the War on Drugs was a success? Not at all. None of this activity had any impact on either drug consumption or the drug market.

Domestic marijuana cultivation took off and the black market in cocaine grew to record size. As a result, prices plummeted. Steven Wisotsky, in *Beyond the War on Drugs*: "In 1980–81, a gram of cocaine cost $100 and averaged 12 percent purity at street level. By 1986, the price had fallen to as low as $80 ($50 in Miami), and the purity had risen to more than 50 percent. It rose to 70 percent purity in 1988. Around the nation, crack was marketed in $5 and $10 vials to reach the youth and low-income markets." In hospitals, cocaine-related emergencies rose from 4,277 in 1982 to more than 46,000 in 1988. That trend began to go down in late 1989, but a new Federal report shows a 13 percent increase in hospital emergencies attributed to cocaine in the third quarter of 1991 and a 10 percent increase in emergency room visits from the use of heroin.

This rapid expansion of supply and decline in price occurred despite President Reagan's increasing the federal antidrug enforcement budget from $645 million in fiscal year 1981 to over $4 billion in fiscal year 1987. A third of that budget was specifically devoted to interdiction. Commenting in 1987 specifically upon the interdiction budget, the Office of Technology Assessment concluded:

> Despite a doubling of Federal expenditures on interdiction over the past five years, the quantity of drugs smuggled into the United States is greater than ever. . . . There is no clear correlation between the level of expenditures or effort devoted to interdiction and the long-term availability of illegally imported drugs in the domestic market.

In 1992, the Bush Administration spent nearly $12 billion on drugs, more than double what was spent in Mr. Reagan's last year in office, two-thirds of it going to interdiction. "It reminds me of that cartoon," says Dr. Herbert Kleber, professor of medicine at Columbia University and a former deputy director of the Office of National Drug Control Policy who quit when he couldn't get more money shifted to treatment. "This king is slamming his fist on the table, saying, 'If all my horses and all my men can't put Humpty Dumpty together again, then what I need is more horses and more men.' "

Why has the government continued to pour money and other resources into a failed policy? For the same reason, I suspect, that we stayed in Vietnam. In *The March of Folly*, Barbara Tuchman suggests that "Woodenheadedness . . . plays a remarkably large role in government. It consists in assessing a situation in terms of preconceived fixed notions while ignoring or rejecting any contrary signs. It is acting according to wish while not allowing oneself to be deflected by the facts."

The War on Drugs has not simply failed. It's made things much worse. Steven Wisotsky writes:

It has spun a spider's web of black-market pathologies, including roughly 25 percent of all urban homicides, widespread corruption of police and other public officials, street crime by addicts, and subversive "narco-terrorist" alliances between Latin American guerrillas and drug traffickers. In the streets of the nation's major cities, violent gangs of young drug thugs armed with automatic rifles engage in turf wars. Federal agents estimated in 1988 that more than 10,000 members of "posses" or Jamaican drug gangs were responsible for about 1,000 deaths nationwide. Innocent bystanders and police officers are among their victims.

Another negative effect of the War on Drugs has been a reduction in civil liberties. The Supreme Court has upheld searches without probable cause, warranted searches of automobiles, adopted a "good-faith exception" to the exclusionary rule, and authorized search of "open fields" adjacent to a residence. The power of the police to stop, question, detain, investigate, and search vehicles has expanded significantly. Wisotsky comments, "The net result of the War on Drugs is gradually, but inexorably, to expand enforcement powers at the expense of personal freedom."

The War on Drugs mentality has prevented doctors from making authorized use of many controlled substances having valuable therapeutic applications. In 1984, the House of Representatives killed a bill that would have made injectable heroin available to dying cancer patients suffering severe, intense and intractable pain, when other drugs were ineffective. In California, patients with extremely debilitating cases of rheumatoid arthritis exhibited remarkable pain-free ability when they smoked freebase cocaine. Nevertheless, the government ended the experiment.

Most recently, the fight has centered around the use of marijuana as a medicinal drug. In March 1992, the Drug Enforcement Administration refused to reclassify marijuana as a Schedule II drug so doctors could prescribe it for patients suffering from glaucoma, cancer, muscular sclerosis, and AIDS. A Federal appeals court had ruled the previous April that the government was using illogical criteria in prohibiting the use of marijuana for medical purposes, because the agency had based a conclusion that marijuana had no "currently accepted medical use" on factors like the drug's general availability, its use by a substantial number of doctors, and recognition of its use in medical texts. Since the drug is illegal, the court said, meeting these criteria would be all but impossible.

Robert C. Bonner, chief of the DEA, said that marijuana had not been shown to be as safe and effective as legal alternatives, such as Marinol, a synthetic form of THC, the active ingredient in marijuana. In his response to the appeals court, Bonner said, "Beyond doubt, the claims that marijuana is medicine are false, dangerous and cruel. Sick men, women and children can be fooled by these claims and experiment with the drug. Instead of being helped, they risk serious side effects." Although made in the guise of scientific information, this is pure moralism. As Dr. Lester Grinspoon, an associate professor of psychiatry at Harvard Medical School who is the author of several books on marijuana's medicinal uses, says, "It's absolutely extraordinary that our government is behaving the way it is toward cannibis. They see legalizing it for medical use as a Trojan Horse for recreational use."

There has been a surge in the last year in requests for medical marijuana by AIDS patients, and some advocates argue that this inspired the recent Government actions. "The government is not doing this to protect patients," said Kennington Wall, a spokesman for the Drug Policy Foundation in Washington, which advocates a liberal national drug policy. "They're doing this to protect their political agenda."

Should Drugs Be Legalized?

If the War on Drugs has been a disaster, should drugs be legalized? A simple "yes" or "no" is impossible, partly because different drugs may require different responses, and partly because there are factual issues yet to be resolved. For example, what would be the effect of legalization on access and consumption? Some argue that legalization would have little impact on access, because illegal drugs are already easily available. More than half the high school seniors questioned by University of Michigan researchers in 1991 said that finding cocaine was "fairly easy" or "very easy." Nearly, 40 percent said the same for crack and about a third for heroin.

Others are convinced that, even if illegal drugs are already easy to obtain, legalization would make drugs even more accessible. This would lead to higher addiction rates, and thus worsen the already massive problems faced by the inner city. Many advocates for inner-city communities view illegal drugs as one aspect of the dominant society's oppression of their communities. Legalization "is construed as an expression of disdain for and dismissal of the misery that drugs bring to inner cities," according to Mosher and Yanagisako.

Advocates of legalization think that it will not increase the number of addicts for three reasons. First, although the price of drugs can be expected to go down, this will have little effect on the behavior of addicts who regard drugs as a necessity, not a luxury. Second, there will be little incentive for addicts to try to "hook" others to support their own habits. Third, even if quantity increases, potency will fall. Prohibition leads to stronger and stronger drugs, which are both more concentrated and have higher value. Therefore, even if greater amounts of drugs are consumed under legalization, they are likely to be less harmful to the population.

Advocates of legalization may be right about . . . its . . . effect on consumption and addiction. Still, it should be remembered that *three times* as many Americans abuse alcohol as use illegal drugs. Why? Because alcohol is legal, it is easy to buy, it is an accepted part of our culture. If addictive drugs were legal, it seems likely that entrepreneurs would cultivate or manufacture them, package them, and advertise them, just as they do alcohol. And it is reasonable to believe that this would result in higher consumption, greater abuse, and a higher rate of addiction. . . .

Sometimes the argument in favor of legalization is based on claims about what we learned from Prohibition. It is often said that Prohibition "didn't work": that people went right on drinking in speakeasies, which facilitated the rise of organized crime and led ordinary citizens to lose respect for the law. In fact, by public-health standards, narrowly construed, Prohibition was a success. Consumption of alcohol fell by more than two-thirds, and cirrhosis rates fell to half the level that obtained in 1910. Two years after repeal, total consumption of alcohol was only one-third of the 1910 level.

Nevertheless, Prohibition was a failure, because it was unduly moralistic, restrictive, and repressive. Moreover, it was unnecessary. As Beauchamp says, ". . . most of what we could accomplish in health and safety under Prohibition could be achieved through more stringent regulation of alcohol. Prohibition is something like ringing a doorbell with a cannon."

It might be argued that it is equally unnecessary to ban addictive drugs, even if one is concerned about their impact on the nation's health and safety. Perhaps we could legalize or decriminalize the sale of addictive drugs, while keeping their availability severely restricted. However, there is an important difference between alcohol and illicit drugs, and that is simply that alcohol is currently legal. Millions of Americans have grown up regarding alcohol as a normal and socially acceptable part of life. Having wine in a restaurant, champagne at weddings, and beer at picnics are pleasures of which many Americans would resent being deprived. Prohibition of alcohol is politically impossible.

Because narcotic and opiate drugs have been illegal since the beginning of this century, they aren't viewed by most people as something to which they have a right. *Keeping* drugs illegal would not engender widespread anger and resentment, as *making* alcohol illegal would. The question faced by policymakers and ordinary citizens is whether we should opt for changing the law, and legalizing addictive drugs. The risks and harms posed by addictive drugs provide a powerful argument against changing the status quo. No doubt it is for this reason that Beauchamp supports "a policy that combines legal suppression of supply, both here and abroad, with more humane and compassionate treatment of users and addicts, even offering some form of maintenance as an alternative to obtaining drugs in illegal settings."

A pragmatic approach also requires us to distinguish between drugs. The case for keeping cocaine and heroin illegal is much stronger than the case for keeping marijuana illegal. Marijuana is not addictive, that is, there is no physical dependence or withdrawal. Psychological dependence appears to be minimal or nonexistent. Sixty-two million Americans have tried marijuana at least once, and roughly 18 million use it regularly. While marijuana is not risk-free (especially for adolescents and pregnant women), there is considerable evidence that it is much less harmful than alcohol. Yet there are approximately one-half million arrests per year for marijuana, almost all for simple possession or petty sale offenses. It is hard to see what social goals require that the criminal justice system be overburdened in this way.

A public-health approach toward drugs would require various measures. First and foremost, it requires continuing education about the benefits and dangers of both legal and illegal drugs. But a public-health approach goes beyond mere education. It supports getting tough on the legal drugs by such measures as getting rid of cigarette vending machines so that cigarettes are not so readily available to minors; restricting the hours of sale of liquor; and levying raising taxes on these items, commensurate with their social cost—billions of dollars in property damage, disease, and lost productivity. At the same time, the respect for individual choice and the rejection of moralism that are part of the public-health approach require that we remain open to the possibility that some currently illegal but comparatively harmless drugs, such as marijuana, should be legalized. And even if we decide to keep cocaine and heroin illegal, the emphasis should be on treatment. For most of the Reagan years, only about 20 percent of the budget went to treatment and education. This rose to about 30 percent under Bush. Despite Clinton's campaign rhetoric, it is still woefully inadequate, according to many experts. Studies indicate that present prevention and treatment efforts reach only 10 percent of alcohol and drug abusers. In addition, there is also very limited research on which prevention and treatment programs work. Dr. Herbert D. Kleber, a former deputy director in the Federal Office of National Drug Control Policy and one of the organizers of the recently created Center on Addiction and Substance Abuse in Manhattan, jokes about the "four-two-one" syndrome in medical school, meaning that in four years of medical school, students get two hours of instruction on the nation's No. 1 health problem, drug abuse. Obviously, this lack of attention must be addressed if we are to combat effectively the drug problem.

CONCLUSION

This paper does not attempt to answer the complex question of whether drugs should be legalized. The answer to that question hinges on various empirical issues, such as whether legalization would increase addiction rates. Instead, my aim has been to show that the right approach to the problem of drug addiction is a public-health perspective, as opposed to a libertarian approach. . . . Whereas the libertarian insists on absolute freedom of choice, regardless of social costs, the public-health approach balances the values of liberty and autonomy against the values of health and safety. It rejects the uncompromising stances characteristic of both moralism and libertarian ideology. Above all, a public-health approach insists that policies must be based on an honest appraisal of the problem and accurate empirical evidence about what does and does not work to solve it.

Controlling Tobacco Advertising:
The FDA Regulations and the First Amendment

LEONARD H. GLANTZ

INTRODUCTION

On August 28, 1996, the Food and Drug Administration (FDA) published regulations designed to reduce the use of tobacco products (meaning cigarettes and smokeless tobacco) by children. Certain parts of the regulations control the sale of tobacco in that they prohibit sales to individuals under 18 years of age and require sales to be made only in direct face-to-face transactions between the retailer and the consumer, thereby prohibiting sales by vending machines with limited exceptions. Other portions of the rule, in an attempt to limit the attractiveness of tobacco use to young people, regulate the way tobacco products are advertised and promoted. All advertising for these products is limited to the use of the black text on a white background. The only exceptions to this restriction are advertisements appearing in adult magazines or posted in facilities that only adults are permitted to enter. An adult publication is defined as a publication that is read by fewer than 2 million persons younger than 18 and whose readers in this age group constitute 15% or less of the publication's total readership. Furthermore, tobacco product manufacturers are prohibited from manufacturing, licensing, marketing, distributing, or selling any product such as hats or shirts that bears the name, logo, or other indicia of product identification; no tobacco manufacturer or distributor may sponsor sporting, cultural, athletic, musical, or cultural events in which any indicia of its to-bacco products are displayed; and no outdoor advertising of tobacco products is permitted within 1000 feet of a playground, elementary, or secondary school. The regulations also require that additional warnings about tobacco's dangers be placed on labels.

These proposed rules raise substantial legal issues. The first is whether the FDA has the jurisdiction to regulate tobacco products at all, a question this

From the *American Journal of Public Health*, 87 (March 1997), 446–451. Reprinted by permission of the American Public Health Association.

paper will not discuss. The second is whether the proposed rules violate the free speech rights of tobacco manufacturers under the First Amendment. This paper will examine the free speech issue in light of recent Supreme Court decisions.

ORIGINS OF THE CONSTITUTIONAL PROTECTION OF COMMERCIAL SPEECH

The specific issue raised by the FDA's regulations is the constitutional protection of commercial speech (speech that proposes a commercial transaction), a murky and evolving area of the law. In 1942 the Supreme Court suggested, without analysis, that commercial speech was not entitled to First Amendment protection. About 3 decades later when the Court next considered this question, it adopted a very different approach. In 1971 (2 years before *Roe v Wade* legalized abortions in all states) a women's health service in New York published an advertisement in a Virginia newspaper stating that abortions were now legal in New York and offering to help women in Virginia obtain abortions. The newspaper publisher was convicted of violating a Virginia law that outlawed the publication of advertisements for abortion services. In *Bigelow v Virginia*, the Court explicitly ruled that commercial speech "enjoys a degree" of constitutional protection. However, it went on to find that the advertisement at issue was not purely commercial; rather, it conveyed information to a diverse audience. For example, the advertisement informed potential law reformers in Virginia that another state had legalized abortion.

The following year the Court dealt squarely with the issue of state regulation of commercial speech. In *Virginia State Board of Pharmacy v Virginia Citizens Consumer Council*, the Court struck down a Virginia statute that outlawed the advertising of prescription drug prices. The issue was "whether speech which does 'no more than propose a commercial transaction' . . . lacks all [constitutional] protection?" The Court answered no, finding that both sellers and buyers have a strong interest in the dissemination of information, and that in a free enterprise economy it is a matter of public interest that commercial decisions be intelligent and well informed. Because commercial speech is constitutionally protected, a state must demonstrate a significant interest to justify abridging the exercise of this right. The state argued that price advertising would reduce the quality of professional pharmacists' services because pharmacists would be forced to reduce their services to meet the prices of discounters. It also argued that price shopping would lead to the loss of the stable pharmacist-customer relationship, making individual attention and monitoring impossible. Finally it argued that advertising would reduce the pharmacist's professional image to that of a mere retailer. In effect, the state argued that drug price advertising was a threat to public health.

The Court was not persuaded by these arguments. It pointed out that professional standards could be better and more directly maintained through direct regulation of pharmacists. The state assumed that low-quality, low-cost pharmacies that advertise would attract unwitting customers. The Court characterized this as a "highly paternalistic approach." Instead, the Court assumed that people would be able to determine where their own best interest lay only if they were well enough informed by opening channels of communication. It pointed out that pharmacists would be allowed to advertise not only the price of drugs but also their superior products and services. The Court concluded, "Virginia is free to require whatever professional standards it wishes of its pharmacists. . . . But it may not do so by keeping the public in ignorance of the entirely lawful terms that competing pharmacists are offering."

The Court also noted that like other speech, commercial speech can be regulated in certain ways. States can regulate the "time, place and manner" of speech in certain circumstances, as well as false or misleading speech.

In subsequent cases, the Court struck down restrictions on lawyer advertising, on the use of "for sale" signs in front of houses, and on contraceptive advertising because these prohibitions infringed on commercial speech. The cases made clear that the Court was giving commercial speech substantial protection while attempting to allow states to regulate it if they could establish a significant enough interest. But the standards to be applied in such a balancing approach were less than clear.

The Court attempted to clarify these standards in *Central Hudson Gas & Electric Corp v Public Service Commission of New York*. In that case, an electric company challenged a New York rule that prohibited electric companies from engaging in any advertising that promoted the use of electricity. The rule's purpose was to further the national policy of conserving energy. The commission also believed that the rule would keep down electric rates because of the way such rates were calculated. The Court applied a four-part test to determine the constitutionality of state restrictions on commercial speech: (1) the speech must concern lawful activity and not be misleading, (2) the asserted governmental interest in restricting the speech must be "substantial," (3) the regulation must "directly advance" the governmental interest, and (4) the regulation must not be more extensive than is necessary to serve the interest.

The Court readily found that selling electricity was a lawful activity and that the proposed advertising was not misleading. It also found that the state's interest in energy conservation and in keeping rates low were substantial, and that there was an immediate connection between advertising and the demand for electricity. Indeed, a monopoly's only reason for advertising would be to increase demand since there are no competitors. However, the Court found that the state's ban on advertising contravened part 4 of the test because it was more extensive than necessary to further the state's energy conservation goals. The electric company argued that the ban prohibited it from advertising products that would lead to more efficient energy use; this included heat pumps, which both sides agreed would greatly improve electric heating. The Court concluded that the state's sweeping ban prevented the company from advertising products that would consume the same amount of energy as alternative sources or actually reduce energy use by diverting demand from less efficient sources.

Several justices who concurred in the outcome questioned the state's authority to ban commercial speech at all. Justices Blackmun and Brennan said, "[We] seriously doubt whether suppression of information concerning the availability and price of a legally offered product is ever a permissible way for the State to 'dampen' demand for or use of the product."

These comments reflect the tension found in these cases. The justices did not disagree that the state has an interest in conserving energy, just as states have an interest in maintaining the quality of pharmacist services. The issue was whether states may further this interest by suppressing speech, which is constitutionally protected, particularly when more direct action can be taken to regulate the activity in ways that would not raise any constitutional problems.

ADVERTISING GAMBLING

The Court gave commercial speech increasing levels of protection, frequently striking down state advertising bans until 1986. That year the case of *Posadas de Puerto Rico v Tourism Company of Puerto Rico* seemed to halt this momentum. Puerto Rico, which permitted casino gambling, prohibited all advertising of the activity that would be accessible to residents of Puerto Rico. Its goal was to reduce residents' demand for casino gambling. In an opinion written by Chief Justice Rehnquist, the Court found that the activity was lawful, the advertising was not misleading, and the state had a substantial interest in reducing the demand for casino gambling by its residents. Further, with regard to part 3 of the *Central Hudson* test, which requires a determination that the advertising ban directly advances the state's interest, the Court found that the legislature's belief that advertising for casino gambling would increase demand was "reasonable" and that such a ban therefore would directly advance the state's interest. The Court also concluded that the ban was no more extensive than necessary to serve the government's interest, and so it also satisfied part 4 of the *Central Hudson* test.

But Justice Rehnquist's majority opinion went further. It argued that the government could ban advertising for any activity that it could prohibit: "It would . . . be a strange constitutional doctrine which would concede to the legislature the authority to totally ban a product or activity, but deny to the legislature the authority to forbid the stimulation of demand for the product or activity through advertising." The Court gave as examples cigarettes, alcoholic beverages, and prostitution. The Court did not seem to require any evidence that the ban on casino advertising would actually have a positive effect. It was willing to defer to the opinion of the legislature without any further evidence, a very low level of review. If this rule were to prevail, governments would have a great deal of latitude to regulate commercial speech because states have wide authority to ban the sale of products and services.

It now appears that the *Posadas* case was an aberration in the Court's commercial speech jurisprudence. After that decision the Court continued to find various bans on commercial speech unconstitutional. In *Rubin v Coors Brewing Company*, the Court struck down a federal law that prohibited beer labels from displaying the alcohol content of the beer. The government contended that such a ban would curb "strength wars" in which brewers would compete for customers on the basis of alcohol content. The Court accepted the government's legitimate interest in trying to prevent excessive consumption of alcohol, but it was not convinced that this approach would directly advance that interest or was no more extensive than necessary. It said that the burden of showing that the regulation furthers the governmental interest in a direct and material way is "not satisfied by mere speculation and conjecture; rather the government body seeking to sustain a restriction on commercial speech must demonstrate that the harms it recites are real and that its restriction will in fact alleviate them to a material degree." The Court rejected the government's concern about strength wars as being based on anecdotal guesses and tidbits. It also rejected the government's argument that the very fact that a brewer brought this type of litigation is proof that advertising increases consumption. The Court said, "Brewers may have many different reasons—only one of which might be a desire to wage a strength war—why they wish to disclose the potency of their beverages." Finally the Court found that there were other, more direct ways to prevent strength wars among brewers, such as the direct regulation of alcohol content in beer, that were "less intrusive" on the manufacturers' First Amendment rights. It is worth noting that in this case the government asked the Court to find that legislatures have broader latitude to regulate speech that promotes "socially harmful activities," and the Court refused to do so.

THE COURT'S 1996 DECISION

The Court's most recent case on commercial speech, *44 Liquormart v Rhode Island*, decided in May 1996, contains a sweeping review of its commercial speech cases and appears to strengthen First Amendment protection for commercial speech. The case concerned the constitutionality of Rhode Island statutes that prohibited publication of the price of any alcoholic beverage in any medium. In previous cases, the Rhode Island Supreme Court upheld the constitutionality of the statute because it served the substantial state interest in "the promotion of temperance." Later, 44 Liquormart, a retail store, placed an advertisement in a newspaper that identified various brands of packaged liquor with the word "WOW" next to pictures of vodka and rum bottles. Concluding that this was a reference to bargain prices, the Rhode Island Liquor Control Administrator assessed a $400 fine.

After paying the fine, the petitioners filed an action in federal district court to have the statutes declared unconstitutional. The judge found that there was a lack of unanimity among researchers regarding the impact of advertising on the consumption of alcoholic beverages. Rhode Island was in the upper 30% of states in the per capita consumption of alcoholic beverages, and alcohol consumption was lower in other states that permitted price advertising. The evidence showed that Rhode Island's ban on liquor price advertising has "no significant impact" on alcohol consumption. Thus, the court ruled that the liquor price ban was unconstitutional because it did not directly advance the state's interest in reducing consumption and was more extensive than necessary.

The case was ultimately appealed to the Supreme Court, which unanimously ruled that the statutes were unconstitutional. While all the justices agreed with the conclusion, not all agreed on the reasons for it. The principal opinion of four justices concluded that the Court developed the commercial speech doctrine to enable states to protect consumers from misleading, deceptive, or aggressive sales practices. In effect, commercial speech is subject to regulation to protect the "fair bargaining process." Thus, it is the state's interest in protecting consumers from "commercial harms" (such as those that would result from false advertising) that justifies regulating commercial speech more than noncommercial speech. But, the opinion said, when the state's purpose for regulating commercial speech has a different goal, the speech involved deserves more First Amendment protection. Restrictions on commercial speech that do not protect consumers from commercial harm often tend to "obscure an 'underlying governmental policy' that could be implemented without regulating speech." The opinion warned, "The First Amendment directs us to be especially skeptical of regulations that seek to keep people in the dark for what the government perceives to be their own good."

The principal opinion found that the Rhode Island price advertising ban "serves an end unrelated to consumer protection." As a result, the ban must be reviewed with "special care." The state must show not only that the ban will advance its interest but that it will do so to a "material degree": that it will "significantly reduce alcohol consumption." The principal opinion then said that the Court can agree with the commonsense notion that lack of advertising would lead to higher prices than would exist if price competition were allowed, and that higher prices might lead to somewhat lower consumption. But in the absence of evidentiary support, the Court cannot find that the advertising ban will "significantly advance" the state's interest in promoting temperance. While the record showed that higher prices might have some effect on the purchasing patterns of temperate drinkers, it did not show that they would "significantly reduce" marketwide consumption or have any effect on abusive drinkers. The liquor stores that brought the suit argued that they would increase their sales by $100 000 per year if they could advertise. The principal opinion interpreted this to mean that the stores would increase their market share by attracting existing alcohol consumers, not by increasing the total number of consumers. The state was not able to identify what price level would lead to a significant reduction in alcohol consumption or how much prices would decline in the absence of a ban. Thus, the Court stated that Rhode Island cannot conclude that advertising leads to increased consumption without engaging in "speculation or conjecture. . . . Such speculation certainly does not suffice when the State takes aim at accurate commercial information for paternalistic ends." Furthermore, the opinion found the restriction on speech to be more extensive than necessary to achieve the state's goal. Accordingly, if the state wished to keep the prices of alcoholic beverages high, it could do so in ways that do not affect speech at all, such as using increased taxation or direct price regulation.

The state, citing *Posadas*, argued that since it could ban the sale of all alcoholic beverages, it could regulate the promotion of the product. The principal opinion conceded that *Posadas* does support the state's argument. However, the opinion found that the *Posadas* case "erroneously performed" the First Amendment analysis and was inconsistent with the rest of the body of law the Court has developed in the commercial speech area. Instead, the opinion said, "in keeping with our prior holdings, we conclude that a state legislature does not have broad discretion to suppress truthful, nonmisleading information for paternalistic purposes that the *Posadas* majority was willing to tolerate." The opinion also explicitly rejected the notion that if a government has the authority to ban an activity it must also have the authority to ban advertising about that activity. The First Amendment forbids government regulation of speech, not conduct. As the opinion put it, "The text of the constitution presumes that attempts to regulate speech are more dangerous than attempts to regulate conduct. . . . As a result the First amendment directs that government may not suppress speech as easily as it may suppress conduct."

The opinion also rejected the state's argument that commercial speech related to "vice" activities should be subject to greater state regulation. Once the state permits products such as alcoholic beverages, lottery tickets, or playing cards to be lawfully purchased, the First Amendment protects speech associated with these items as much as with any other items.

Justice Thomas, who wrote the majority opinion in the 1995 *Coors* case, wrote a concurring opinion even more strongly protecting commercial speech.

He rejected the *Central Hudson* analysis because the principal opinion would seem to uphold the ban on alcohol advertising if it could be proven to be effective. Justice Thomas argued that a state may not further its legitimate interests by "keeping would-be recipients in the dark." He also argued that advertising bans would virtually always fail the fourth prong of the *Central Hudson* test because directly banning, taxing, controlling the price, or otherwise restricting the sale of a product would always be as effective as restricting advertising. This very conservative justice adopted the view of liberal Justice Harry Blackmun in his concurring opinion in *Central Hudson* "that all attempts to dissuade legal choices by citizens by keeping them ignorant are impermissible." Justice Thomas' views on this matter are important because he appears to be the "swing vote" on commercial speech cases.

Four concurring justices took a more limited approach to the issue. They simply noted that the Rhode Island restrictions fail the *Central Hudson* test because the state failed to demonstrate a "reasonable fit" between its ban on alcoholic beverage advertising and its temperance goal. But even these justices said that courts must not accept a state's proffered justification for regulating speech at face value but rather must "examine carefully" or "more searchingly" the state's justification. They made clear that a "closer look" than that taken in *Posadas* is required.

TOBACCO ADVERTISING AND THE FIRST AMENDMENT

The justices' different approaches make it difficult to ascertain definitively the constitutional limits on governmental authority to regulate commercial speech. However, it appears that the commercial speech doctrine is evolving in the direction of affording such speech increased protection. How would the Court view the regulation of tobacco promotion as proposed by the FDA?

The FDA proposal is a combination of bans and restrictions. The distribution of clothing and other paraphernalia with tobacco indicia is entirely banned. Outdoor advertising within 1000 feet of locations frequented by children is banned, but outdoor advertising in other locations is permitted. Advertising in certain publications is limited to black and white text and is therefore regulated but not banned.

In the recent Supreme Court cases, the government has attempted to ban information such as the price of alcoholic beverages or the alcoholic content of the product. These are objective facts that consumers might wish to use in making purchasing choices. Tobacco promotion, however, tends to be more emotive than factual. Joe Camel, people running on the beach, or a hat with the name of a chewing tobacco on it does not provide *information*. Therefore it could be argued that these restrictions do not deprive consumers of information needed to make an informed purchasing choice, a major purpose underlying the protection of commercial speech. The Court, however, has not addressed the relevance of this distinction in the past and has protected advertising that simply lets the consumer know of the existence of a particular product, such as contraceptives.

It is also noteworthy that the Court has been particularly hostile to bans apparently because consumers would not have ready access to the information in question. For example, if alcoholic beverage prices cannot be advertised, the consumer has no easy way to obtain that information. Even with the FDA restrictions, however, tobacco companies will have ample opportunity to make the general public aware of their products.

Further, the FDA's proposal is directed at advertising that might affect children. In all states it is unlawful to sell tobacco products to children, and if it can be shown that the restricted advertising and promotions are directed at children, the restricted speech would be directed at products that are *unlawful* for the target audience to purchase. The First Amendment protects commercial speech only for products that may be lawfully purchased.

There is no doubt that the government can restrict advertisements for tobacco products that are intended for an exclusively child audience. Thus, the government can outlaw such advertisements in the *Weekly Reader*. The issue is whether the proposed regulations are crafted narrowly enough so that the child audience is protected without any undue infringement on the adult audience. Some attempt was made to define the type of publication that the FDA considers to be read by children. However, the agency prohibits the use of other indicia of tobacco products in *all* athletic, artistic, and cultural events, and in many instances this may have virtually no impact on children's use of tobacco. It is unlikely, for example, that substantial numbers of children attend the opera in the evening. Moreover, under these regulations, shirts, hats, and similar promotional items may not be sold or given to adults, not just children. Similarly, the black and white text requirement applies to publications that have adults as the vast majority of readers.

In the past the Court has recognized that states have considerably more authority to protect children than they do adults from what they consider to be offensive material. For example, in *Ginsburg v New York* the Court found that states could adopt different definitions of obscenity for minors and adults. They could also outlaw the sale of material to children under 16 years of age that they could not outlaw for sale to adults without violating the First Amendment. However, the Court did not permit states to outlaw adults' access to such material in order to protect minors. In perhaps a more apt case, the federal government outlawed the mailing of unsolicited advertisements for contraceptives. One argument the government made to support this law was that it would aid parents who desired to keep their children from seeing such mailings. In striking down this statute in *Bolger v Youngs Drug Products Corp*, the Court said,

> This marginal degree of protection is achieved by purging all mailboxes of un-
> solicited material that is entirely suitable for adults. We have previously made clear
> that a restriction of this scope is more extensive than the Constitution permits, for
> the government may not 'reduce the adult population . . . to reading only what is
> fit for children'. . . . The level of discourse reaching a mailbox simply cannot be
> limited to that which would be suitable for a sandbox.

As a result, the government's ability to protect children by regulating advertising that mostly reaches adults is limited.

The prohibition against outdoor advertising as a means of reducing alcohol
and tobacco use by children has been litigated. The US Court of Appeals for
the Fourth Circuit has upheld the constitutionality of a Baltimore ordinance
that bans, with certain limited exceptions, outdoor advertising for alcoholic
beverages. The same court also upheld a similar ordinance restricting outdoor
tobaco advertising. In upholding these restrictions, the court applied the *Central Hudson* standards. There is no doubt that the state has a substantial interest in reducing the use of alcohol and tobacco by minors. The dispute centered on the means with which to achieve the clearly desirable ends. This
court was satisfied that there is a "logical nexus" between the means and the
ends chosen by the government to address the problem, and that the proper
standard for approval of legislative action is the "reasonableness of the legislature's belief that the means it selected will advance its ends." This, however,
is a much lower standard of review than that recently applied by the Supreme
Court. Indeed, both of these cases were appealed to the Supreme Court, which
vacated and remanded them back to the appeals court for further consideration in light of the *44 Liquormart* case.

On remand, the Fourth Circuit again upheld Baltimore's restrictions on outside advertising for alcoholic beverages. This court, in a two to one decision,
upheld the ordinance for three reasons: it was targeted at restricting ads directed
at persons under 18 who could not legally buy alcoholic beverages; the state
has more power to protect children than adults; and the ordinance was not an
outright ban but, in the court's opinion, merely restricted the time, place, and
manner of such restrictions. Based on this conclusion, the court also upheld
Baltimore's ordinance restricting tobacco advertising. The dissenting judge argued that the *Liquormart* case required a further remand to the trial court for
findings of fact to determine if the restrictions on speech would actually further
the goal of reducing teenage drinking and whether it would do so to a material
degree. It is likely that these cases will return to the Supreme Court.

The standard of review that the principal opinion adopted in *44 Liquormart*
presents a serious challenge to the proposed regulations on tobacco advertising
and promotion. These regulations are designed to further a governmental policy
rather than to protect consumers from commercial harm. This is the regulatory
category the principal opinion said should be subject to heightened scrutiny. It

is clear from the principal opinion that the Court will no longer assume that there is a connection between advertising and consumption or passively accept the governmental judgment on the matter. In *44 Liquormart*, the Court required evidence that the ban on liquor price advertising would "significantly reduce alcohol consumption," thereby advancing the state's interest to a "material degree." Will the government be able to demonstrate that its proposed regulations will have this sort of impact on underage smoking?

There is considerable evidence that tobacco advertising has an effect on the brand of tobacco that children use. However, the evidence that advertising has a significant impact on smoking initiation is much more equivocal. Even studies that show that there are some effects where tobacco advertising is *totally banned* demonstrate that those effects are relatively small. For the FDA's proposed restrictions to be found constitutional, the FDA will need to demonstrate that restrictions that are not total bans will have a significant effect. For example, it will need to show that restricting billboards within 1000 feet of areas where children congregate but not elsewhere, that prohibiting colorful advertising while permitting black and white advertising, and that prohibiting the indicia of tobacco products on clothing will significantly reduce the use of tobacco by minors. This will be difficult, if not impossible, given the current state of knowledge.

The final hurdle the FDA will need to overcome is to demonstrate that the restriction on speech is no more extensive than necessary to meet its goal. If there are alternative ways to meet the state's goal that would not restrict speech, such restrictions would appear to be more extensive than necessary. The principal opinion in *4 Liquormart* suggested that if the state wished to keep the price of alcoholic beverages high, it should not ban price advertising but rather should increase taxes or directly regulate prices. Tobacco control advocates have already convinced states and the federal government to take action against smoking by minors. Cigarette sales to minors are outlawed, additional taxes have increased prices, educational strategies are used in schools, and anti-tobacco advertising campaigns have been launched. Furthermore, there is some evidence that counteradvertising more effectively reduces rates of smoking than advertising bans. Ironically, the success of such measures is an argument against the need for advertising restrictions as a way of reducing tobacco use by children.

CONCLUSION

The FDA's regulations that affect commercial speech will face a significant constitutional challenge. Whether they will be upheld by the Supreme Court is not clear. The regulations do not totally ban tobacco advertising, which is the type of regulation subject to the Court's strictest scrutiny. It could be argued that they regulate only the "time, place and manner" of tobacco promotion, the type of regulation the Court is more inclined to uphold. On the other hand, the regulations are sweeping, affecting all advertising media, including those that are primarily directed at adults. Furthermore, the effect the regulations will have on children's smoking behavior is far from clear. The trend has been for the Court to be increasingly hostile to governmental restrictions on commercial speech even when the governmental goal is clearly beneficial, such as reducing alcohol consumption.

For those in public health, the protection of commercial speech may be seen as a mixed blessing. The doctrine protects the promotion of alcohol and may well restrict the government's ability to control tobacco advertising. On the other hand, it also protects advertisements for contraceptives, abortion services, and prescription drug prices, all of which were banned by states in the past. The lesson of the constitutional protection of free speech is that one cannot protect speech one approves of and ban speech one dislikes. Those who advocated bans on advertising for contraceptives and abortions felt strongly enough about these issues to convince legislatures and governors to act in their favor. But popular disapproval of speech with a particular content is the reason why there is a First Amendment to protect it. Popular speech needs no protection.

Should the Court strike down the FDA's regulations, there are still many weapons left in the antitobacco arsenal. Certainly the non-speech-related portion of the rule raises no constitutional questions. No constitutional right is invaded by prohibiting vending machine sales, for example. Furthermore, government can act in at least one new way to try to reduce tobacco advertising: it can eliminate tax deductions for the expenses associated with tobacco promotion. It is quite remarkable that the same federal government that is attempting to restrict a particular type of speech indirectly subsidizes that speech by permitting tobacco companies to deduct advertising and promotional expenses from their taxable revenue. There is no doubt that the government could change this rule without raising any substantial constitutional issue. There is no right to a tax deduction. The tobacco industry might argue that such an action would be a deprivation of their rights to equal protection under the law because other industries are permitted to deduct advertising expenses. But such an argument would border on the frivolous. Since there would be no invasion of a fundamental constitutional right, the government would need to demonstrate only that its act was reasonably related to a legitimate goal, a much lower standard than that found in the commercial speech cases. Certainly it would be rational for the government to rescind the indirect subsidization of the promotion of a product that endangers public health as much as cigarettes do. If advertising were made more expensive, there might well be less of it.

If the FDA has jurisdiction over cigarettes, it could also mandate the reduction or elimination of nicotine from this product. This would be a direct means by which it could reduce the negative effects of the drug it wishes to regulate. This move would have a much more direct impact than advertising restrictions, and it also would not raise any constitutional issues.

None of this will come as a surprise to the FDA. The comments accompanying the regulations discuss the First Amendment issue and conclude that the regulations are consistent with the Constitution. The FDA has done a superb job of creating a record to support its position. The Supreme Court will ultimately decide whether that record is good enough to justify the FDA's regulation of commercial speech.

5

INJURY AND VIOLENCE

During the Great Society period, Ralph Nader, William Haddon, Jr., and others argued for transforming injury from a field that viewed injuries as accidents, unpredictable and even inevitable (as "acts of God"), to one that views injuries as exposure-related, predictable, and controllable by communal measures. This transformation focused attention on the field of injury as a communal interest, as one producing savings in lives and prevented injury that benefited the whole community. Again, this shift in focus redefined injury as more than just an individual problem; it was also a community problem. Although specific injuries are a relatively rare occurrence for the individual in a given year (injury is a far more lethal threat when spread over a lifetime), they are common within a community. Most injuries arise from activities that are frequently engaged in by millions of people (like driving an automobile); risks that are, in the short run relatively safe, yet yield overall death and injury tolls that merit public action.

The first selection in this chapter, "Energy Damage and Ten Countermeasure Strategies," is by William Haddon, Jr., a state and federal health official, physician and epidemiologist. (Haddon's term *countermeasure strategy* roughly translates to *preventive strategy.*) Extending the paradigm of communicable disease prevention to chronic disease, Haddon encourages students and practitioners to take a fresh look at just what the range of options might be to prevent a wide range of health problems.

Haddon's typology of injury prevention will strike many as odd. He speaks of humans as *hosts* and hazards as *agents* and of both as they exist in a mediating environment. This shift in orientation is congruent with a shift in contemporary public health and prevention thought, a shift to the notion of *exposure causality.* By stressing the individual as host and by using the idea of *exposure,* which formerly meant infectious expsure to a biological agent, Haddon and others have shifted attention to the field, or environment of risk, that humans together face—risks from exposure to such hazards as the automobile, poorly designed highways, and dangerous work sites containing threats like cotton dust or coal dust. This shift in focus to exposure causality has moved attention away from the exclusive focus on the individual agent and his or her miscalculations or foolishness.

Haddon served as Lyndon Johnson's head of the new National Highway Traffic Safety Administration, one of the first of a whole series of new institutions created during the Great Society to carry public health far beyond the boundaries of the traditional (and conservative) U.S. Public Health Service. Today, injury control is a major component of the field of public health. We have made dramatic progress in cutting the levels of injury, especially on the highways, and even for the category of alcohol-related automobile crashes. For the first time in decades, alcohol-related crashes have fallen below 40% among all crashes, when for decades they remained immovably associated with roughly half of all crashes.

In our second selection, James A. Mercy and his colleagues review the paradigm of injury and suggest extending this model further, to control injuries resulting from violence against persons. Violence is defined as interpersonal violence, "a threatened or actual use of physical force against a person or group that either results or is likely to result in injury or death." They note the high rates of violence committed against young persons. Of primary concern is the high rate of violence associated with homicide in the United States when compared to other nations and the role that firearms play in establishing these rates. Mercy and his colleagues argue that a scientific approach to preventing injuries and death from firearms (as opposed to what he terms the sterile debate over firearm control) will help lower these rates. They suggest that developing "'prosocial' attitudes or beliefs" by the nation's youth will help lower rates of violence in neighborhoods where violence is epidemic, while also seeking to attack the social inequality that may be the fundamental cause of violence. This drive among injury experts is accompanied by a call to lower the role of the criminal sanction as the primary instrument of policy in limiting violence. This focus on controlling violence through controlling the harms associated with handguns and other guns has produced a furious reaction by the National Rifle Association, which is seeking to use its allies in the U.S. Congress to defund that part of the Centers for Disease Control that focuses on handgun violence.

There is little doubt that extending the injury paradigm to interpersonal violence will remain hugely controversial in the years to come, and not the least because it brings public health into collision with perhaps its most potent opponent, the gun lobby.

Regarding limiting the use of the criminal justice system to control violence, Mark Moore in our third selection is skeptical. He welcomes the entry of public health experts into the arena of violence prevention. He notes the usefulness of this new perspective in reshaping our perceptions of how to prevent violence and says that this reshaping is already underway in the notion of "community policing." But he doubts that a public health response can mostly replace the criminal justice sanction. Prevention, he says, is most successful when the causes of a problem are specific and not widespread; however, when they are, this results in an impossibly large landscape on which government must act. The virtue of the criminal justice sanction is that it can be tailored to the actual problem or criminal act of violence itself. Moore's views are especially of interest because, as a national expert on criminal justice, he also chaired a National Academy of Sciences panel in the late 1970s and early 1980s that strongly endorsed implementing a public health perspective for alohol problems and their prevention.

Energy Damage and the Ten Countermeasure Strategies

WILLIAM HADDON, JR.

An important landmark is reached in the evolution of a scientific field when classification of its subject matter is based on the relevant, fundamental processes involved rather than on descriptions of the appearances of the phenomena of interest. In illustration, a fundamental turning point was reached when the debilitation and progressive susceptibility to bruising of shipboard scurvy could for the first time be classified as the process resulting from a deficiency of consumption of something variously present in fruits and vegetables (much later identified as ascorbic acid, vitamin C). In fact, such transition from classifications consisting essentially only of a description of appearances to those based on fundamental processes is basic to scientific progress generally; hence, examples abound from the full gamut of scientific concerns.

Additonal illustrations, among the many, include the classificatory and conceptual transitions that followed recognition:

a. That rocks could be grouped on the basis of the processes involved in their formation—as sedimentary, igneous, metamorphic.
b. That the variations among the Galapagos finches studied by Darwin were the result of differential ecologic processes.
c. That earthquakes were one aspect of tectonic processes.
d. That the epidemic disease of the young which could for decades be described only as 'infantile paralysis' was a rare variant of a commonplace process initiated by infection with one of several similar and previously unknown viruses.
e. That plague was a process in which a specific pathogen, *Pasteurella pestis*, rats, fleas, and people interacted.

From the *Journal of Trauma*, 13 (1973), 321–326. Reprinted by permission of Williams & Wilkins.

EXTRARATIONAL EXPLANATIONS IN THE ABSENCE
OF PROCESS KNOWLEDGE

Before such conceptual and hence classification advance, lacking an understanding of process, and therefore of the possibility of human intervention or
avoidance, phenomena of concern to people have commonly been attributed to
extrarational factors. 'Luck', 'chance', 'accident', 'fate' and similar terms are
the hallmarks of such ignorance, and perhaps of a human necessity for explaining it away. The distinction between the way in which people tend to deal with
the understood as opposed to the merely known-about is illustrated nicely by
the renowned anthropologist Malinowski. He found that Trobriand natives
viewed the hazards outside the reef, which they did not understand, in ways
more supernatural than they viewed those inside the reef, which they did understand. As he wrote, 'It is most significant that in the lagoon fishing, where man
can rely completely upon his knowledge and skill, magic does not exist, while
in the open-sea fishing, full of danger and uncertainty, there is extensive magi-
cal ritual to secure safety and good results'.

DIVINE PUNISHMENT AS AN EXPLANATION IN
THE ABSENCE OF PROCESS UNDERSTANDING

The Book of Job epitomizes another commonplace aspect of human response to
undesirable happenings not yet understood—and therefore not yet cate-
gorized—in process terms. The events are explained as divine retribution for
shortcomings. The suffering of oneself, someone else, or some group occurs
because it is divine and well-deserved punishment. Therefore, unless the sin can
be expiated by appropriate change in behavior, it may be 'too bad', but there is
nothing else to be done to ameliorate the personally or societally undesirable
happening unless it is an increase in efforts at human reform.

EXPANDED CLASSIFICATORY SETS AND DIFFERENT SETS

The transition to understanding of underlying, relevant processes commonly
results in more than just a relabeling of past groupings. Usually the phenomena
previously recognized have been 'the tip of the iceberg', and the recognition of
underlying process adds much more. Thus, in the case of what was originally
termed 'infantile paralysis', it was found that the infectious process routinely
involved hundreds of individuals subclinically for each person ill enough to be
diagnosed. Moreover, parallel illustrations are legion, not only from medicine
but also widely from other sciences.

For example, understanding the actual nature of earthquakes is to classify them conceptually as one aspect of a far broader range of tectonic processes; and understanding the origins of a butterfly or a clam is to identify it in terms of its life cycle, a process classification. Understanding the process involved in eclipses is to classify them as one aspect of celestial mechanics.

Another frequent result of transition to process-based understanding is re-grouping of phenomena not merely in expanded sets, but in new sets that do not bear a one-to-one correlation with the old. As process (or, to use a related [medical] term, etiologic) understanding advanced, the set of phenomena for-merly referred to as 'wasting' was in effect, parcelled out to such process-defined sets as tuberculosis, amebiasis, protein deficiency, and a host of others.

More relevant here is to view the process in reverse; that is, from the stand-point of the etiologic or process sets in picking up pieces of many pre-existing descriptive sets.

Thus syphilis, the etiologic set based on the infectious agent, *Treponema pallidum*, picked up parts of previous descriptive sets, such as paresis, gummas, penile lesions, rashes, certain gastric lesions, certain abnormalities of the growing ends of bone, and many others, but not all of those in any one of the earlier descriptive sets. Again, an important point is that there is usu-ally not in such transitions, a one-to-one relationship between the earlier, de-scriptive ways of looking at the phenomena and those process-based which are substituted for them.

The foregoing is brief background for that which follows, an introduction to the classification of certain widespread, important phenomena defined and grouped in terms of a small number of closely parallel processes. Most of the included phenomena are not yet regarded in process terms by the implicit and explicit classifications still applied to them by most professionals and laymen. Yet there is widespread, implicit, and at least qualitative recognition of the processes themselves, because cultures, past and present, abound in actions di-rected at changing the outcome of these processes through interventions at spe-cific points in their sequences.

ENERGY DAMAGE PROCESSES

The phenomena of concern are those involved when energy is transferred in such ways and amounts, and at such rates, that inanimate or animate structures are damaged. The harmful interactions with people and property of hurricanes, earthquakes, projectiles, moving vehicles, ionizing radiation, lightening, confla-grations, and the cuts and bruises of daily life illustrate this class.

TEN STRATEGIES FOR REDUCING THESE LOSSES

Several strategies, in one mix or another, are available for reducing the human and economic losses that make this class of phenomena of social concern. In their logical sequence, they are as follows:

The *first* strategy is to prevent the marshalling of the form of energy in the first place; preventing the generation of thermal, kinetic, or electrical energy, or ionizing radiation; the manufacture of gunpowder; the concentration of U-235; the build-up of hurricanes, tornadoes, or tectonic stresses; the accumulation of snow where avalanches are possible; the elevating of skiers; the raising of babies above the floor, as to cribs and chairs from which they may fall; the starting and movement of vehicles; and so on, in the richness and variety of ecologic circumstances.

The *second* strategy is to reduce the amount of energy marshalled: reducing the amounts and concentrations of high school chemistry reagents, the size of bombs or firecrackers, the height of divers above swimming pools, or the speed of vehicles.

The *third* strategy is to prevent the release of the energy: preventing the discharge of nuclear devices, armed crossbows, gunpowder, or electricity; the descent of skiers; the fall of elevators; the jumping of would-be suicides; the undermining of cliffs; or the escape of tigers. An Old Testament writer illustrated this strategy in the context both of the architecture of his area and of the moral imperatives of this entire field: 'When you build a new house, you shall make a parapet for your roof, that you may not bring the guilt of blood upon your house, if any one fall from it'. This biblical position, incidentally, is fundamentally at variance with that of those who, by conditioned reflex, regard harmful interactions between man and his environment as problems requiring reforming imperfect man rather than suitably modifying his environment.

The *fourth* strategy is to modify the rate of spatial distribution of release of the energy from its source: slowing the burning rate of explosives, reducing the slopes of ski trails for beginners, and choosing the re-entry speed and trajectory of space capsules. The third strategy is the limiting case of such release reduction, but is identified separately because in the real world it commonly involves substantially different circumstances and tactics.

The *fifth* strategy is to separate, in space or time, the energy being released from the susceptible structure, whether living or inanimate: the evacuation of the Bikini islanders and test personnel, the use of sidewalks and the phasing of pedestrian and vehicular traffic, the elimination of vehicles and their pathways from community areas commonly used by children and adults, the use of lightning rods, and the placing of electric power lines out of reach. This strategy, in a sense also concerned with rate-of-release modification, has as its hallmark the elimination of intersections of energy and susceptible structure—a common and important approach.

The very important *sixth* strategy uses not separation in time and space but separation by interposition of a material 'barrier': the use of electrical and thermal insulation, shoes, safety glasses, shin guards, helmets, shields, armor plate, torpedo nets, antballistic missiles, lead aprons, buzz-saw guards, and boxing gloves. Note that some 'barriers', such as crash padding and ionizing radiation shields, attenuate or lessen but do not totally block the energy from reaching the structure to be protected. This strategy, although also a variety of rate-of-release modification, is also separately identified because the tactics involved comprise a large, and usually clearly discrete, category.

The *seventh* strategy, into which the sixth blends, is also very important—to modify appropriately the contact surface, subsurface, or basic structure, as in eliminating, rounding, and softening corners, edges, and points with which people can, and therefore sooner or later do, come in contact. This strategy is widely overlooked in architecture, with many minor and serious injuries the result. It is, however, increasingly reflected in automobile design, and in such everyday measures as making lollipop sticks of cardboard and making some toys less harmful for children in impact. Despite the still only spotty application of such principles, the two basic requisites, large radius of curvature and softness, have been known since at least about 400 BC, when the author of the treatise on head injury attributed to Hippocrates wrote: 'Of those who are wounded in the parts about the bone, or in the bone itself, by a fall, he who falls from a very high place upon a very hard and blunt object is in most danger of sustaining a fracture and contusion of the bone, and of having it depressed from its natural position; whereas he that falls upon more level ground, and upon a softer object, is likely to suffer less injury in the bone, or it may not be injured at all . . . '.

The *eighth* strategy in reducing losses in people and property is to strengthen the structure, living or nonliving, that might otherwise be damaged by the entry transfer. Common tactics, often expensively underapplied, include tougher codes for earthquake, fire, and hurricane resistance, and for ship and motor vehicle impact resistance. The training of athletes and soldiers has a similar purpose, among others, as does the treatment of hemophiliacs to reduce the results of subsequent mechanical insults. A successful therapeutic approach to reduce the osteoporosis of many postmenopausal women would also illustrate this strategy, as would a drug to increase resistance to ionizing radiation in civilian or military experience. (Vaccines, such as those for polio, yellow fever, and smallpox, arc analogous strategies in the closely parallel set to reduce losses from infectious agents.)

The *ninth* strategy in loss reduction applies to the damage not prevented by measures under the eight preceding—to move rapidly in detection and evaluation of damage that has occurred or is occurring, and to counter its continuation and extension. The generation of a signal that response is required; the signal's transfer, receipt, and evaluation; the decision and follow-through, are all elements here—whether the issue be an urban fire or wounds on the battlefield or highway. Sprinkler and other suppressor responses, firedoors, MAYDAY and SOS calls, fire alarms, emergency medical care, emergency transport, and related tactics all illustrate this countermeasure strategy. (Such tactics have close parallels in many earlier stages of the sequence discussed here, as, for example, storm and tsunami warnings.)

The *tenth* strategy encompasses all the measures between the emergency period following the damaging energy exchange end the final stabilization of the process after appropriate intermediate and long-term reparative and rehabilitative measures. These may involve return to the pre-event status or stabilization in structurally or functionally altered states.

SEPARATION OF LOSS REDUCTION AND CAUSATION

There are, of course, many real-world variations on the main theme. These include those unique to each particular form of energy and those determined by the geometry and other characteristics of the energy's path and the point or area and characteristics of the structure on which it impinges—whether a BB hits the forehead or the center of the cornea.

One point, however, is of overriding importance: subject to qualifications as noted subsequently, there is no logical reason why the rank order (or priority) of loss-reduction countermeasures generally considered must parallel the sequence, or rank order, of causes contributing to the result of damaged people or property. One can eliminate losses in broken teacups by packaging them properly (the sixth strategy), even though they be placed in motion in the hands of the postal service, vibrated, dropped, piled on, or otherwise abused. Similarly, a vehicle crash, per se, need necessitate no injury, nor a hurricane housing damage.

Failure to understand this point in the context of measures to reduce highway losses underlies the common statement: 'If it's the driver, why talk about the vehicle?' This confuses the rank or sequence of causes, on the one hand, with that of a loss-reduction countermeasure—in this case 'crash packaging'—on the other.

There are, nonetheless, practical limits in physics, biology, and strategy potentials. One final limit is operative at the boundary between the objectives of the eighth and ninth strategies. Once appreciable injury to man or to other living structure occurs, complete elimination of undesirable end results is often impossible, though appreciable reduction is commonly achievable. (This is often also true for inanimate structures, for example, teacups.) When lethal dam-

age has occurred, the subsequent strategies, except as far as the strictly secondary salvage of parts is concerned, have no application.

There is another fundamental constraint. Generally speaking, the larger the
amounts of energy involved in relation to the resistance to damage of the structures at risk, the earlier in the countermeasure sequence must a strategy lie. In
the ultimate case, that of a potential energy release of proportions that could not
be countered to any satisfactory extent by any known means, the prevention of
marshalling or of release, or both, becomes the only approach available. Furthermore, in such an ultimate case, if there is a finite probability of release,
prevention of marshalling (and dismantling of stockpiles of energy already marshalled) becomes the only, and essential, strategy to assure that the undesirable
end result cannot occur.

FOR EACH STRATEGY AN ANALOGOUS OPPOSITE

Although the concern here is the reduction of damage produced by energy
transfer, it is noteworthy that to each strategy there is an opposite focused on
increasing damage. The latter are most commonly seen in collective and individual violence—as in war, homicide, and arson. Various of them are also
seen in manufacturing, mining, machining, hunting, and some medical and
other activities in which structural damage, often of a very specific nature, is
sought. (A medical illustration would be the destruction of the anterior pitu-
itary with a beam of ionizing radiation as a measure to eliminate pathologic
hyperactivity.) For example, a maker of motor vehicles or of aircraft landing-
gear struts—a product predictably subject to energy insults—could make his
product more delicate, both to increase labor and sales of parts and materials,
and to shorten its average useful life by decreasing the age at which commonplace amounts of damage increasingly exceed in cost the depreciating value
of the product in use. The manufacturer might also design for difficulty of
repair by using complex exterior sheet metal surfaces, making components
difficult to get at, and other means. . . .

A SYSTEMIC ANALYSIS OF OPTIONS

It has not generally been customary for individuals and organizations that influence, or are influenced by, damage due to harmful transfers of energy to analyze systematically their options for loss reduction, the mix of strategies and
tactics they might employ, and their cost. Yet it is entirely feasible and not
especially difficult to do so, although specific supporting data are still often
lacking. In fact, unless such systematic analysis is done routinely and well, it is

generally impossible to maximize the pay-offs both of loss-reduction planning and of resource allocations.

Such analysis is also needed to consider properly the problems inherent in the use of given strategies in specific situations. Different strategies to accomplish the same end commonly have different requirements; in kinds and numbers of people, in the disciplines involved, in material resources, in capital investments, and in public and professional education, among others. In the case of some damage-reduction problems, particular strategies may require political and legislative action more than others. And, where the potential or actual hazard exists across national boundaries, correspondingly international action is commonly essential.

The types of concepts outlined in this note are basic to dealing with important aspects of the quality of life, and all of the professions concerned with the environment and with the public health need to understand and apply the principles involved—and not in the haphazard, spotty, and poorly conceptualized fashion now virtually universal. It is the purpose of this brief note to introduce the pathway along which this can be achieved.

Public Health Policy for Preventing Violence

JAMES A. MERCY, MARK L. ROSENBERG, KENNETH E. POWELL, CLAIRE V. BROOME, AND WILLIAM L. ROPER

A new vision for how Americans can work together to prevent the epidemic of violence now raging in our society has emerged from the public health community. This vision arises from the recognition that, by any measure, violence is a major contributor to premature death, disability, and injury. Fundamental to this vision is a shift in the way our society addresses violence, from a focus limited to reacting to violence to a focus on changing the social, behavioral, and environmental factors that cause violence. From a public health perspective, effective policies for preventing violence must be firmly grounded in science and attentive to unique community perceptions and conditions. Scientific research provides information essential to developing such policies and prevention strategies and methods for testing their effectiveness. Equally critical is the full participation of communities to engender a sense of ownership of this problem and its solutions. Public health seeks to empower people and their communities to see violence not as an inevitable consequence of modern life but as a problem that can be understood and changed. . . .

IMPACT OF INTERPERSONAL VIOLENCE ON THE PUBLIC'S HEALTH

Interpersonal violence can be defined as threatened or actual use of physical force against a person or a group that either results or is likely to result in injury or death. Public health approaches violence as a health issue and consequently uses injuries—both fatal and nonfatal, psychological and physical—to quantify the impact of violence.

On an average day in the United States, sixty-five people die from and more than 6,000 people are physically injured by interpersonal violence. The violent acts appear to be occurring with greater frequency and severity in our society.

From *Health Affairs*, 12 (1993), 7–26. Copyright © 1993 The People-to-People Health Foundation, Inc. All rights reserved. Reprinted by permission.

In fact, the 1980s were arguably the most violent decade of this century, if not in U.S. history. More than 215,000 people died and twenty million more suffered nonfatal physical injuries from violence. Violence also exacts a huge economic toll. The average annual financial costs of medical and mental health treatment, emergency response, productivity losses, and administration of health insurance and disability payments for the victims of assaultive injuries occurring from 1987 to 1990 were estimated at $34 billion, with lost quality of life costing another $145 billion. These grim statistics obscure the disproportionate impact of violence on specific subgroups within our society—most notably, young men, women and children, and the poor.

Youth and Violence

Young people are disproportionately represented among the perpetrators of violence. Arrest rates for homicide, rape, robbery, and aggravated assault in the United States peak among older adolescents and young adults. During the 1980s more than 48,000 people were murdered by youths ages twelve to twenty-four. Interviews with assault victims indicate that offenders in this age range committed almost half of the estimated 6.4 million nonfatal crimes of violence in 1991.

Adolescents and young adults also face an extraordinarily high risk of death and injury from violence. Homicide is the second leading cause of death for Americans ages fifteen to thirty-four and is the leading cause of death for young African Americans. Homicide rates among young American men are vastly higher than in other Western industrialized nations (Exhibit 1). In addition, persons ages twelve to twenty-four face the highest risk of nonfatal assault of any age group in our society. The average age of both violent offenders and victims has been growing younger and younger in recent years.

Violence Against Women and Children

Women are frequent targets of physical and sexual assault by partners and acquaintances. Many of these assaults are fatal. In 1990, 5,328 women died as the result of homicide. Six of every ten of these women were murdered by someone they knew, about half of them by a spouse or an intimate acquaintance. In addition, homicide is the leading cause of death for women in the workplace, accounting for 41 percent of all occupational injury deaths among women during the 1980s. More than 99 percent of assaults on women, however, result not in death but rather in physical injury and severe emotional distress. In 1985 an estimated 1.8 million women were physically assaulted by male partners or cohabitants. In addition, it has been estimated that 1,871 women are forcibly raped each day in the United States. The consequences for women include an

EXHIBIT 1 International Variation In Homicide Rates For Males Ages Fifteen To Twenty-Four, 1988–1991.

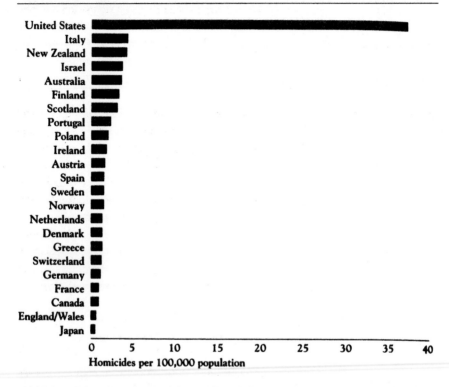

Sources: National Center for Health Statistics, *Vital Statistics,* 1990; and World Health Organization Statistics Annuals, 1990 and 1991.

increased risk of attempted suicide, abusing alcohol and other drugs, depression, and abusing their own children.

Children also are all too frequently the targets of abuse in our society. In 1988 an estimated 1,016 to 2,026 children died from abuse and neglect in the United States. In 1986 a minimum of 1.6 million children experienced some form of nonfatal abuse or neglect. The long-term consequences for abused children include an increased likelihood of depression, poor self-esteem, alcohol and substance abuse, self-destructive behavior, and aggression. These patterns often persist through adolescence and into adulthood. Some, but not all, adults who were abused as children are more likely than other adults to abuse their children and intimate partners and to be arrested for violent crime.

The Impact of Violence on the Poor

The evidence is consistent and compelling that poor people bear a disproportionate share of the public health burden of violence in our society. Homicide victimization rates consistently have been found to be highest in those parts of cities where poverty is most prevalent. In 1991 the risk of becoming a victim of a nonfatal violent assault in the United States was three times greater for persons from families with incomes below $7,500 than for those with family incomes above $50,000.

The Contribution of Firearms

Firearms play a central role in interpersonal violence. In 1990 alone, firearms were used to commit more than 16,000 homicides; an additional 239,400 persons were nonfatally injured duing assaults with firearms. Further, firearms were involved in more than 18,000 suicides, approximately 1,500 unintentional deaths, and an undetermined number of suicide attempts and nonfatal accidents. The lifetime cost of all firearm-related injuries occurring in 1990 was estimated to be $20.4 billion. Firearm-related death rates for women, teenage boys, and young adults are higher now than they ever have been. For young people ages ten to thirty-four, firearms are the second leading cause of death, and one out of five deaths to U.S. teens is due to firearms. In fact, in 1990 more U.S. teenagers died from firearm-related injuries than from all natural diseases combined.

PUBLIC HEALTH CONTRIBUTIONS TO VIOLENCE PREVENTION

Despite the magnitude of this problem, daily reminders in the media, and the imprisonment of an unprecedented proportion of our population, this American tragedy continues largely unabated. We need new solutions. Public health's contributions include placing prevention at the forefront of our efforts, making science integral to identifying and developing effective policies and programs, and integrating the efforts of diverse scientific disciplines, organizations, and communities. Each of these contributions speaks to an existing deficit in our society's response to this problem.

Focus on Prevention

The public health approach brings a strong emphasis and commitment to identifying policies and programs aimed at preventing violent behavior, injuries, and deaths. America's predominant response to violence has been a reactive one— to pour resources into deterring and incapacitating violent offenders by apprehending, arresting, adjudicating, and incarcerating them through the criminal justice system.

This approach, however, has not made an appreciable difference. Although the average prison time served for a violent crime in the United States tripled between 1975 and 1989, there was no concomitant decrease in the level of violent crimes. Removing violent offenders from society by tripling the average sentence for a violent crime, on the other hand, may have prevented 10 to 15 percent of the violent offenses that would have been committed had these prisoners been on the streets. One can only conclude that other forces must be driving the violent crime rate upward. We can either continue to apply increasingly severe penalties and hope to hold our own, or search for additional preventive methods. Even within the criminal justice community there is a movement toward looking for new approaches through community- or problem-oriented policing.

Underlying the public health approach is the strong conviction that violence can be prevented. The wide variation in the homicide rate among developed nations supports this stance. The rate of homicide among males ages fifteen to twenty-four living in developed nations with accurate vital statistics data was more than eight times higher in the United States than in the next-highest country, Italy (37.2 versus 4.3 homicides per 100,000 population in 1988–1991). Even the rate for young white males in the United States—a group more comparable with young Italian males—was more than three times the rate in Italy. The relatively high rates of violence in the United States, therefore, are not an inevitable consequence of economic development. The potential for much lower rates of violence than we are now experiencing also is evident in our own history. Within the United States the homicide rate has varied more than twofold since 1950, ranging from a high of 10.7 per 100,000 in 1980 to a low of 4.5 in 1956.

Perhaps most importantly, although most violence prevention efforts have not been adequately evaluated, at least a few show promise of being successful. Regular visits to the homes of unmarried, poor, teenage mothers by health practitioners have been shown to reduce the incidence of child abuse in a controlled random trial. Providing training in communication, negotiation, and problem solving to middle school youth with behavioral problems has reduced the number of suspensions attributed to violence. The Perry Preschool Project, an educational program directed at the intellectual and social development of preschool children, has been credited with reducing the cost of delinquency and crime, including violence, by approximately $2,400 per child. Laws that prohibit carrying guns in public and that impose a mandatory sentence for crimes perpetrated with a firearm have been found to have small but positive effects on reducing firearm homicides. After passage of the 1977 Washington, D.C., restrictive licensing law that prohibited handgun ownership by everyone but police officers, security guards, and previous gun owners, firearm suicides and homicides declined by 25 percent. Homicide rates remain high and have increased in Washington, D.C., however, indicating that other actions besides restricting handgun ownership are necessary. Thus, despite the fact that we have a great deal more to learn about how to prevent violence, epidemiologic patterns and preliminary evaluation research clearly indicate that it can be prevented.

There exists a broad array of potentially effective intervention strategies through which violence might be prevented. Exhibit 2 presents a listing of examples of these interventions grouped by whether their primary goal is to change knowledge, skills, or attitudes; the social environment; or the physical environment. The efficacy of most of these interventions has not been demonstrated. Nevertheless, they are among the many options to be considered as part of a broad-based, sustained strategy to prevent violence. Among these options, strong emphasis must be placed on addressing the role of social and economic

EXHIBIT 2 Strategies For Preventing Violence And Its Consequences.

STRATEGY TYPE	DESCRIPTION	INTERVENTION EXAMPLES
Change individual knowledge, skills, or attitudes	Deliver information to individuals to Develop prosocial attitudes and beliefs Increase knowledge Impart social, marketable, or professional skills Deter criminal actions	Conflict resolution education Social skills training Job skills training Public information and education campaigns Training of health care professionals in identification and referral of family violence victims Parenting education Mandatory sentences for crimes with guns
Change social environment	Alter the way people interact by improving their social or economic circumstances	Adult mentoring of youth Job creation programs Respite day care Battered women's shelters Economic incentives for family stability Antidiscrimination laws enforced Deconcentrated lower-income housing
Change physical environment	Modify the design, use, or availability of Dangerous commodities Structures or space we move through	Restrictive licensing of handguns Prohibition or control of alcohol sales at events Increased visibility of high-risk areas Disruption of illegal gun markets Metal detectors in schools

deprivation in causing violence. Recent research points to numerous dimensions of poverty that are related to high community rates of violence: high concentrations of poverty, transiency of the population, family disruption, crowded housing, weak local social structure (for example, low organizational participation in comunity life, weak intergenerational ties in families and communities, and low density of friends and acquaintances), and the presence of dangerous commodities or opportunities associated with violence (for example, gun availability and drug distribution networks). If we are to be successful in preventing violence, these fundamental social and economic factors must be addressed.

Public Health Science in Action

Although many scientific disciplines have advanced our understanding of violence, the scientific basis for developing effective prevention policies and programs remains rudimentary. Public health brings something that has been missing from this field: a multidisciplinary scientific approach that is explicitly directed toward identifying effective approaches to prevention.

This approach starts with defining the problem and progresses to identifying associated risk factors and causes, developing and evaluating interventions, and implementing interventions in programs (Exhibit 3). Although the exhibit suggests a linear progression from the first step to the last, in reality many of these steps are likely to occur simultaneously. Information systems used to define the problem also may be useful in evaluating programs. Similarly, information gained in program evaluation and implementation may lead to new and promising interventions.

The first step, defining the problem, includes delineating related mortality and morbidity and goes beyond simply counting cases. This step include obtaining information on the demographic characteristics of the person involved, the temporal and geographic characteristics of the incident, the victim/perpetrator relationship, and the severity and cost of the injury. These additional variables may be important in defining discrete subsets of injuries for which different interventions may be appropriate. For example, prevention of violence between intimate acquaintances is likely to require a different approach than prevention of violence among strangers.

The second step in the public health approach involves identifying risk factors for and causes of injuries. Whereas the first step looks at "who, when, where, what, and how," the second step looks at "why." This step also may be used to define populations at high risk for injury and to suggest specific interventions. Risk factors can be identified by a variety of epidemiologic studies, including rate calculations, cohort studies, and case-control studies.

The next step is to develop interventions based in large part upon information obtained from the previous steps and to test these interventions. Methods for

EXHIBIT 3 Public Health Model Of A Scientific Approach To Prevention.

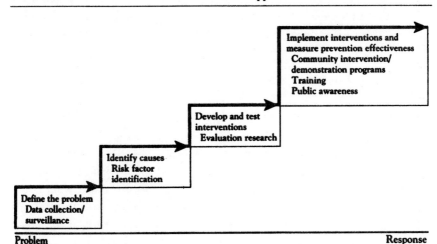

testing include prospective randomized controlled trials, controlled comparisons of populations for occurrence of health outcomes, time series analyses of trends in multiple areas, and observational studies such as case-control studies.

The final stage is to implement interventions that have been proved or are highly likely to be effective. In both instances it is important that data be collected to evaluate the program's effectiveness, particularly since an intervention that has been found effective in a clinical trial or an academic study may perform differently at the community or state level. Another important component is determining the cost-effectiveness of such programs. Balancing the costs of a program against the cases prevented by the intervention can be helpful to policymakers in determining optimal public health practices.

The public health model for a scientific approach to prevention has been applied to a wide range of noninfectious as well as infectious public health problems, with a remarkable record of success. Smallpox has been eradicated, smoking rates have been drastically reduced, and the number of people who die in car crashes has been reduced by tens of thousands. We believe that this time-tested, goal-oriented approach will yield similar benefits in the area of violence prevention. . . .

PRIORITIES FOR PUBLIC HEALTH ANALYSIS AND ACTION

Public health priorities for violence prevention include preventing injuries from firearms, interrupting the "cycle of violence," developing and evaluating community approaches to violence prevention, and changing public attitudes and beliefs toward violence. It is believed that attention to these areas offers the greatest chance of saving lives, preventing injuries, and reducing the overall impact of violence on our society.

Preventing Firearm Injuries

Public health has come to see the need for preventing firearm injuries as central to preventing violence, for several reasons. First, firearms are involved in a high proportion of deaths associated with interpersonal violence. In 1990, 65 percent of the more than 24,000 homicides that occurred involved firearms. Further, firearms are involved in approximately 20,000 deaths associated with suicide and unintentional injury each year. Second, studies indicate that firearms have played a key role in the increasing rates of violent death, particularly among youth. For example, recent increases in youth homicide and suicide are almost entirely attributable to increases in homicides and suicides involving firearms. Third, scientific evidence clearly indicates that the presence of a gun in a violent interaction dramatically increases the likelihood that one or more of the participants will be killed; the implication here is that guns are more lethal than other weapons. Fourth, scientific evidence is mounting that access to firearms poses significant risks to owners and their families. For example, in a well-designed study that controlled for other known risk factors, the presence of a gun in a household was found to increase the risk of suicide almost fivefold and the risk of homicide almost threefold. Finally, as previously noted, evaluation research suggests that certain regulatory approaches can prevent deaths involving firearms.

Public health's major contribution in this area has been to advance the scientific understanding of ways in which firearm injuries can be prevented. In fact, public health scientists have been credited with bringing about a "sea-change" in firearm injury research over the past ten years. This scientific approach has spanned the first three stages of the public health model outlined in Exhibit 3. To define the problem, public health scientists have used existing surveillance data to assess the magnitude, characteristics, and impact of the problem on a national, state, and local basis. They are exploring ways to improve the national surveillance of fatal and nonfatal firearm injuries and the monitoring of risky behavior associated with firearm injuries, such as weapon carrying among youth. State and local public health agencies also are developing city and statewide systems for collecting data on firearm injuries. Public health scientists have helped to identify risk factors by quantifying the risks of gun ownership, looking not only at the risks from guns in the hands of criminals, but also at the risks to gun owners and their families. This research has shown, for example, that for every time a gun kept in the home is used to kill someone in self-defense, it is used forty-three times to kill someone in a criminal homicide, suicide, or unintentional shooting; and if a gun is used in an incident of domestic violence, then the likelihood of one of the two disputants' being murdered is twelve times greater than if another type of weapon were used.

Public health scientists also have been involved in carrying out the third stage of the public health model: testing the effectiveness of interventions. For example, a Detroit ordinance prohibiting the carrying of firearms in public was evaluated and found to have a dampening effect on increases in firearm homicides occurring outside the home. In another example, researchers examining the impact of more restrictive policies toward handgun ownership in Canada found that between 1980 and 1986 the rate of homicide in Seattle, Washington, was 65 percent higher than in Vancouver, British Columbia, and that virtually all of this difference was due to an almost fivefold higher rate of handgun homicide in Seattle. They concluded that a regulatory policy that restricts access to handguns may reduce the rate of homicide in a community.

Although our understanding of the role of firearms in violence has advanced substantially, many questions remain: How frequently are guns used to successfully ward off potentially violent attacks? Do the risks and benefits of firearm possession vary, depending on whether one lives in a rich or poor neighborhood or whether one has children? How do adolescents get guns, and why do they want them? In addition, few interventions to prevent firearm injuries have been evaluated. There is a critical need to assess the value of the numerous intervention strategies that can be, and in some cases are being, adopted. Exhibit 4 lists interventions that focus solely on firearms, grouped by four major prevention strategies.

Addressing firearm-related injuries from a public health perspective helps to reshape the public discussion on firearms in several ways. First, with a firm scientific understanding of the role of firearms in violence, public discussion shifts from a criminal justice debate on "gun control" to a public health discussion of "preventing firearm injuries." The gun-control debate has become so polarized that neither side really seeks to understand the other. As result, there is no middle ground and very little constructive dialogue. By reframing the debate, public health can help to engage many more people in this critically important issue. Second, if scientific information on the health risks of firearms is developed and disseminated, people are empowered to take responsibility and make decisions to reduce the risks for themselves, their families, and their communities.

A third element in reframing the issue of firearm injuries is shifting the focus from an "all-or-none" solution to a broad array of diverse strategies and policies. The remarkable success of public health in preventing motor vehicle injuries exemplifies this approach. Over the past thirty years the United States has invested more than $250 million to discover ways to create safer cars, safer

EXHIBIT 4 Strategies For Preventing Firearm Injuries.

STRATEGY	INTERVENTION
Change how guns are used/stored	Restriction of gun carrying in public Mandatory sentences for gun use in crimes Owner liability for damage by guns Metal detectors in vulnerable places Safety education
Affect who has guns	Permissive licensing (for example, all but felons, minors, mentally ill, and so on) Waiting periods Forbid sales to high-risk purchasers Disrupt illegal gun markets Combination/electronic locks on guns
Reduce lethality of guns	Protective clothing Reduce barrel length/bore size Reduce magazine size Ban dangerous ammunition
Reduce number of guns	Restrictive licensing (for example, only police, military, guards, and so on) Buy back guns Increase taxes on guns Restrict imports Prohibit ownership

Source: Adapted from A.J. Reiss Jr. and J.A. Roth, eds., *Understanding and Preventing Violence* (Washington: National Academy Press, 1993), 272–273.

roadways, and safer drivers. Because of this effort cars now have steering wheels that protect the driver, front ends that crush to absorb impact, safety belts, and air bags; also, many highway systems have eliminated unsafe intersections. All drivers must pass licensing examinations, and we have made great progress in removing drunken drivers from the roads. As a result, the highway driving death rate has decreased markedly, saving more than 243,000 lives. Firearm injuries can be reduced similarly without banning all guns. As with motor vehicle safety, progress can be made by using a variety of approaches that include changes in behavior and environmental modification. . . .

Changing Public Attitudes and Beliefs

Recent experience with public health information and education campaigns for reducing smoking and cardiovascular disease and preventing acquired immunodeficiency syndrome (AIDS) suggests that similar efforts can be important parts of the public health approach to preventing violence. Within the field of injury control, there has been a long-standing debate over the effectiveness of educational efforts to prevent injuries. Early in the history of injury control, many people felt that injuries could be prevented just by telling people to "be careful." Soon, however, critics showed that it was much more effective to change the environment than it was to try to change individual behavior. As a result, many injury-control advocates felt that behavioral change was an ineffective way to prevent injuries. It is clear now, however, that effective injury-control programs—and preventing injuries from violence is no exception—take advantage of both behavioral changes and changes in the environment. For example, to realize the benefits of child safety seats, parents must purchase them and use them correctly.

Public health has now become much more sophisticated in the use of marketing techniques to bring about change. We know that we need to formulate precise objectives, identify target audiences, carefully develop culturally competent messages, and then measure the impact of these marketing efforts on the outcomes of interest. Public health information campaigns for violence prevention must achieve a number of goals. First, they must make people aware of the magnitude and characteristics of the problem of violence today. Second, they must give hope to individuals and communities, informing them that there are things that work and things that people and communities can do to prevent violence. Third, they must mobilize individuals, organizations, and communities to act. Fourth, they must provide information about what works and how to conduct effective prevention programs. And fifth, they must be designed so that we can measure their effectiveness and use that information to constantly improve them.

Most recent attention to violence and the media has been limited to the negative impact of violence in the movies and on television. This has had at least two adverse results. First, opportunities to develop positive uses of the media through social marketing have not been adequately considered. Second, false expectations have been raised about the potential of reducing violence in life by reducing violence in the media.

Popular movies and television contain high levels of violence, and large organizations such as the American Psychological Association and the American Academy of Pediatrics have publicly stated their conviction that violence in the media causes acts of violence in real life. Research has shown that viewing violence on television or in the movies can make children more aggressive and irritable. Researchers have suggested that children today see so much violence on television that they are desensitized to it and may even be encouraged to commit violent acts because of their viewing. There seems little doubt that violence in the media conributes to violence in society. Violence in the media, however, is but one segment, of uncertain size, of the full scope of influences that produce violence in our society. Efforts to reduce media violence should be part of a larger effort to change the many factors contributing to frequent violent behavior in American society. . . .

Violence Prevention: Criminal Justice or Public Health?

MARK H. MOORE

It is difficult to resist being swept up in the enthusiasm for public health approaches to preventing violence. Current levels of violence certainly demand a
response. The ones we have made in the past, rooted primarily in the philosophy and practices of criminal justice, seem old, tired and stale—even bankrupt.
In contrast, public health approaches seem fresh, optimistic, and full of potential. Most importantly, public health approaches have been extremely successful
in engaging new actors—community groups, private enterprise, medical establishments, and social service agencies—in the effort to reduce violence. So, I
feel both churlish and counterproductive in raising questions about something
that is generally so helpful.

Nonetheless, in the interest of ensuring that society makes the best possible
response to violence over the long run, I want to do precisely that: to raise
some questions about the public health approach to violence. . . .

PUBLIC HEALTH: SUBSTITUTE FOR OR COMPLEMENT
TO CRIMINAL JUSTICE?

Exactly what public health claims in nominating itself to help to solve the
nation's violence problem is a little unclear. Sometimes it seems to claim that it
represents a comprehensive alternative to criminal justice responses to violence.
Thus, James Mercy and colleagues write:

> A new vision for how Americans can work together to prevent the epidemic of
> violence now raging in our society has emerged from the public health commu-
> nity. . . . Fundamental to this vision is a shift in the way our society addresses
> violence, from a focus on reacting to violence after it occurs to a focus on changing
> the social, behavioral, and environmental factors that cause violence.

From *Health Affairs*, 12 (1993), 34–46. Copyright © 1993 The People-to-People Foundation,
Inc. All rights reserved. Reprinted by persmission.

This is perhaps the grandest claim and does seem to suggest that the public health approach could replace, or at least subsume, the criminal justice approach to reducing violence. At other times the claims are more modest. They seem to suggest a world in which public health attempts to prevent violence stand alongside criminal justice attempts to respond to the violence that continues despite the best efforts of the public health community to prevent it. . . .

DIFFERENT KINDS OF VIOLENCE

One important limitation of the current public health approach is that it does not focus on all components of the violence problem. For example, Mercy and colleagues begin with a broad definition of "interpersonal violence" and present startling statistics about the total number of people touched by violence each year in the United States. They then move to a more detailed analysis of some particular forms of violence—that involving youth (both as offenders and as victims), and that inflicted on women and children.

The emphasis on these particular kinds of violence is typical of the public health approach. Moreover, it is an important corrective to the traditional focus of the criminal justice system. That system has long neglected the violence occurring in the intimate settings of family and involving either spouses or children. The reasons are that this kind of violence is not always reported to criminal justice agencies and that even if it is reported, the criminal justice response of arrest and prosecution may be neither possible nor desirable to deal with the situation at hand. Thus it has been left to doctors in emergency rooms to reveal the extent of this kind of violence, and to the public health community to develop a wider variety of preventive and crisis responses than are typically imagined by criminal justice agencies. It also has been left to the public health community to increase the priority given to this kind of violence by observing the connection between preventing child abuse and reducing adult criminal violence a generation into the future.

Similarly, although the police certainly will see youth violence, it has been left to the public health community both to establish its importance as the principal threat to the health of young men and to stress preventive rather than control responses. For these reasons, the public health emphasis on these particular forms of violence is helpful.

Yet a person with a criminal justice background cannot help but notice that the focus on youth, women, and children excludes the kind of violence that is in fact most common: the violence that occurs among adult men in robberies, in bars, and in organized criminal enterprises. The simple fact is that the majority of people killed or injured in interpersonal violence in the United States in any given year are adult males—not youth, not women, and not children. These forms of violence attract much of the attention of the criminal justice system; criminal justice responses often seem most appropriate for them.

Thus, in facing the whole problem of violence in society, there is an important complementarity in criminal justice and public health approaches. Each approach sees and emphasizes a somewhat different piece of the violence problem. Either alone would be incomplete.

PREVENTIVE VERSUS REACTIVE APPROACHES

A second claim made by the public health community is that it brings a preventive approach to violence that might replace the reactive approach of the criminal justice system. This is fine rhetoric, useful for mobilizing a crusade. But in important ways it is false.

For one thing, this rhetoric obscures the potential advantages of relying on a reactive rather than a preventive approach. The difficulty with preventive approaches is that precisely because they are preventive, they force one to act on problems and situations that are related only probabilistically to the problem one is really trying to solve. This often means that one has to act in many more places and situations than would be necessary if one were reacting to the essential problem. That poses no difficulty, of course, if the number of places where violence could occur is not all that great, and where the preventive intervention one makes in those places is neither expensive nor intrusive, and is effective in preventing violence in both the short and long runs.

Unfortunately, it is by no means obvious that these conditions always exist. Sometimes the number of people or places where one must intervene to prevent violence increases by several orders of magnitude. Sometimes the need to be in so many places where violence might occur stretches resources so thinly that preventive interventions become too superficial to produce much of a preventive impact at all. . . .

The criminal justice system also has long been interested in intervening early in the lives of those who seem headed for future violence and in doing so through providing assistance and care as well as close control. The juvenile justice system is an old invention of the criminal justice system designed precisely to provide a different, more preventive response to violent acts committed by children and to the conditions in which they live that put them at risk of serious criminal offending in the future. Similarly, for several generations police officers have tried to reduce violence among young males by acting as positive role models, organizing youth athletic leagues, and establishing gang liaison officers.

Somewhat more recently, police departments have adopted some important new tactics designed to prevent crimes through mechanisms other than arrest and prosecution. The idea of "community policing" seeks to use police officers to help communities mobilize their own capacities for self-defense in an attempt to reduce the opportunities and occasions for violence. Similarly, the idea of "problem-solving policing" seeks to identify "hot spots" where violence is particularly likely to occur and to invent responses that make them more peaceable. Typically, the responses do not involve making arrests but instead involve altering the conditions that seem to favor disorder and violence.

Finally, many preventive mechanisms the public health movement imagines relying on to reduce violence may depend on, or be strengthened by, parallel criminal justice efforts. For example, the public health community would like to reduce a particularly important risk factor for violence: children possessing and carrying guns in cities. Achievement of this goal will in all likelihood depend not only on teaching parents to lock up any guns they might have and to keep checking on whether their kids are carrying weapons to school, and not only on regulating licensed gun dealers more closely to ensure that they do not sell guns to children, but also on police efforts to arrest fences who will sell stolen guns to children and gang members whose gun carrying on the streets is forcing other kids to carry guns in self-defense. Similarly, the effort to prevent youthful traffic fatalities associated with drunken driving depended not only on selling the concept of the "designated driver" to youth and on regulating liquor stores more closely, but also on setting up sobriety checkpoints at times and places where drunken driving seemed particularly likely and dangerous. . . . Again, then, the public health approach is seen as an important complement to rather than a substitute for criminal justice approaches to violence. It is not true that one is preventive and the other reactive. They both may be required to produce the desired preventive and control effects.

THE PRACTICAL POTENTIAL OF PUBLIC HEALTH APPROACHES

The ultimate question about the role of public health approaches in dealing with violence is how much of the burden of effective control of violence we can expect them to shoulder. To build confidence in the public health approach, Mercy and colleagues offer several bits of evidence.

First, they point to the fact that the United States has a much higher rate of violence than do other advanced, industrialized nations and that its current level of violence is higher than it has been in the past. These facts are used as "benchmarks" indicating the potential of achieving much lower levels of violence than we now accept. The benchmarks certainly make it plausible that violence can be reduced. But simply observing these facts falls well short of either demonstrating that such levels are now plausible or showing how to produce them. One must make the assumption that the public health approach has the tools to transform the current U.S. culture to that of other countries or to what it once was in this country. That is a fairly large claim.

To make that claim possible, public health advocates produce a second kind of evidence: They point to the success that public health approaches have had in dealing with such problems as smallpox, smoking, and auto accidents. These examples, too, are reassuring and hopeful. But they also fall short of demonstrating that public health methods alone could deal effectively with violence. Indeed, the example of automobile accidents (which is in many ways the closest analogue) might be used to show the potential of public health and criminal justice approaches working together. It may be that the reduction in traffic fatalities owes as much to the criminalization of drunken driving as to safer cars, safer roadways, or increased education about the dangers of drunken driving. . . .

Again, my point is not to deny the essential value of the public health approach. Obviously, there is an enormous difference between programs that reduce violence by saving the lives of both victims and offenders (which the public health approaches tend to do) and programs that reduce violence by saving only the lives of victims (which is how the criminal justice interventions tend to work). My point is simply to tone down the claims of what can be accomplished by public health on its own and to remind people of the continuing need for a criminal justice response. We cannot dismantle the police, prosecutors, and prisons quite yet.

THE INTERNAL COHERENCE OF THE PUBLIC HEALTH APPROACH

What is genuinely exciting about the public health approach (even to a jaded old criminal justice guy like me) is the fact that it does seem to provide a framework for analyzing and acting on the problem that simulates new ideas and, perhaps even more importantly, draws new people into thinking about and acting on the problem of violence. It is significant, I think, that this approach appeals to women and to people of color and gives them a way to participate in the conversation that makes them feel more hopeful, more empowered, and less vulnerable to the suspect machinations of the criminal justice system. It is also wonderful that it attracts people who are trained in the methods of science—who like data, information, and research. And its pragmatic spirit—the resourceful, determined search for anything that will work—is a breath of fresh air into the sterile ideological debates that are strangling the current discussion within criminal justice circles. As a movement, then, the public health initiative is extraordinarily welcome. Still, for all the strengths of the ideas, some important issues will need to be worked out. . . .

THE IDEOLOGICAL BASIS OF BOTH APPROACHES

In the background of the discussion about public health and criminal justice approaches to violence are some important questions about values and ideology that must be acknowledged and discussed openly if practitioners in both fields are to be able to exploit the potential of their diverse approaches. The essential question concerns the role of individual blame and accountability in responding to incidents of "intentional violence."

Obviously, the ideas of individual guilt, blame, and accountability are central to the criminal justice approach to "intentional violence." The moral (as opposed to practical) justification for punishment depends on assuming that individuals are accountable for their own actions and that their degree of culpability depends on whether or not they intended to inflict injury on their fellow citizens. That is generally what is at issue in a criminal trial—not the question of what would be effective in controlling future offending by the particular offender being tried or by the general population. Moreover, that is often an important issue in the mind of the victim of violence and his or her relatives. In short, the criminal justice approach recognizes that society is interested in producing morally appropriate as well as practically effective responses to intentional violence.

In contrast, the public health approaches want to deemphasize and make unnecessary these difficult judgments of moral accountability. They would prefer to get at the problem by attacking the antecedent causes or the risk factors that shape the context of offending rather than the motivations and values of individual offenders. They would prefer to find the causes of violence in society than in the evil intentions of individual offenders. They would prefer to see the problem as one of science and technique rather than of morality and passion. That, at least, is often the way it seems to criminal justice practitioners.

To the extent that these different moral intuitions exist, or seem to exist, they tend to widen the differences between the two communities. Criminal justice practitioners see the public health community as apologists for misbehavior. Public health practitioners see the criminal justice practitioners as wrathful avengers, more interested in venting their emotions than in achieving practical effects.

To get over this hurdle, it is important for each side to acknowledge the truth of what the other side has to say. It is true that intentionally injuring a fellow citizen is morally offensive and should be responded to with moral indignation as well as with a practical plan for reducing violence in the future. It also is true that some offenders are bad and dangerous. And although society or cruel fate may have played an important role in making them that way, there is precious little that can be done about it now. This much must be granted to criminal justice practitioners by public health practitioners.

On the other hand, it also is true that many instances of violence that turn up in the criminal justice system, including some of the most serious, are produced by relatively ordinary citizens who find themselves in extremely provocative circumstance, not by dangerous, determined offenders. This in no way excuses the conduct. But it does temper society's just response. It also is true that there may be some important ways that society could work on the conditions that give rise to violence and, through that work, save both the offender and the victim. To the extent that such interventions are possible, they should be pursued enthusiastically, for they are always to be preferred to the sad business of prosecuting offenders after the fact. That much must be granted to public health practitioners by criminal justice practitioners.

Indeed, this latter point is particularly urgent, for it is the public health approach that now needs encouragement. And it is the public health approach that constitutes the new and promising frontier. For all my quibbles, I am delighted that it has arrived when it has. We need it desperately.

6

AIDS AND OTHER NEWLY
EMERGENT DISEASES

With the appearance of the HIV and AIDS epidemic, many were caught by surprise. The age of epidemics was thought to be ending. Smallpox had been eradicated throughout the world. Tuberculosis was on the decline in many places. Polio had been defeated in the industrial societies. While tuberculosis, plague, polio and other threats like malaria and cholera still raged throughout the world, many experts expected that these scourges would be eliminated or sharply reduced in the near future. AIDS should have served as a warning against this optimism, but for most experts, it did not. This was because AIDS in the West and especially in the United States was an epidemic first among the gay and intravenous drug-taking communities. Because HIV infection and AIDS were seen as a disease transmitted through the sexual practices of gay men, or by injecting drugs with contaminated needles, the fight against it was seen as being as much a battle against discrimination and moralism as a battle against a frightening new epidemic.

The use of the law to proscribe behavior on moral grounds, even if the behavior does not harm individuals, is known as *legal moralism*. Legal moralism has cultural and religious origins but its deepest roots are in purity rituals: avoidance rituals designed to make the environment and the community safe from the threat of uncleanness and contamination. Modern public health, which uses laws and regulations to save lives and prevent disease, has long been entangled with legal moralism, which uses the same measures to protect society against behavior that is viewed in some quarters as "offensive, degrading, vicious, sinful, corrupt, or otherwise immoral."[1] These morals offenses "included mainly sex offenses, such as adultery, fornication, sodomy, incest and prostitution, but also a miscellany of nonsexual offenses,"[2] such as the desecration of a corpse. From the first the debate over AIDS and HIV policy has been entangled with the controvesies surrounding the belief that society is entitled to proscribe behavior regarded as sinful or wicked.

Moralism is opposed to a public health perspective because it believes epidemics to be the result of moral dissolution. It makes the victims of epidemics, rather than the disease itself, the threat to society. Camus said it well, in the words of Dr. Rieux in *The Plague*: "All I maintain is that on this earth there are pestilences and there are victims, and it is up to us as much as possible, not to join forces with the pestilences."[3]

In the campaign to forge a coherent, nonmoralistic policy against the AIDS epidemic in the United States, a number of states—New York, New Jersey, and Massachusetts among them—constructed elaborate protections for people with HIV and AIDS which prevented traditional public health notification procedures and partner notification from coming into play. In general, AIDS was treated as an "exception" to the regime normally used by state and local public health agencies to monitor the outbreak and spread of communicable diseases such as tuberculosis or other sexually transmitted diseases. These laws were passed over the objections of many medical groups and other segments of the public who pointed out that such policies left many spouses and others unprotected.

In the first selection for this chapter, Chandler Burr notes the contradictions inherent in AIDS exceptionalism. For example, it has been argued that partner notification would be ineffective, in the case of HIV and AIDS, because those who were infected had so many partners. Yet partner notification has been used for many other sexually transmitted diseases where the infected individuals had hundreds of sexual contacts. Another reason for treating HIV as an exception to the communicable disease regime was the absence of effective treatment. With the arrival of new drug treatment therapies that seem to slow the progression of the disease, this rationale no longer holds. For these and other reasons, Burr urges an end to AIDS exceptionalism, a suggestion which appears to be taking hold. For example, in New York, mandatory reporting legislation has recently been passed.

In the second selection, Bayer and Dupuis review traditional public health policies such as testing, case reporting, and partner notification in the context of the resurgence of tuberculosis. Unless TB patients faithfully take their medications, even after they are no longer symptomatic, it will be impossible to suppress the disease, prevent its spread, and prevent the appearance of drug-resistant strains of tuberculosis. Treating those with active tuberculosis is especially difficult because many are without symptoms. Further, because they are so often poor, homeless, or addicted to intravenous drugs, it is difficult to maintain contact with them and assure that they are following their treatment regime. This has led some to advocate the use of coercive measures, including confinement, as necessary to combat this new public health menace. As new drugs and treatment regimens are developed, the same arguments may be used with regard to people with HIV and AIDS. However, given the many infected people who desperately want treatment but are unable to pay for it or to get into clinical trials, it seems unlikely that coercive measures are the solution to the AIDS epidemic.

We may come to a different conclusion about the dangers of coercion with the emergence of a whole new cast of epidemic diseases. We have noted the optimism of the 1960s and 1970s about the prospect of eliminating epidemics altogether, at least in the coming decades. AIDS was the great exception. But then, suddenly, new diseases (or at least diseases little known in the West) came tumbling out of the back closets of the world: the Hanta virus, Lassa fever, the Ebola virus, mad cow disease, a new variant of bubonic plague in India, the return of cholera to South America, and the reemergence of dengue fever, malaria, and yellow fever. Of course, many of these diseases had remained major killers in the world outside of the western developed one, but they hadn't received much attention in the western news media. When virologists began to speak of newly emergent viruses, "new" often meant something old that turns up in a new place.

Joshua Lederberg, in the third selection for this chapter, offers a powerful if short analysis of the precarious position humans occupy within the ecosystem. He says that "[W]e have too many illusions that we can, by writ, govern the remaining vital kingdoms, the microbes, that remain our competitors of last resort for dominion of the planet." He argues that "The opening of wild lands to human occupation also has exposed people to unaccustomed animal viruses, to zooneses," and that we should not let our preoccupation with the AIDS epidemic "obscure the multiplicity of infectious disease that threaten our future." He goes on to say that "we share a common vulnerability to these scourges. No matter how selfish our motives, we can no longer be indifferent to the suffering of others."

In our fourth selection, Paul R. Epstein provides a more detailed discussion of the environmental stresses and instability that are likely underlying the appearance of new diseases or old diseases in new places, and of our common vulnerability to new threats. Cholera likely arrived in the Americas because of discharges of bilge water from southeast Asian freighters. Once here, cholera found great algal blooms ready to amplify and broadcast the threat, along with ships that moved goods to the U.S. gulf coast. Some experts warn that the appearance of vast algal blooms throughout the world signal a fundamental ecological threat for the spread of disease and ecosystem instability. Weather shifts such as El Niño events likely have led to periods of intense rains in desert regions and consequent upsurges in vectors (deer mice) for Hanta virus and plague, and the subsequent infection and deaths from these diseases among U.S. residents. Epstein argues for increased monitoring of precarious environmental regions and close cooperation among climatological, wildlife, and public health experts, groups that seldom have coordinated in the past.

It remains to be seen how these new diseases and epidemics will alter the balance of power in the struggle to protect the community and to preserve the rights of individuals. Many will argue that these new threats will never be conquered unless and until the basic human rights of decent housing, clean water, the ability to limit family size, and basic medical care are secured for all humans everywhere, and until growth and the despoiling of the ecology is checked. Others will argue that, in addition to these basic protections, communities will of necessity have to protect themselves against infected individuals and groups through the classic public health methods of reporting of cases, notification, and the provision of treatment where available.

NOTES

1. Edwin M. Schur and Hugo Bedau, *Victimless Crimes* (Englewood Cliffs, NJ: Prentice-Hall, 1974, p. 90).
2. Joel Feinberg, *Social Philosophy* (Englewood Cliffs, NJ: Prentice-Hall, 1973).
3. *The Plague*, trans. Stuart Gilbert (New York: Modern Library, 1948, p. 229).

The AIDS Exception: Privacy vs. Public Health

CHANDLER BURR

Epidemiology, which encompasses both the systematic study of infectious disease and the implementation of the means to contain it, is something of a medical oddity. As dependent on statisticians and politicians as it is on medical-care providers, and often used at times of desperation, by practitioners who have been accorded police and in certain cases military powers, epidemiology has sometimes had to strike a balance between the harshness that may be required to control infectious diseases and the civil liberties of people whose rights may be subject to abridgement.

Since the turn of the century, with the introduction in this country of bacteriological testing and the establishment of boards of health, standard public-health measures have been deployed against infectious diseases. These measures, leaving aside the extreme step of holding people in quarantine, have typically included at least some of the following: *routine testing* for infection, often undertaken without explicit patient consent; *reporting* to local health authorities of the names of those who test positive for infection; *contact tracing*, or the identification of any people who may have been exposed to infection; and *notification* of these possibly infected people that they may have been exposed. Some combination of these four practices has been commonly applied against outbreaks of infectious diseases, including typhoid, diphtheria, and tuberculosis, and against upsurges in sexually transmitted diseases. It would be surprising if, out of all the viruses and bacteria that can do us significant harm, one was exempted from the scope of these measures. It would be even more surprising if the one chosen pathogen was responsible for an epidemic that today constitutes the leading cause of death among all Americans aged twenty-five to forty-four.

This very thing has, of course, happened, largely in order to accommodate civil-rights concerns. The practie of traditional public health has been to a great degree suspended for acquired immune deficiency syndrome and for human immunodeficiency virus, the virus that causes it. Although various

From *The Atlantic Monthly*, June (1997), 57–67. Reprinted by permission of the author.

traditional public-health steps are being taken against AIDS and HIV, in differing combinations from state to state, the result is a chaotic patchwork—one that is inadequate, a growing number of critics say, to the task of containing and eradicating AIDS.

"We have convinced ourselves," Ralph Frerichs, a prominent epidemiologist at the University of California at Los Angeles, wrote in a recent issue of the journal *Epidemiology*, "that the fight for survival can be waged in a way that is socially acceptable but not always biologically credible." Many public-health officials, he contended, "have remained steadfast in their commitment to programs and approaches that have hidden the identity of HIV carriers but have failed to halt viral transmission"—a commitment that is in the end bound to prove self-defeating, "making winners of the virus but losers of people."

THE PRICE OF COOPERATION

What is known in the field of public health as AIDS exceptionalism has been maintained in legally and programmatically direct ways and also in complex and subtle ways. Its origins are not difficult to ascertain.

When AIDS first surfaced, in the early 1980s, it was indisputably a disease of urban male homosexuals (and, to a far lesser extent, of intravenous-drug users). Public-health authorities, faced with a fatal, communicable disease whose method of transmission they did not understand, desperately needed the cooperation of the infected—as they would in any epidemic. In the case of AIDS, however, the infected eventually became disinclined to cooperate. "In the first months and years of the epidemic," the journalist Elinor Burkett, the author of *The Gravest Show on Earth* (1995), recalled not long ago, "people with AIDS died in the hallways of hospitals, where nurses wouldn't touch them. They were kicked out of their apartments. Insurance companies canceled their policies. Their bosses fired them. They had no idea how to get Social Security disability payments or Medicaid."

The discovery of HIV, and the development of a test that could detect it, brought matters to a head. In the aftermath of anti-gay persecution and even violence, the price exacted by a terrified gay community for cooperation in even a rudimentary public-health effort was ironclad anonymity. In 1985, shortly before the federal government was to announce the licensing of the first test for detecting HIV, the National Gay Task Force and the gay civil-rights group Lambda Legal Defense and Education Fund filed a petition in federal court to delay this action, pending a legal guarantee that the test would not lead to widespread screening aimed at gay men. They then put pressure on the Food and Drug Administration, which along with the federal Centers for Disease Control (now the Centers for Disease Control and Prevention, and henceforward referred to as the CDC) had been made aware of eager queries from school districts hoping to use the HIV test to identify and fire gay teachers. The FDA quickly acceded to the demand that the HIV test be used not to screen and identify *people* for HIV infection in systematic campaigns but only to screen the blood in blood banks.

Out of the threat that the HIV test posed to privacy grew a rigid resistance to almost all HIV testing without consent—and a public-health approach to combating AIDS characterized by considerable delicacy. The FDA's agreement to restrict how the HIV test could be used resolved, temporarily, a political problem. Left unanswered, as Randy Shilts, in his book *And the Band Played On* (1987), observed, was "the broader public health question of how you can control a disease if you decline to find out who is infected." Shilts went on, "In this poisoned atmosphere, the nuances of long-term consequences for control of the infection fell low on the list of gay concerns."

The result, ultimately, was the effective suspension of traditional public-health procedures for AIDS, which is to say, there would be no routine testing for HIV; the reporting of the names of the HIV-infected would be required only in some places, and would miss the epidemic's hotspots; and contact tracing and notification would as a result be greatly handicapped, and in many places pursued in desultory fashion if at all, often in the face of opposition. All efforts were to be voluntary—dependent on educational outreach and persuasion rather than on systematic procedures. "U.S. officials had no alternative but to negotiate the course of AIDS policy with representatives of a well-organized gay community and their allies in the medical and political establishments." Ronald Bayer, a professor at the Columbia University School of Public Health, wrote in a critical retrospective some years ago, "In this process, many of the traditional practices of public health that might have been brought to bear were dismissed as inappropriate."

A number of opportunities present themselves for the routine testing of people for various diseases by public institutions, routine testing being defined as testing that can be performed without a person's explicit consent. Pregnant mothers are routinely tested for tuberculosis, hepatitis B, and syphilis; testing for chlamydia and group-B streptococcus is also common under certain circumstances. Newborn babies are routinely tested, without the mothers' permission, for phenylketonuria and hypothyroidism. Patients admitted to hospitals may undergo a variety of blood tests, depending on their symptoms, the tests being performed as a matter of course, without necessarily informing the patient or asking explicit permission. Although a patient can at any time refuse to undergo a routine test, he or she does not have to be specially notified that the test is being done or given a specific opportunity to refuse.

HIV testing, in contrast, is almost always voluntary—which means it is done either at an anonymous-testing site or with a person's explicit permission (and which usually means also that the person being tested must sign a release). At the federal level HIV testing is required only of immigrants entering the country, foreign-service and military personnel, and federal-prison inmates. At the state level routine testing is prohibited everywhere except under narrowly defined circumstances. Marcia Angell, the executive editor of *The New England Journal of Medicine*, and a proponent of routine testing in some form, says, "Having to ask specifically has a huge effect, and it is a clear difference between AIDS and many other diseases."

Making even certain subpopulations the target of routine testing would turn up large numbers of infected people who currently escape detection. In a 1992 *New England Journal of Medicine* article Robert Janssen and his colleagues at the Division of HIV/AIDS at the National Center for Infectious Diseases recommended voluntary targeted testing for HIV in certain hospitals, a policy well short of routine testing and yet one that has been implemented virtually nowhere. They wrote,

> We estimate that about 225,000 HIV-positive persons were hospitalized in 1990, of whom only one third were admitted for symptomatic HIV infection or AIDS. Routine, voluntary HIV testing of patients 15 to 54 years old in hospitals with 1 or more patients with newly diagnosed AIDS per 1,000 discharges per year could potentially have identified as many as 110,000 patients with HIV infection that was previously unrecognized.

Testing that is merely voluntary may also miss populations that disproportionately need to be reached. The people least likely to have the virus are the most likely to say yes to a test, and the people most likely to have it are the most likely to say no. In one study infection rates were 5.3 times as high among people who refused HIV testing as among people who consented to it.

One might ask, How could a study give the infection rate of those who refused the HIV test? The answer demonstrates the methods that researchers—in this case, at the New Mexico Health and Environment Department—must employ in order to obtain data without violating personal rights as protected by law. Voluntary, anonymous HIV tests were offered over a three-month period to all patients visiting a sexually-transmitted-disease clinic. Eighty-two percent of the patients consented to being tested for HIV. To determine the rate of HIV infection among those who did not consent to testing, researchers located serum that had been taken from these patients for syphilis testing, removed all identifying information, and then tested the serum for HIV.

Exceptionalists argue that routine testing will "drive AIDS underground"— make people avoid the health-care system altogether. There is no empirical proof that this will or won't occur to a greater extent than it already does, under a voluntary regime. Ultimately one must ask whether people who would go underground because of perceived self-interest should dictate policy—and also whether such people would cooperate in disease-prevention efforts under any circumstances.

Why does testing matter? The most basic epidemiology holds that early knowledge of where a virus is moving—into which populations—is essential to slowing its spread. Even if a disease cannot be cured, knowing who the infected people are may help prevent the transmission of the disease to other people. Geneviève Clavreul, a California-based consultant to the International Cancer and AIDS Research Foundation, says that because of testing and reporting restrictions the California Department of Public Health is in essence "flying blind" in its epidemiological tracking. By law or regulation, cases of certain sexually transmitted diseases and of many other infectious diseases must be reported to state departments of health, and the names of the infected are in most cases provided and are always held in confidence. HIV is the exception. Although the disease called AIDS must be reported by name in all fifty states, infection with HIV, the virus that causes AIDS, need not be; only twenty-six states mandate the (confidential) reporting by name of positive test results for HIV, and these states tend to be ones with modest caseloads. Twelve states— including California and New York, by far the two worst-afflicted states—have no broad reporting requirements for HIV.

Requiring the reporting of AIDS but not HIV seems equivalent to requiring, say, that full-blown cases of hepatitis B be reported but not any newly detected infections with the hepatitis virus. Actually, it is worse. The incubation period for hepatitis B is usually two or three months, whereas the period between infection with HIV and a diagnosis of AIDS is often longer than ten years. This means that during all this time HIV-positive people can be both infectious and outside the public-health system. The disease is further privatized by the HIV home-testing kits now on the market, which to yet one more degree put testing and reporting into the hands of individuals.

As noted, state public-health practices mandate that certain sexually transmitted diseases be reported; in part to avoid reporting HIV some states have decided not to classify HIV as a sexually transmitted disease—even though the primary mode of HIV infection is, of course, sexual. As of 1995 only twelve states had classified AIDS and HIV infection as sexually transmitted diseases. Only sixteen states had even classified them as communicable diseases. Treating AIDS and HIV infection as exceptions, twenty-three states, including New York and California, had classified them as a separate category of disease. A report prepared for the CDC by Georgetown University and Johns Hopkins University's Program on Law and Public Health observes of this situation: "Disease-specific legislation may thwart public health goals by generating separate policies, programs, and procedures for diseases that may share common behavioral risk factors and require a unified approach for treatment and prevention."

Beyond issues of testing and reporting lies the issue of partner notification. "Partner notification" is the term used by the CDC to describe a spectrum of outreach efforts. One such effort is contact tracing, also called "provider referral," in which doctors or public-health officials locate partners of infected people (if the infected people are willing or able to provide names) and notify them of possible infection; the name of the known infected person is always kept confidential. At a further remove on the spectrum is "patient referral," in which infected people locate and notify partners on their own. Only thirty-three states have laws that explicitly allow doctors or public-health officials to notify the sex or needle-sharing partners of those with AIDS or infected with HIV. Only four states (Arkansas, North Carolina, South Carolina, and Oregon) have statues requiring notification.

All states technically have something that they can point to as a "partner-notification program," having such a program being a prerequisite for obtaining certain federal funds. But the effectiveness of partner-notification programs varies widely, for reasons relating as much to how the programs are implemented as to what specific steps they call for: the real difference is between states, such as Colorado and North Carolina, that actively strive to find and notify partners primarily through provider referral, and states, such as New York and California, that tend to rely on patient referral, deferring the responsibility of notification of the infected.

As one would expect, there seems to be a marked contrast between the effectiveness of well-established partner-notification programs in which provider-referral services are made available, and that of programs in which infected people themselves do the notifying if they are so inclined. One study found that active partner-notification programs offering provider-referral services get 30 to 90 percent (depending on the city or state) of people who have tested positive to cooperate in contacting those they may have infected. Ninety percent or more of those contacted agree to be tested. However, programs in which notification is left up to the infected achieve a cooperation rate of less than 10 percent. It should be noted also that by virtue of the fact that trained public-health personnel in most instances make the notifications in provider-referral cases, testing information and counseling are made readily available to possibly infected contacts. Programs that notify primarily through provider referral find a larger proportion of other infected people, and find them earlier. The sooner a person knows of his or her infection and begins treatment, and the higher that person's T-cell count when treatment begins, the better the prognosis. In a recent study conducted at a Los Angeles AIDS clinic the average T-cell count in HIV-positive women who entered the clinic through active provider-referral partner notification was found to be 411; the average for all other women entering the clinic was 157. ("T-cell count" refers to the number of T-helper cells, a kind of white-blood cell that is essential to the proper functioning of the cellular immune system; HIV attacks and kills these cells. The T-cell count is closer to 1,000 in a healthy person, though the healthy range is subject to considerable variability. A T-cell count under 200 is one of the criteria for a diagnosis of AIDS.)

Does an absence of routine testing, reporting, and notification mean that a lot of undiscovered AIDS and HIV cases are festering in the larger society? Yes. According to the CDC, the number of Americans infected with HIV is as high as 900,000; of these, the CDC estimates, perhaps half are unaware of their infection. At least a quarter of all people in whom AIDS was diagnosed from 1990 to 1995 in Los Angeles County first became aware of their infection when they came to hospitals or clinics with advanced symptoms, having never previously been tested for HIV. In all likelihood such people had been HIV-positive for years. Most cancer, diabetes, or high-blood-pressure patients have been tested for these medical problems, know their status, and have begun treatment well before admission to a hospital with advanced symptoms. The situation with AIDS means, as one Los Angeles AIDS clinic director observed during a recent interview, that "something is really wrong." Because the lifetime cost of treating HIV is so high (estimated in 1993 to be $119,000 per patient), the CDC has concluded that AIDS and HIV notification programs pay for themselves if only one in eighty notifications prevents a new HIV infection by indicating to the notified person that a change in behavior is warranted.

AIDS has been so thoroughly exempted from traditional public-health approaches that civil libertarians have defeated in court attempts by health authorities to notify the spouses of people who have died of AIDS that their husbands or wives were HIV-infected. During the first years of the disease, legislation urged by civil libertarians prohibited physicians and public-health officials from notifying even the spouses of living people who had tested positive for HIV, some of whom continued to have unprotected sex with their partners. In some states laws have been enacted making partner notification by a physician at best discretionary under tightly defined circumstances.

National legislation on spousal notification, passed last year, mandates that states make a "good-faith effort" to notify at-risk spouses. However, in effect the law applies only to states that already require the names of infected people to be reported. And in any event, the matter of partner notification when the partners are (or were) married addresses, of course, only a small part of the AIDS problem.

WRONGHEADED RATIONALES

How has AIDS exceptionalism been justified? In the mid-1980s four arguments were regularly heard for exempting AIDS from standard public-health practices. 1) There had never before been a disease that seemed to constitute a de facto marker for homosexuality, with all the social stigma that this label carries. 2) The confidentiality of testing would inevitably be violated, precisely because AIDS is more stigmatized than any other disease. 3) Given the large number of sex partners of many of those who have become HIV-infected, contact tracing would be ineffectual. 4) Because there is no cure for AIDS, and no treatment to render the infected uninfectious, it was pointless to report HIV infection as is done for other infections.

However legitimate the civil-liberties issues it sought to address may have been more than a decade ago, the exceptionalist orthodoxy is now fundamentally wrongheaded as a matter of good public health and medicine.

The argument that AIDS is a unique marker for homosexuality is incorrect, and always was so. Rectal gonorrhea in men has been almost exclusively a disease of the gay population, and is a more reliable marker for homosexuality, if anyone were looking for such a marker, than AIDS ever was. And yet cases of rectal gonorrhea have appeared for decades, by name and date, in confidential case reports sent to state public-health departments.

The argument that confidentiality will inevitably be violated has met a serious counter-argument in the form of reality: the experience of Minnesota and Colorado, which have since 1985 mandated the confidential reporting by name of both HIV and AIDS cases. As of the end of last year, for example, Colorado health authorities had received the names of 5,723 people with AIDS and of 5,137 additional people infected with HIV. There have been no breaches of confidentiality. As noted, twenty-six states now require confidential reporting of all HIV cases by name. A single intentional breach of confidentiality in the CDC's AIDS surveillance system is known to have occurred (in Florida).

As for discrimination, the federal Americans with Disabilities Act (ADA), passed in 1990, a decade after the beginning of the AIDS epidemic, prohibits discrimination based on HIV status. In addition, the federal Vocational Rehabilitation Act of 1973, state discrimination laws, and state constitutions have all been interpreted by courts as protecting people from exactly the sort of discrimination that AIDS exceptionalists claim is inevitable. And courts have in most cases ruled that being infected with HIV constitutes a disability according to the legal definition of the term, even when the infected person is asymptomatic. "We've done more or less everything that can be done on the legislative front to protect people from discrimination on the basis of HIV status," says Chai Feldblum, an associate professor at Georgetown University Law School and one of the principal architects of the ADA. "The laws are there."

The argument that contact tracing will prove to be ineffectual because many of those infected with HIV have had a large number of sex partners ignores the fact that many of those infected with syphilis and gonorrhea, other diseases for which gay men are at increased risk, have also had a large number of sex partners, and yet contact tracing has been standard procedure for these diseases for decades.

The argument that name reporting is pointless because there is no treatment has always been open to question on a number of grounds. Yes, the statement may have a certain logic from the perspective of a given infected individual concerned only about his or her fate. But if infected people can be identified, education and counseling may at the very least prompt changes in their behavior which will diminish the risk that they go on to infect others: contact tracing, in turn, extends the possibility of risk-diminishing behavioral change even more widely. Knowing who is infected is essential in helping to prevent new infections, even if the infected person himself cannot be helped.

In any event, evidence shows that new medical treatments are making HIV less infectious than ever. The latest treatments are astonishingly promising for at least some of the infected population.

Some 15 to 30 percent of HIV-infected pregnant women pass the virus on to their infants. Early treatment with zidovudine, or AZT, for the woman during pregnancy and for the infant after birth, can cut the proportion to eight percent. A new class of drugs called protease inhibitors is likely to cut the rate even further, if the drugs are used early. The key word is "early"—which means testing pregnant mothers, not just newborn babies. The American Medical Association now recommends that HIV testing be made mandatory for pregnant women. Gay and AIDS activists have denounced this recommendation.

Protease inhibitors, which in some cases have reduced the level of HIV in the bloodstreams of the infected to undetectable levels, have revolutionized care for many patients. "I think we already have the capability to make HIV infection a chronic, manageable disease like diabetes in patients who can afford the therapy and who can take it with one-hundred-percent compliance," says Joel Gallant, the director of the Moore HIV Clinic at the Johns Hopkins University School of Medicine. Protease inhibitors have provoked debate as to their long-term effectiveness, their ability to withstand viral resistance, and their price (the protease inhibitor Invirase costs approximately $7,000 for a year's supply), and also, as Gallant has noted, because of the fastidiousness required for effective administration. But the fact remains that the exceptionalist argument that no treatment is possible is losing whatever force it had.

The benefits of knowing who is infected are still more compelling today than they were in 1992, when the CDC AIDS laboratory chief Donald Francis, writing in the *Journal of the American Medical Association* in favor of more aggressive testing and the channeling of the infected into prevention and counseling programs, brought up "the ability to deliver important new products produced by scientific research." He wrote,

> Should the day come when a vaccine or therapeutic drug becomes available, a system for immediate delivery to those in greatest need would be required. There is no system by which to do that now. But if all infected persons were being followed

up in an early intervention program, delivery would be straightforward. In my opinion, early intervention should be given the highest national priority.

The fact that AIDS is not easily transmissible (it is a hundred times less infectious than hepatitis B, and incomparably less contagious than an airborne disease like tuberculosis) provides further impetus to discover who is and is not HIV-infected. The knowledge that a given person is infected, if it means that the person takes any preventive measures at all, is much more valuable in the case of AIDS than it is for other diseases.

REMEDY-RESISTANT POLITICS?

Despite such developments, attempts to alter the public-health approach to AIDS, though on occasion successful, have met with fierce opposition. A case in point occurred in the spring of 1995, when Gary Ackerman, a liberal Democratic congressman from New York, introduced a bill with 220 co-sponsors to "unblind" a national infant-testing program for HIV run by the CDC as a way of monitoring HIV-infection rates in women. Since 1988 the CDC had been "blind-testing" infants for HIV in forty-five states—using blood samples, collected at birth, from which all identifying tags had been removed. Testing for HIV in this way meant that the CDC knew how many infants carried their mother's HIV antibodies but not who they or their infected mothers were. Mothers, therefore, were being sent home without being informed that they and in some cases their children were infected with a fatal virus. The CDC had no choice in the matter, being legally prevented from testing without informed consent. Under the Ackerman bill mechanisms were to be instituted so that if an infant tested positive, those doing the testing would have a way of knowing who that infant was, and its mother could be informed.

The response to this proposed legislation was immediate. Virtually every gay and AIDS group, including Gay Men's Health Crisis, the AIDS Action Council, and the National Association of People With AIDS, along with the ACLU and prominent public-health experts at leading universities, opposed the bill, largely on the grounds that unblinding the tests would do nothing to help prevent HIV transmission from mothers to their infants and would violate the privacy inherent in such an anonymous surveillance study, potentially scaring pregnant women away from seeking proper prenatal care. The intensity of feeling with which such measures have been opposed should not be underestimated. Ackerman's bill was modeled on a bill introduced in the New York State Assembly by the Democratic legislator Nettie Mayersohn to unblind the anonymous infant-testing program in New York. Mayersohn, a pro-choice, feminist old-line liberal who in 1989 had been named Legislator of the Year by the New York State chapter of the National Organization for Women, was labeled a "fascist" by individuals associated with the AIDS lobby. (Last June, three years after Mayersohn introduced her original legislation, the New York legislature passed a bill allowing the state to institute mandatory HIV testing of newborns and to notify parents of the test results. Newborn testing began last February.)

In the matter of the Ackerman legislation, the head of the CDC informed Ackerman that if the bill were not withdrawn, the CDC would suspend the infant-testing program altogether. Ackerman gave no credence to this threat by a public-health agency, because the infant-testing program was demonstrably useful in tracking the prevalence and trajectory of heterosexual AIDS. But the CDC program was indeed suspended. Public-health authorities thus lost even this imperfect means of monitoring one aspect of the epidemic.

In response to the CDC's suspension of testing, Ackerman joined forces with Tom Coburn, a Republican congressman and a Christian conservative from Oklahoma, to draft new legislation that has become known as the "Baby AIDS Compromise." The legislation was enacted last May as part of a larger bill, the Ryan White CARE Reauthorization Act. The compromise requires state health-care workers to offer counseling and voluntary HIV testing to pregnant women who have not previously been tested for HIV. States that by March of 2000 do not meet certain goals with respect to the voluntary HIV testing of pregnant women or to HIV incidence among newborns will have to implement a mandatory infant-testing program or lose some federal AIDS funding.

The ultimate question for AIDS exceptionalism is this: Do the disease-containment and disease-prevention measures of traditional public health—the measures from whose full force AIDS has been significantly shielded—work? The answer given to this question by AIDS exceptionalists as well as traditionalists seems to be yes. Joel Gallant, for example, opposes routine involuntary testing for HIV and aggressive partner notification, but not on medical grounds; rather, he fears the potential for employment and insurance discrimination, domestic abuse, and breaches of confidentiality. He maintains that he would otherwise favor traditional public-health procedures for the fight against AIDS, particularly routine testing.

Lee Reichman, the executive director of the National Tuberculosis Center and a physician on the staff of the New Jersey Medical School who cares for AIDS patients, cautions that given the course that the evolution and politics of the disease have taken, traditional public-health measures by themselves may no longer be feasible, in part because of the possibility that they will drive the infected underground. As noted, this is an exceptionalist article of faith. But Reichman goes on: "Traditional public health is absolutely effective at controlling infectious disease. It should have been applied to AIDS from the start, and it wasn't. Long before there was AIDS, there were other sexually transmitted diseases, and you had partner notification and testing and reporting. This was routine public health at its finest, and this is the way STDs were controlled."

In the months ahead a national debate may well be joined over rescinding the exceptional public-health status of AIDS, owing in part to a bill introduced by Tom Coburn, the Oklahoma congressman. Coburn's bill, the HIV Prevention Act of 1997, would establish confidential HIV reporting nationwide. It would require states to inform anyone who has been exposed to HIV. It would require that all people accused of sexual offenses be tested for HIV. And it would allow health-care providers to test a patient for HIV before performing a risky invasive medical procedure. The Coburn bill contains a number of other provisions and also two nonbinding "sense of the Congress" resolutions, one urging states to criminalize the intentional transmission of HIV, the other affirming the principle that strict confidentiality must be observed in carrying out the bill's provisions. (A companion bill has been introduced in the Senate.) "The fact is that epidemiology works," Coburn says, "and public-health policies work to control disease, and they work by identifying vectors of infectious disease, and you notify people at risk. If you don't do that, you can't control the disease. And that's what we've not done with HIV."

The AIDS Action Council—a group "dedicated solely to shaping fair and effective AIDS policy," in the words of its literature—has denounced the Coburn bill as "an attempt to federalize policies that do nothing but stigmatize and punish people living with HIV/AIDS." The act, in the view of the council, "replaces education and personal responsibility with 'Big Brother' intrusion and control." In previous statements the council has characterized measures like the ones now proposed as "failed policies that do nothing to prevent any more Americans from becoming infected with HIV."

It is hard to see how traditionalist policies can be said to have "failed" with AIDS, since they have not been systematically tried. Be that as it may, some skepticism toward legislation like Coburn's is warranted. Conservatives representing themselves as public-health advocates are certainly vulnerable to a charge of hypocrisy. Coburn's bill does not address one of the exceptionalists' central criticisms: that although traditional procedures will identify more infected people, conservatives are not prepared to offer any plan for helping those infected people (many of whom have no health insurance and little education, and many of whom are homeless) after they have been identified. The Coburn bill offers no new funds for the state public-health departments that would be obliged to carry out its testing and reporting provisions. A traditionalist approach to AIDS will cost money, and those who advocate such an approach should be making the case that more money is needed.

Exceptionalists also point out, correctly and bitterly, that the hatred directed against homosexuals, and the discrimination they experience at the hands of anti-gay conservatives, among others, are responsible in the first place for the very exceptionalist policies that conservatives like Coburn now so strongly oppose. Coburn's own outlook gives one pause. It was Coburn who elicited condemnation and ridicule when he criticized the airing on network television last winter of *Schindler's List,* complaining about the depiction of violence and frontal nudity.

As noted, epidemiology has sometimes had to weigh the issue of civil rights against the issue of effective disease control. The time has come to consider anew how these factors should tip the scales. We do not, of course, have an absolute guarantee that traditional epidemiology applied to AIDS and HIV would markedly bolster the success of public-health, efforts. But such a guarantee is hardly required. Marcia Angell, of *The New England Journal of Medicine,* observes, "Nobody can document or prove that traditional methods of control would work better at containing AIDS, because nobody has done what would be necessary to get such proof—studying two populations, one in which traditional methods are applied and one in which they aren't. The reason no one has done this is that it is impossible. It is impossible because it's unethical and logically unworkable. So, as in many things in life, the default position is common sense. And I have no doubt, given the track record of these methods in controlling other diseases that if, for example, we screened all expectant mothers, we could prevent AIDS in many cases. And if we traced partners, we would prevent AIDS in many cases. And if we routinely tested in hospitals, we would prevent AIDS in many cases."

Ralph Frerichs, of UCLA, framed the matter like this in the course of an interview: "Historically, public health has always transcended the legal system, much like the military. When you have an outside threat, you can suspend the normal rules of society. Traditionally, we epidemiologists have been granted full responsibility, but society has eroded that and we now talk about respecting the rights of human individuals who have disease-causing viruses, bacteria, and so on, which makes it increasingly difficult to stop the spread of these diseases. This is society's choice. But this is de facto granting rights to the viruses and to the bacteria. And when epidemics are presented this way, as a matter of rights, the public has a harder time distinguishing the infection from the infected. The virus is our enemy, not the person with the virus, but at the same time that person harbors the virus, and we need to take a series of steps to prevent that virus from moving to another person.

"In AIDS, as in all epidemics, there is a tradeoff between emphasizing detection of the virus and the civil-rights violations that detection engenders. Given that we have not pushed for aggressive testing, reporting, and partner notification, it appears that our society is willing to accept a higher amount of HIV infection to avoid interfering with the rights of HIV-infected people."

Earlier this year the Centers for Disease Control and Prevention reported that largely because of gains in life expectancy among the infected, annual deaths from AIDS had registered a significant decline for the first time since the onset of the epidemic. That they have done so is hardly grounds for complacency. It is evidence, however, that medical interventions make a palpable difference—and is all the more reason to start subjecting AIDS, from a public-health perspective, to more systematic procedures.

In the end AIDS would be unlikely to prove resistant to good basic public-health policies. It may survive if it can circumvent good sense.

Tuberculosis, Public Health, and Civil Liberties

RONALD BAYER AND LAURENCE DUPUIS

INTRODUCTION

Tuberculosis, a scourge referred to in the seventeenth century as the "captain of all these men of death," has returned to plague contemporary America, just when medical and public health measures seemed poised to consign the disease to the pages of history. In 1989, the Center for Disease Control's Advisory Council for the Elimination of Tuberculosis established a goal of eliminating tuberculosis in the United States by 2010. But as early as 1985, the long trend of declining tuberculosis cases had already reversed itself, and by 1992, there were 52,000 more cases than would have been expected had the downward trend continued.

The dramatic return of this disease poses serious questions about the failures of public health policy during the 1970s and 1980s. The new epidemic has also forced a reappraisal of the legal and ethical implications of disease-control measures that might be marshaled to combat the spread of contagious disease. This selection first briefly reviews the medical and epidemiological background of the current tuberculosis epidemic and the influence of AIDS on traditional approaches to disease control. The remainder . . . focuses on the specific ethical and legal questions surrounding tuberculosis control, with a particular emphasis on the civil-liberties implications of four approaches to disease control: the provision of supportive services to encourage patients to complete therapy; the use of directly observed therapy to monitor adherence to therapy; the involuntary detention of noncompliant patients; and the forced administration of tuberculosis medications.

THE RETURN OF TUBERCULOSIS

Tuberculosis is a communicable disease caused by *Mycobacterium tuberculosis,* an organism that is most commonly transmitted by inhaling airborne droplets expelled by the cough of a person with infectious tuberculosis. In most cases, people infected with *M. tuberculosis* do not develop clinical disease, but remain noninfectious, asymptomatic carriers. Among infected persons with noncompromised immune systems, there is an estimated 5–10% *lifetime* risk of developing clinical disease. People with both *M. tuberculosis* and HIV infection, by contrast, have a 5–10% *annual* risk of developing clinical disease. Clinical disease most commonly affects the lungs, but may affect other sites as well. Treatment of active disease ordinarily involves taking several drugs, at least two to three times per week, for a period of 6–9 months. Such treatment is generally highly effective, and results in long-term cure in about 95% of cases. Treatment of HIV-infected tuberculosis patients, however, is complicated by the unusually rapid progression from initial infection to active disease, which results in a high incidence of treatment failure and mortality.

Tuberculosis was among the leading causes of death in western society throughout the nineteenth century and remains one of the most common infectious diseases worldwide. Approximately one third of the global population carries *M. tuberculosis,* 8 million new cases are reported annually, and each year nearly 3 million die from the disease. In the United States, however, the prevalence of the disease declined steadily, beginning in the early part of the century and continuing until the mid-1980s. The historical decline in TB morbidity and mortality has been attributed to a number of factors. Prior to the introduction of antibiotic therapy in 1946, the decline in tuberculosis probably was the result of improvements in nutrition and housing that accompanied rising wages and improved living standards in the first half of the century, as well as specific public health interventions—such as education, isolation, and quarantine—that contained the spread of the disease. From 1953, the year after the introduction of the antituberculosis drug, isoniazid, through 1984, the number of tuberculosis cases reported decreased from 84,304 to 22,255, an average decline of 5% per year.

Despite the overall decline in tuberculosis in the United States, the disease continued to be a significant problem among people of color and in low-income communities. For example, in 1984, when the tuberculosis case rate had dropped to 9.4 new cases per 100,000 population in the United States, the case rate in central Harlem—a predominantly African-American community with high rates of poverty—was 90.7 per 100,000.

Beginning in 1985, the downward trend in reported cases of tuberculosis in the United States was reversed. From 1985 through 1991, the number of reported TB cases increased 18%. The HIV epidemic is certainly a major factor in the resurgence of tuberculosis. In New York City, nearly 50% of tuberculosis patients in 1988–89 were also infected with HIV; this suggests that many reported cases are the result of reactivation of latent infection in immune-suppressed individuals. While reactivation of latent disease has contributed to the increase in reported tuberculosis cases, recent studies indicate that more than one third of active cases in New York City and San Francisco are the result of recent transmission. Dramatic cutbacks in public funding and in facilities for TB control and treatment, as well as increasing poverty, homelessness, over-crowded housing and drug abuse have all played critical roles in the emerging epidemic.

The resurgence of tuberculosis is primarily afflicting those disadvantaged communities where the disease had persisted despite the overall national de-cline. From 1985 through 1990, the number of tuberculosis cases increased dramatically among Hispanics, African-Americans, and Asian/Pacific Islanders, while reported cases among non-Hispanic whites continued to decline. By 1990, the TB case rate in central Harlem approached 200 per 100,000, approx-imately 4 times the New York City rate and 20 times the national rate. These are also the communities, that have borne much of the weight of the continuing HIV/AIDS epidemic.

Exacerbating the ominous increase in tuberculosis is the emergence and pro-liferation of strains of the disease that resist one or more of the medications typically used to treat TB patients. In a national survey of culture-positive TB cases reported in the first quarter of 1991, investigators found that 9.5% of cases were resistant to rifampin and/or isoniazid, two of the safest and most effective first-line antituberculosis drugs, and that 3.5% of cases were resistant to both drugs. A study in New York City found that 19% of culture-positive cases during April 1991 were resistant to both rifampin and isoniazid. Multi-drug-resistant tuberculosis (MDR-TB) is considerably more difficult and expen-sive to treat than nonresistant disease, and is associated with much greater mor-tality, particularly among patients infected with HIV. In a report on 171 carefully treated and monitored non-HIV patients with multidrug-resistant dis-ease, only 56% of the patients had successful drug-therapy outcomes (negative sputum cultures without relapse) and 37% died, about half from tuberculosis. In investigations of nine outbreaks of multidrug-resistant tuberculosis in hospitals and prisons, the CDC found mortality rates ranging from 72% to 89%. Between 20% and 80% of the cases in those outbreaks were HIV infected.

The rise of multidrug-resistant tuberculosis is ultimately attributable to in-adequate drug therapy, which results either from inappropriate treatment by the physician or poor adherence to recommended therapy by the patient. Al-though the current system for tracking rates of treatment completion is inade-quate, available data indicate that in some of the cities hardest hit by drug-resistant strains of tuberculosis, completion rates have been dismally low. For example, in New York City between 1986 and 1990, only 53.6% of patients completed six continuous months of therapy, whereas San Francisco, Dallas, and El Paso all had completion rates above 90% during the same period. At one location in New York, 89% of tuberculosis patients were lost to follow-up before they had completed therapy. Although drug-resistant strains initially develop as a result of inadequate therapy, it must be underscored that such strains can be transmitted directly to previously healthy individuals. One study in New York concluded that most patients with drug-resistant tuberculosis did not acquire drug-resistant disease through inadequate treatment of a susceptible strain, but were initially infected with a drug-resistant strain transmitted to them by another person.

DISEASE CONTROL AFTER AIDS

Responses to the resurgence of tuberculosis must be understood in the context of the AIDS epidemic, which has shaped popular as well as professional conceptions of the appropriate public health approaches to epidemic disease.

As the public policy responses to AIDS took shape in the United States and in other democratic nations, a consensus emerged against using coercive state interventions long associated with the practice of public health. Rather, a voluntaristic strategy took hold that focused on eliciting the cooperation of those at risk for HIV infection. Mass education, voluntary testing and counseling, the protection of the rights of privacy of those with HIV, and the prohibition against unwarranted acts of discrimination were essential elements of this approach. The roots of this strategy, broadly endorsed by public health officials at the federal, state, and local levels, were many. HIV transmission typically takes place in intimate or secretive settings between consenting adults during sexual intercourse or drug use, not through casual contact. Public health and clinical medicine have no magic bullet to cure the disease; only voluntary personal risk-reduction behavior is effective in preventing further transmission. AIDS primarily affects marginalized populations—gay and bisexual men, intravenous drug users, social and ethnic minorities—with a long history of suspicion about the intentions and practices of government. The shaping of AIDS policy was singularly affected by the capacity of one of these groups—urban, middle-class gay men—to articulate their concerns about the dangers of using the AIDS epidemic as a pretext for undermining their hard-won, but still fragile, rights of privacy and liberty.

But tuberculosis is not AIDS. It is an airborne disease that can be transmitted to contacts who may be largely unaware that they are being placed at risk, or who may be unable to take precautions to protect themselves. Unlike AIDS, tuberculosis is generally curable. Even drug-resistant tuberculosis may be treated effectively, particularly in cases where the disease is susceptible to at least one of the first-line medications. The availability of effective therapy makes it possible to interrupt the spread of infection to the general population through medical intervention with the individual patient. Finally, while legislation and practice surrounding AIDS reflected the transformation that had occurred in American constitutional law over the previous three decades, which had expanded the rights of the individual to challenge the exercise of state authority, TB surveillance and control were still governed "by antiquated laws that predate modern concepts of constitutional law and the need for a flexible range of public health powers."

It is an unfortunate irony that AIDS and tuberculosis—the former a new threat that has evoked a radical rethinking of public health practices stressing principles of voluntarism, the latter an ancient threat, the control of which epitomized the coercive tradition in public health—have been superimposed upon each other for epidemiological and biological reasons. The resurgence of tuberculosis in the midst of the AIDS epidemic challenges us to revisit the legal and ethical principles that guide public health practices and to navigate a course between a return to broad and relatively unfettered coercive state action and a reliance on solely voluntary measures that may not prove sufficient to protect vulnerable communities.

THE ETHICAL AND LEGAL FOUNDATIONS OF TUBERCULOSIS CONTROL

The threat of tuberculosis to the public health provides the ethical and legal basis for government intervention in decision-making regarding an individual's health care. In contemporary ethical theory, and in biomedical ethics, strong emphasis is placed on the rights of the individual and on principles of autonomy and self-determination. But as central as those values are, the legitimacy of limiting them has long been recognized. Although conflict does exist about the nature and justification of those limits, there is no controversy in liberal democratic cultures over the principle that when the exercise of one person's freedom may result in harm to another, the state may intervene. Known as the "harm principle," this universally recognized limitation on autonomy was given its most potent expression by the nineteenth-century philosopher John Stuart Mill:

> [T]he only purpose for which power can be rightfully exercised over any member of a civilized community, against his will, is to prevent harm to others. His own good, either physical or moral, is not a sufficient warrant.

This principle clearly provides an ethical foundation for establishing public health programs designed to require those with communicable diseases to behave in ways that are likely to reduce the risk of transmission. It is sufficiently robust to justify requiring those with infectious tuberculosis to avoid public places where exposure to others would occur, and to authorize state action to enforce such requirements.

The public health authority to limit individual freedom when disease threatens has long been recognized in constitutional jurisprudence. Nearly ninety years ago, in *Jacobson v. Massachusetts,* a case that centered on the question of compulsory vaccination, the Supreme Court held that the U.S. Constitution permitted states to enact "such reasonable regulations . . . as will protect the public health and the public safety" as long as such efforts did not "contravene the Constitution of the United States, nor infringe any right granted or secured by that instrument." *Jacobson* also reiterated the rule that courts should give deference to a state's exercise of the police powers designed to protect the public health. Such measures could be invalidated only if they had "no real or substantial relation" to their ostensible goals. This extraordinary deference to government action prevailed throughout much of the 20th century, persisting as late as the 1960s. The past three decades of constitutional development, however, particularly in the area of involuntary confinement of psychiatric patients, have seen increased scrutiny of the exercise of the police powers, raising questions about the constitutionality of statutes relating to communicable disease and tuberculosis control, many of which were enacted before the profound shift in the balance between individual liberties and state authority.

Although the law gave considerable latitude to public health officials, virtually all TB control measures were focused on the necessity of identifying, treating, and limiting the activity of those whose tuberculosis was infectious. In 1992, the Centers for Disease Control undertook a broad review of state laws governing tuberculosis control, and found that 43 states provided for the quarantine of TB patients within their own homes, 35 specifying that the quarantine should last until the person was no longer infectious. Forty-two states permitted the commitment of TB patients to treatment facilities, 24 permitting such confinement until the individual no longer posed a health threat to others.

The resurgence of tuberculosis and the emergence of drug-resistant strains among inadequately treated patients have compelled public health officials to recognize the necessity of efforts to assure that patients with tuberculosis be treated beyond the period of infectiousness until they are cured. In 1992, a panel meeting under the auspices of the United Hospital Fund of New York made the attainment of "treatment until cure" the centerpiece of its recommendations. The Advisory Council for the Elimination of Tuberculosis underscored the necessity of treatment until cure in its 1993 report on the status of TB control laws throughout the United States.

The ethical, legal, and constitutional principles that justify public health efforts to control tuberculosis seem broad enough to justify efforts to assure that all patients with tuberculosis are treated until cured. Legal commentators have endorsed the goal of treatment until cure, as have advocates acting on behalf of individuals with HIV infection and AIDS. There has been sharp controversy, however, over the nature of the public health interventions that might be employed to achieve the goal of treatment completion, and the extent to which the legal and ethical principles that guide medical and public health practice should constrain the exercise of those interventions.

ETHICAL AND LEGAL ISSUES IN ENHANCING PATIENT ADHERENCE TO TREATMENT

Although there may be exceptions, patients diagnosed with acute infectious tuberculosis tend to be compliant with treatment because of the desire to be rid of the unpleasant symptoms of the disease—weakness, fever, cough, and night-sweats. Much more complex is the attainment of compliance during the post-acute phase of tuberculosis, when symptoms no longer motivate the patient to take his or her medication. Poor patient compliance with treatment is not unique to tuberculosis, although failure to complete therapy for many other diseases does not have the same dire individual and public health consequences.

Any effective approach to improving adherence to therapy must be sensitive to the obstacles to treatment that face the economically disadvantaged and socially marginalized people among whom tuberculosis is most common. The prevalence of homelessness, drug abuse, alcoholism, and psychiatric comorbidity are factors that must be considered in shaping policies to enhance treatment completion. Brudney, who has been particularly concerned with tuberculosis among the homeless, has written:

> Homelessness, by definition, means lack of permanent shelter. Whether a person lives on the streets, wanders from one SRO to another, or moves in and out of a congregate facility, medical care is rarely his or her first priority. The daily search for food and shelter belie the possibility of an organized schedule, appointment keeping or routine medical ingestion as is necessary with TB treatment. Alcoholism, drug dependence and psychiatric disturbances affect anywhere from 50 to 90 percent of the homeless, and the notion that persons so affected can remember and comply with clinic appointments and medication regimens is laughable.

In ethics there is a dictum that states "ought implies can." A person cannot be held morally accountable for failing to adhere to ethical or legal standards if he or she cannot do so, or if he or she faces insuperable obstacles to adherence. This ethical principle compels us to recognize that the elimination of impediments that impinge on the capacity of an individual to cooperate in his or her own care for tuberculosis is essential. This is especially so given the prospect of the imposition of compulsory measures and the potential loss of liberty for those who are not compliant. What are the practical implications of "ought implies can"?

The goal of treatment completion and the ethical norms that should shape the measures used to attain that goal require that homeless individuals not be discharged from hospitals to the streets or to chaotic and often dangerous mass shelters after treatment for their acute infectious tuberculosis. They cannot reasonably be expected to comply with their care unless they are provided with a secure residence and, in many instances, with other social supports. That is also true of prisoners with tuberculosis whose sentences come to an end before their treatment has been completed. Individuals with drug or alcohol addiction must be provided with referrals and access to treatment programs. So too must individuals with psychiatric illnesses that could impair their capacity to comply with long-term, often complex, treatment regimens. Unfortunately, hospital discharge plans rarely, if ever, assure access to such supportive services that facilitate treatment. The provision of such services will be costly, but will ultimately be less costly than the consequences of treatment failure—the spread of tuberculosis and the potential development of drug-resistance. Furthermore, effective outpatient services are less costly than the confinement of patients in secure facilities.

The ethical requirement that the government provide supportive services to enhance the prospect of compliance may find legal expression in the constitutional principle that requires the state to use the least restrictive means possible to achieve its goals when individual liberties are at stake. More than three decades ago the U.S. Supreme Court held in *Shelton v. Tucker:*

> Even though the governmental purpose be legitimate and substantial, that purpose cannot be pursued by means that broadly stifle fundamental personal liberties when the end can be more narrowly achieved. The breadth of legislative abridgment must be viewed in the light of less drastic means for achieving the same basic purpose.

In *Lessard v. Schmidt,* a Federal District Court decision handed down in 1972, the implications of this standard were further defined. The state "must bear the burden of proving (1) what alternatives are available; (2) what alternatives were investigated; and (3) why the investigated alternatives were not deemed suitable."

Public health authorities now generally recognize that it is preferable, from both an ethical and a practical perspective, to make affirmative efforts to encourage voluntary compliance with health precautions before resorting to coercive action. In the context of tuberculosis, federal, state, and local health authorities acknowledge the importance of providing social supports and other "enablers"—such as car fare, meals, and even small cash payments—for undergoing care. However, it remains unclear whether what is accepted in principle will be put into practice by health officials. Also unclear is whether a court would *legally* require the state to expend public resources to enhance the prospect of compliance with TB therapy before taking more coercive action.

For some advocates for patients with tuberculosis, the case for requiring the provision of services before depriving a patient of liberty is clear. The New York City Tuberculosis Working Group, for example, has argued:

In deciding whether the prescription against forced detention had been overcome by clear and convincing evidence, the court would consider any evidence of mitigating circumstances including failures by the City to provide services or benefits to which the patient was entitled. . . . It is unethical, illegal, and bad public policy to detain "non-compliant" person's before making concerted efforts to address the numerous systematic deficiencies that make adherence to treatment virtually impossible for many New Yorkers.

From the perspective of the Working Group, the government that fails to provide adequate social supports for the most vulnerable loses the legal as well as the moral authority to threaten with a deprivation of liberty those whose behavior poses a health risk.

However, poor public policy—even unethical public policy—is not necessarily unconstitutional. A court would have to consider whether a failure on the part of the government to provide a particular service—for example, a stable apartment, as opposed to a bed in a dangerous shelter—renders an effort to impose restrictions on individual liberty constitutionally suspect. At a time when government resources are limited, a court would also have to consider whether the claims of those with tuberculosis, who are threatened with a deprivation of liberty, are always to be given precedence over those who are equally needy but who do not have tuberculosis. Must the state always give priority to those with tuberculosis who find themselves on long waiting lists for drug treatment? Or for minimally decent living conditions? Must they be given priority over those who may have waited for extended periods and who may be quite desperate, perhaps even more desperate? The legal question posed here is whether the doctrine of the least restrictive alternative, which initially served as a negative limit on government action (i.e. the state cannot hospitalize if outpatient care would have been as effective), can also be interpreted to impose positive obligations on government, such as an obligation to provide social supports that may facilitate compliance? . . .

DIRECTLY OBSERVED THERAPY

Among the strategies designed to enhance patient compliance is directly observed therapy (DOT), a practice that involves having the patient take his or her medications in the presence of a health care provider or other responsible third party. First proposed for individuals with poor records of treatment adherence and for those whose demographic or psychological profile suggested a high risk of treatment failure, directly observed therapy has emerged as a standard of care. Recently, the Centers for Disease Control and Prevention, a number of prominent physicians, and others have recommended that all tuberculosis patients be placed on a regime of directly observed therapy, at least in localities where rates of completion fall below an acceptable level. Indeed, the Advisory Council for the Elimination of Tuberculosis calls for DOT in areas where treatment completion falls below 90%.

The primary rationale for the administration of medications under direct supervision is the recognition that nonadherence is common among patients who must take medication over an extended time period. In the case of tuberculosis, such noncompliance has the grave consequence of leading to drug resistance and reactivation of clinical disease. The CDC recommends that DOT "be considered for all patients because of the difficulty in predicting which patients will adhere to a prescribed treatment regimen." In addition, the recommendation for universal, rather than selective, DOT is motivated by a desire to avoid discrimination based on race, social class, and other factors that providers may perceive to have an effect on compliance.

The practice of directly observed therapy has been efficacious from a public health perspective. It has contributed to increasing rates of treatment completion. In addition, a recent study in Texas found substantial declines in the rates of drug resistance and relapse after the institution of a county-wide program of universal directly observed therapy. The rate of primary drug resistance (i.e. the patient contracted a drug-resistant strain from another person) decreased from 13.0 percent to 6.7 percent, while the rate of acquired resistance (i.e. a patient's initially drug-sensitive strain became resistant, probably due to a treatment failure) declined from 14.0% to 2.1 %. The relapse rate declined from 20.9% to 5.5%.

From an ethical, legal, and constitutional perspective, the important question is not who should be *offered* the support of DOT, but rather, when may DOT be *imposed* by the state.

Faced with the dramatic rise of multidrug-resistant tuberculosis and data that suggested very high rates of treatment failure, Iseman, Cohn & Sbarbaro put forth a public health argument for universal directly observed therapy.

> We believe it is time for entirely intermittent directly observed treatment programs to be used for all patients. Some will argue that it will be impossible to treat every patient with directly observed therapy and that many people with tuberculosis do comply with treatment and would be offended by having to submit to direct observation while they swallow-medications. Unfortunately, the literature is replete with studies demonstrating . . . that professionals are not able to distinguish the compliant from the noncompliant in advance.

Given the price of failure, in morbidity, mortality, and the cost of treating resistant strains of TB, they conclude, "we cannot afford not to try it." The case for universal directly observed therapy, at least at the outset of treatment, has also been made by the United Hospital Fund Working Group on Tuberculosis and HIV. It too was concerned by the failure of other approaches to achieve high rates of treatment completion and by the inability of professionals to predict treatment adherence. Though fully aware of the burdens that DOT would entail for some individuals, the working group concluded that, on ethical and legal grounds, universal DOT was desirable:

> The fact that all start their post-hospitalization treatment under a common program of supervision should help to reduce the stigma of treatment and create an effective public health plan for the control of TB. Such an approach will also limit the extent to which initial treatment decisions violate the principle of justice which seeks to preclude acts of invidious discrimination.

The call for universal directly observed therapy has provoked sharp opposition. First, it has been argued that such an effort would entail an enormous waste of scarce resources. Funds that could best be used to provide services to those most in need would be diverted to the supervision of those who would be compliant on their own. But most critically, universal directly observed therapy has been challenged as an unethical intrusion upon autonomy, as "gratuitously annoying"; as a violation of the constitutional requirement that the least restrictive alternative be used; and as contrary to the requirements of the Americans With Disabilities Act that decisions involving restrictions on those with disabilities be based on an individualized assessment. The Policy Director for the Gay Men's Health Crisis, D. Hansel, has written:

> I cannot see how mandatory directly observed therapy can be reconciled with the principle of the least restrictive alternative in the exercise of governmental power, since it would require the imposition of a coercive treatment regime in a class of people without any showing that they, as individuals will fail voluntarily to follow a course of medical treatment. Nor does it comport with basic Constitutional due process principles, which require an individualized determination before state sanctions are imposed.

Legal commentators too have generally rejected mandatory, DOT as overly broad and thus violative of constitutional principles. However, this opposition to *universal* DOT should not be construed as a rejection of *mandatory* DOT in all cases. Even advocates for patients' civil liberties accept mandatory, court-ordered DOT in cases of clear noncompliance, especially when the alternative appears to be involuntary confinement.

In its 1993 revision of the New York City Health Code, the City's Board of Health rejected universal mandatory DOT and instead authorized the Commissioner of Health to impose DOT on patients who were noncompliant with treatment during the noninfectious stage of their illness.

DETENTION OF NON-COMPLIANT PATIENTS

As noted earlier . . . ethical, legal, and constitutional principles have long recognized the authority of the state to confine individuals with infectious tuberculosis when they pose a threat to the health of others. This power to deprive an individual of his or her liberty in the name of public health has vested public health officials with an authority that, from the perspective of the individual, may be indistinguishable from that wielded by the criminal justice system. Yet until relatively recently, the protections accorded to defendants in criminal prosecutions have not been extended to those viewed as a threat to the public health. As late as 1966, a California appellate court upheld the confinement of a TB patient pursuant to a law that provided virtually no procedural protections for the patient. In its ruling, the court, quoting an earlier case, stated:

> Health regulations enacted by the state under its police power and providing even drastic measures for the elimination of disease . . . in a general way are not affected by constitutional provisions, either of the state or national government.

This broad deference to the legislature and to the exercise of public health powers would come to look archaic just a few years later, as the jurisprudence of confinement underwent a radical revision in the wake of a series of far-reaching constitutional challenges to the power of the state to confine patients with psychiatric disorders to mental hospitals. By 1979, Chief Justice Burger would state in *Addington v. Texas:*

> This Court has repeatedly recognized that civil commitment for any purpose constitutes a significant deprivation of liberty that requires due process protection. Moreover, it is indisputable that involuntary commitment to a mental hospital . . . can engender adverse social consequences to the individual. Whether we label this phenomena "stigma" or choose to call it something else is less important than that we recognize that it can occur and that it can have a very significant impact on the individual.

It was on the basis of such developments in mental health law, rather than as a result of challenges to the actions of public health officials in responding to tuberculosis cases, that it became possible to assert successfully that TB patients be accorded the procedural protections guaranteed by the Constitution. In 1980, in the only reported appellate court decision to date upholding the procedural rights of a tuberculosis patient, the Supreme Court of Appeals in West Virginia articulated a standard that expressly followed the developments in mental health law. The state's Tuberculosis Control Act was ruled unconstitutional because it did not guarantee the right to counsel, did not provide for the right to cross examine, confront and present witnesses, and failed to hold the state to the stringent "clear and convincing" standard of proof required by *Addington.*

Although the West Virginia decision is not controlling in other states, the social transformation in the legal and political context within which issues of confinement were considered in the 1970s and 1980s did shape policy and practice in the United States. . . .

This expansion on the conceptions of who posed a threat to the public health, driven by concerns about MDR-TB, represented a move of great significance. No longer did the person to be confined have to represent an immediate threat of transmission. Rather it was the *prospect* of reactivation and the *prospect* of the development of drug-resistance that provided the grounds for state intervention. Here the concept of "threat" was informed by the population-based concerns of public health. It was concern about the collective consequence of permitting many individuals to conduct themselves in a way that posed some threat that motivated the extension of public health powers to reach noninfectious TB patients. But this was a calculus far different from one that would center on the potential risk posed by a given individual. Nevertheless, legal commentators have, by and large, agreed that "confinement until cure would probably be found constitutional for noninfectious patients who did not adhere to treatment."

A striking reflection of the expansion of the concept of what constitutes a public health threat was the adoption in 1993 of treatment until cure regulations by the New York City Board of Health. Under the newly enacted Section 11.47 of the City's Health Code, the Commissioner may confine an individual for whom there is a "substantial likelihood, based on such person's past and present behavior, that he or she cannot be relied upon" to complete treatment. Under the amended code, a court review must be accorded to a confined patient within five business days, and even if the individual does not request release, the Department of Health must seek judicial review within the first 60 days of detention, and subsequently at 90-day intervals. Upon requesting release, the confined individual is entitled to a lawyer, and, if too poor to afford counsel, must be provided with one at public expense. . . .

FORCED MEDICATION

Remarkably, the very New York Health Code that extended the scope of the Commissioner's authority to isolate noncompliant patients despite their noninfectious status states that the regulations are "not to be construed to permit or require the forcible administration of any medication without a prior court order." In part, this restraint is simply a reflection of prevailing constitutional doctrines that recognize the rights of psychiatric patients, even criminally or civilly committed patients, to refuse treatment. It also reflects the importance of general principles of autonomy and informed consent. At the heart of judicial rulings that have established the right to refuse medication is the assumption that individuals may retain the right to some self-determination even when confined because they pose a risk to themselves or others. In *Rivers v. Katz,* the

New York Court of Appeals held that a civilly committed patient can be compelled to accept medication only after a judicial determination that the individual lacked the capacity to make a reasoned decision about the particular treatment. The determination of capacity was to be made at a hearing at which the patient was afforded representation by a lawyer.

What holds for a patient whose mental capacities are impaired is certainly true for those who are confined for tuberculosis, where no assumption about such impairment can be made. A decisionally capable patient may choose to forgo treatment even at the risk of death. That is the bedrock of the principle of informed consent. But such a patient does not have the right to endanger others. That is the bedrock of the statutory authority to confine noncompliant TB patients. It is, of course, possible that in a given case the refusal to accept medication may reflect psychiatric impairment. Under such circumstances, and after appropriate judicial review, compulsory treatment of the psychiatric disorder might be undertaken to enhance the prospect that the patient would be able to make an informed judgment about whether to cooperate in the treatment of his or her tuberculosis. But the ultimate paradox may remain: The state may confine a noncompliant individual because of the failure to undergo treatment, but may not impose treatment on the confined patient. This paradox underscores the fundamental limits of state power in a liberal society: The government may act to protect the public, but not to protect the competent individual from, his own willful, perhaps foolish, choices.

CONCLUSION

From both an ethical and legal perspective, the state has an obligation to assure that the population is protected against the ravages of infectious disease. That responsibility in the context of tuberculosis is best exercised by the development of programs and strategies designed to facilitate the identification and treatment of those with disease. In large measure, the central public health goals can be achieved by encouraging the cooperation of patients with tuberculosis. The expanded provision of directly observed therapy, indeed the establishment of directly observed therapy as a standard of care, may also be crucial. There will, however, be occasions when recourse to coercion will be necessary to protect the public health. Such occasions come at a price both because of the public costs of confinement and the individual's loss of liberty. But acknowledging that it may be necessary to rely on coercion should not be confused with making compulsion the centerpiece of a tuberculosis program. For pragmatic and principled reasons, coercion must be viewed as a last resort.

Much has been learned since the resurgence of tuberculosis took a place on the national agenda in the early 1990s. It has become clear that the rise in the number of cases, and, more centrally, the increase in the number of multidrug-resistant cases stemmed, at least in part, from the erosion of the public health infrastructure and the intensification of poverty and overcrowding in urban areas. With public alarm providing the motivation, governmental expenditures on TB control rose sharply. Those funds made possible a rapid expansion of local health department initiatives, including the broadening of voluntary directly observed therapy. In New York City, for example, the number of TB patients receiving directly observed treatment increased from fewer than 100 in 1991 to more than 1200 in 1993. The fruits of those efforts may be reflected in 1993 statistics, which for the first time in eight years on a national level and the first time in 14 years in New York City indicate that new cases of tuberculosis declined. It is too soon to know whether these numbers represent a trend or a statistical adjustment. But what is certain is that if stabilizing or declining tuberculosis cases provoke another cycle of budgetary retrenchment, the foundations for yet another upsurge in cases will have been laid. This time history will repeat itself not as tragedy but as farce.

Medical Science, Infectious Disease, and the Unity of Humankind

JOSHUA LEDERBERG

The ravaging epidemic of acquired immunodeficiency syndrome has shocked the world. It is still not comprehended widely that it is a natural, almost predictable, phenomenon. We will face similar catastrophes again, and will be ever more confounded in dealing with them, if we do not come to grips with the realities of the place of our species in nature. A large measure of humanistic progress is dedicated to the subordination of human nature to our ideals of individual perfectability and autonomy. Human intelligence, culture, and technology have left all other plant and animal species out of the competition. We also may legislate human behavior. But we have too many illusions that we can, by writ, govern the remaining vital kingdoms, the microbes, that remain our competitors of last resort for dominion of the planet. The bacteria and viruses know nothing of national sovereignties. In that natural evolutionary competition, there is no guarantee that we will find ourselves the survivor.

Some of the great successes of medical science, including the "miracle drugs," the antibiotics of the 1940s, have inculcated premature complacency on the part of the broader culture. Most people today are grossly overoptimistic with respect to the means we have available to forfend global epidemics comparable with the Black Death of the 14th century (or on a lesser scale the influenza of 1918), which took a toll of millions of lives.

Visualize human life on this planet as mirrored in the microcosm of a culture of bacteria; a laboratory test tube can hold ten billion cells, twice the human population of the globe. More than 70 years ago, Frederick William Twort and Felix d'Herelle discovered that bacteria have their own virus parasites, the bacteriophages. It is not unusual to observe a thriving bacterial population of a billion cells undergo a dramatic wipeout, a massive lysis, a sudden clearing of the broth following a spontaneous mutation that extends the host range of a single virus particle. A hundred billion virus particles will succeed the bacteria;

From the *Journal of the American Medical Association,* 260 (August 5, 1988), 684–685. Reprinted by permission of the American Medical Association.

but their own fate now is problematic, as they will have exhausted their prey (within that test tube). Perhaps there are a few bacterial survivors: mutant bacteria that now resist the mutant virus. If so, these can repopulate the test tube until perhaps a second round, a mutant-mutant virus, appears.

Such processes are not unique to the test tube. The time scale, the numerical odds, will be different. The fundamental biologic principles are the same.

Humans are more dispersed over the planetary surface than are the "bugs" in a glass tube; there are more diverse sanctuaries, and we have somewhat fewer opportunities to infect one another. The culture medium in the test tube is more hospitable to virus transmission than is the space between people (with the exceptions of sexual contact and transfusion). The ozone shield still lets through enough solar ultraviolet light to hinder aerosol transmission, and most viruses are fairly vulnerable to desiccation in dry air. The unbroken skin is an excellent barrier to infection; the mucous membranes of the respiratory tract are much less so. Our immune defenses are a wonderfully intricate legacy of our own evolutionary history. This enables machinery for producing an indefinite panoply of antibodies, some one of which is (we may hope) a specific match to the antigenic challenge of a particular invading parasite. In the normal, immune-competent individual, each incipient infection is a mortal race between the penetration and proliferation of the virus within the body and the evolution and expansion of antibodies that may be specific for that infection. Previous vaccination or infection with a related virus will facilitate an early immune response. This in turn provides selective pressure on the virus populations, encouraging the emergence of antigenic variants. We see this most dramatically in the influenza pandemics, and every few years we need to disseminate fresh vaccines to cope with the current generation of the flu virus.

Many defense mechanisms, inherent in our evolved biologic capabilities, thus mitigate the pandemic viral threat. Mitigation also is built into the evolution of the virus; it is a Pyrrhic victory for a virus to eradicate its host! This may have happened historically, but then both the vanquished host and the victorious parasite will have disappeared. Even the death of the single infected individual is relatively disadvantageous, in the long run, to the virus compared with a sustained infection that leaves a carrier free to spread the virus to as many contacts as possible. From the perspective of the virus, the ideal would be a nearly symptomless infection in which the host is oblivious of providing shelter and nourishment for the indefinite propagation of the virus' genes. Our own genome carries hundreds or thousands of such stowaways. The boundary between them and the "normal genome" is quite blurred. Not much more than 1% of our DNA can be assigned specific physiological functions; most of it is assumed to be a "fossil" legacy of our prior evolutionary history, DNA that is today parasitic on the cell. Further, we know that many viruses can acquire genetic information from their hosts, which from time to time they may transfer to new ones. Hence, intrinsic to our own ancestry and nature are not only Adam and Eve, but any number of invisible germs that have crept into our chromosomes. Some confer incidental and mutual benefit. Others of these symbiotic viruses or "plasmids" have reemerged as oncogenes, with the potential to mutate to a state that we recognize as the dysregulated cell growth of a cancer. This is a form of Darwinian evolution that momentarily enhances the fitness of a cell clone at the expense of the entire organism. Still other segments of "nonfunctional" DNA are available as reserves of genetic potential for further evolution, in a sense more constructive for the individual and the species.

At evolutionary equilibrium we would continue to share the planet with our internal and external parasites, paying some tribute, perhaps sometimes deriving from them some protection against more violent aggression. The terms of that equilibrium are unwelcome: present knowledge does not offer much hope that we can eradicate the competition. Meanwhile, our parasites and ourselves must share in the dues, payable in a currency of discomfort and precariousness of life. No theory lets us calculate the details; we can hardly be sure that such an equilibrium for earth even includes the human species even as we contrive to eliminate some of the others. Our propensity for technological sophistication harnessed to intraspecies competition adds a further dimension of hazard.

In fact, innumerable perturbations remind us that complex systems often fluctuate far from equilibrium—each individual death of an infected person is a counterexample. Our defense mechanisms do not always work. Viruses are not always as benign as they would be if each particle had the intelligence and altruism to serve the long-term advantage of the group.

Fears of new epidemics as virulent as those of the past have been modified by the expectation that modern hygiene and medicine would contain any such outbreaks. There is, of course, much merit in those expectations. Influenza in 1918 was undoubtedly complicated by bacterial infection that now can be treated with antibiotics; vaccines, if we can mobilize them in time, can help prevent the global spread of a new flu. However, the impact of technology is not all on the human side of the struggle. Monoculture of plants and animals has made them more exposed to devastation. The increasing density of human habitations as well as inventions such as the subway and the jet airplane that mix populations all add to the risks of spread of infection. Paradoxically, improvements in sanitation and vaccination sometimes make us the more vulnerable because they leave the larger human herd more innocent of microbial experience.

The opening of wild lands to human occupation also has exposed people to unaccustomed animal viruses, to zoonoses. Yellow fever has sustained reservoirs in jungle primates, and the same source is the probable origin of the human immunodeficiency virus in Africa. It is mystifying that yellow fever has not become endemic in India, where competent mosquitoes and susceptible people abound. We will almost certainly be having like experiences from the "opening" of the Amazon basin.

Our preoccupation with acquired immunodeficiency syndrome should not obscure the multiplicity of infectious diseases that threaten our future. It is none too soon to start a systematic watch for new viruses before they become so irrevocably lodged. The fundamental bases of virus research can hardly be given too much encouragement. Recombinant DNA, still a scare word in some quarters, is our most potent means of analyzing viruses and developing vaccines. Such research should be done on a broad international scale to both share the progress made in advanced countries and amplify the opportunities for field work at the earliest appearance of outbreaks in the most afflicted areas.

The basic principles of vaccination were established long ago, but practical means of production of vaccines for viral afflictions like polio had to await the cell and tissue culture advances of the 1950s. The most celebrated example, smallpox, also has the oldest historical roots. That success has encouraged other proposals for the eradication of other infectious agents. Rarely do we have the understanding of its natural history needed to calibrate the feasibility of the goal. This will strain our basic knowledge of the genetics and evolution of the etiologic agents.

For example, our stratagems on malaria, gonococcus, and human immunodeficiency virus are all confounded by the poorly understood capacity of the viruses to undergo further antigenic evolution. We know a bit more about influenza, but not enough to give us more than a few weeks or months of lead time merely to respond to its perennial variations.

As one species, we share a common vulnerability to these scourges. No matter how selfish our motives, we can no longer be indifferent to the suffering of others. The microbe that felled one child in a distant continent yesterday can reach yours today and seed a global pandemic tomorrow. "Never send to know for whom the bell tolls; it tolls for thee."

Emerging Diseases and Ecosystem Instability: New Threats to Public Health

PAUL R. EPSTEIN

INTRODUCTION

The 1980s marked the return of infectious diseases to front stage. Of course, infectious diseases never disappeared outside the West. Today, many direct contagions, such as tuberculosis, multidrug resistant tuberculosis, pertussis, and diphtheria, and those involving vectors and animal reservoirs such as yellow fever, malaria, and dengue, are undergoing redistribution. Indeed, the present period of unprecedented ecological change and the growing economic and social crises that are driving vast movements of hosts are together contributing to the resurgence of old pests and the appearance of new ones. Important components in this rapid evolution are the vulnerabilities of ecosystems and instabilities in climate.

The Centers for Disease Control and Prevention (CDC) has launched a program to monitor and mitigate emerging diseases by focusing on the evolution of new pathogens and the reemergence or redistribution of old ones. The range of issues involved were recently reviewed and were the subject of an interdisciplinary workshop in Woods Hole, Mass, sponsored by Harvard School of Public Health New Disease Group in November 1993.

Two new diseases of 1993—a virulent viral strain appearing in the United States and a novel cholera variant bursting upon the scene in Asia—are cause for alarm and demand pause for reflection. But once the precise agents have been identified, a deeper comprehension of the web of environmental, social, and host factors from which they have emerged, and of the breakdowns in "natural" controls on species abundance that they represent, can reveal a great deal about the "health"—the stability, resilience, diversity, and vigor—of Earth's life-support systems.

From the *American Journal of Public Health*, 85 (1995), 168–170. Reprinted by permission of the American Public Health Association.

THE HANTAVIRUS

In the southwestern United States, hantavirus infection has been confirmed in 94 persons in 20 states with 48% mortality (Dr J. Woodall, New York State Department of Health, personal communication, October 10, 1994). In Louisiana, a variant close to but distinct from the "four-corners" strain killed a bridge worker; a "cousin" hantavirus was found in a Floridian (who survived) and remains present in local cotton rats (*Sigmodon hispidus*); another variant was found in Indiana; and in February 1994, a 22-year-old student in Rhode Island died of possibly another variant.

The sudden appearance of an unexpected and lethal clinical presentation (hantavirus pulmonary syndrome), caused by viruses that have perhaps long existed at low levels in rodent populations and were previously associated with distinctly different clinical entities, raises important questions. Was the related virus that was identified in 1983 by serology and polymerase chain reaction in similar mouse populations in the Southwest as virulent then for humans as it is today, or is the current high mortality indicative of a new strain? Are the extreme virulence and new cell tropism (pulmonary versus renal and hemopoietic) also signs of a novel variant? Or has an extant viral agent been amplified through changes in rodent ecology, and have conditions helped select and disseminate a highly virulent variant?

An Evolving Agent?

In the past, hantaviruses have been associated with hemorrhagic fever with renal syndrome and perhaps with chronic nephropathy. Four distinct hantaviruses of the family *Bunyaviridae*—Hantaan, Puumala, Seoul, and Prospect Hill—have been identified, and several others have been described in Southeast Asia and in Europe. In the 1950s, Hantaan virus caused Korean hemorrhagic fever with renal syndrome in thousands of United States and United Nations troops, although the etiology remained obscure until 1976. Puumala virus, carried in the European bank vole (*Clethrionomys glareolus*), produces a milder neuropathia epidemica in Scandinavia and the Balkans, as does Seoul virus in Asia. During the 1980s, hantaviruses were isolated from domestic rats in Texas; from deer mice (*Peromyscus maniculatus*) and humans in California, Colorado, and New Mexico; and from a meadow vole captured on Prospect Hill, Md. To date, this last has been unassociated with human disease. The current variant was named Muerto Canyon virus after the locale of recognition, which prompted some Native Americans to contest the name; it has been since designated "Sin Nombre."

Hantaviruses, apparently asymptomatic in rodents and transmitted in their saliva and excreta, may be associated with hypertension and chronic renal disease in the United States. However, the 1993 appearance was the first outbreak of acute illness associated with the hantavirus in the United States, and its flulike presentation, followed swiftly by acute respiratory distress syndrome, is unique. In the four-corners area, *P. maniculatus,* which is widespread in North America, appears to be the primary reservoir host (as it is for Lyme disease [*Borrelia burgdorferi*]), while another close relative may harbor the Louisiana strain. The CDC has issued guidelines for minimizing indoor and outdoor exposure to all rodents.

Reports of new *Hantavirus* isolates from new areas of Europe suggest that other hantaviruses are present in other geographically isolated rodent populations (Dr S. S. Morse, Rockefeller University, personal communication, March 1994). The identification of Puumala virus (normally found in voles) in the house mouse (*Mus musculus*) in Yugoslavia suggests that interspecies transfer of hantaviruses can occur under suitable conditions. Because emerging infections often arise in areas undergoing ecological or demographic change, the former Yugoslavia, beset by war and economic breakdown, is a critical region and deserves close monitoring.

A Changing Environment

A likely scenario in the southwestern United States is that heavy rains following 6 years of drought caused pine nuts and grasshoppers to flourish, thereby nourishing deer mice. Then, driven from underground burrows by flooding, a swollen population of natural hosts (a 10-fold increase from May 1992 to May 1993) enhanced the chance for the virus to thrive and be passed on. Thus, whatever the hantavirus' route of entry into the human population, alterations in nutrient supplies and in the ratio of prey with *Peromyscus* predators (owls, snakes, coyotes, and cats) created selection pressures for the emergence or amplification of an apparently new variant of *Hantavirus.*

A Navajo chief reflected, "We suffer for we have not taken better care of the earth" and "our people have lost harmony with nature." The landscape and diversity of animals in the region, where rainwater channeled from rocky outcrops once irrigated the fields, have declined from overgrazing and deforestation. But large climatological swings and a year of great storms (witness the blizzards and the floods of 1993 and 1994) may reflect even greater instability in Earth's natural systems.

Weather patterns and jet streams across North and South America, western Europe, Asia, and Africa are strongly influenced by the Pacific Ocean warming center. El Niño events, which begin at Christmastime, determine patterns for a year and have, until recently, occurred about twice a decade. Warmer seas evaporate quickly, yielding greater precipitation over some areas and drought in others. The strength of the 1992/93 El Niño was unexpected, and the endurance of $+2$ to $3°C$ anomalies in ocean temperatures into summer was unprecedented. Because the persistence of negative South Pacific sea-level pressures that drive El Niño now spans over 4 years (an occurrence without analogue in the historical record), and warming is predicted to continue at least through the 1994/95 winter, weather patterns have become particularly erratic and volatile (i.e., unstable).

Leading climatologists have projected more frequent El Niño events, with greater variation in storm frequency, onset, intensity, and duration, accompanying a continued increase in greenhouse gases. The ocean is a "global thermostat," explains Rachel Carson in *The Sea Around Us,* and the warming atmosphere transfers heat to the oceans for worldwide distribution. It is the global "conveyor belt" of warm Gulf Streams moving north, and of deep, cold southward currents, that may have stalled (or reversed directions) to produce the rapid climate swings of the past, as disclosed in Greenland ice-core records.

Monitoring El Niños, temperature, wind, and precipitation patterns, and biodiversity has enormous implications for surveillance of disease vectors and reservoirs; indeed, the widespread resurgence of infections may have profound implications for future fossil fuel and forestry policies.

A NOVEL VARIANT OF CHOLERA

In India and Bangladesh, a new variant of cholera erupted in January 1993. By mid-April, the novel form of *Vibrio cholerae*—armed with cholera enterotoxin plus a colonizing gene and bearing a previously undetected antigen (O139)—had invaded Calcutta (15 000 cases, 230 dead) and saturated Dhaka (600 cases per day at peak). The novel strain, dubbed "O139 Bengal," which is considered more hardy than biotype El Tor in terms of its environmental adaptation (Dr R. B. Sack, Johns Hopkins University School of Hygiene and Public Health, personal communication, April 1994), is spreading in Thailand and Pakistan and is present in 10 Southeast Asian nations (R. Cash, MD, Harvard School of Public Health, personal communication, May 1994). Its epidemiological spectrum, infecting adults and children, indicates the absence of cross-immunity between it and El Tor, the agent of the ongoing seventh pandemic that left Asia in 1961. One case has been imported into the United States, but the "anastomoses" between water supplies and sanitation requisite for endemicity are largely absent, save for the Mexico-US border region.

The Algal Reservoir

Aquatic plants, seaweeds, and freefloating phyto- and zooplankton can harbor vibrios in viable but nonculturable, sporelike forms, as demonstrated by fluorescent antibody and polymerase chain reaction techniques. (Note that O139 Bengal has not been tested in this regard, but there is no reason to suspect that its affinity for algae and weeds is different from that of other O1 and non-O1 vibrios.) The growth of marine and freshwater photosynthesizers is prompted by nitrogen-rich wastewater, fertilizers, acid rain, and runoff soil (eutrophication). Wetlands and mangroves ("nature's kidneys") filter out nitrates and phosphates. While inputs are increasing, the filtration systems are being lost to development and aquaculture, diking and drilling. Concurrently, fish stocks (predators of plankton) are in decline in 14 of the world's 17 major fishing grounds. In addition, climate-related warmer sea surface temperatures also increase algae growth by (1) augmenting photosynthesis and algal metabolism, (2) increasing nutrient-rich coastal upwelling, and (3) shifting the community of organisms toward more toxic species ("red tides," fish and shellfish poisoning), which are in turn less palatable to grazers. Indeed, planktonologists postulate a "global epidemic" of coastal algal blooms that may well represent one of the first biological signals of global change (Dr T. J. Smayda, University of Rhode Island School of Oceanography, personal communication, June 1994).

Other Vibrios

El Tor *V. cholerae* may have arrived in the Americas in the ballast and bilge-water of ships coming from Asia, there finding abundant algal blooms for amplification; from there it hitchhiked in Latin American ship hulls to the US Gulf Coast. And in the Gulf, another vibrio (*Vibrio vulnificus*), found in oysters, has caused deaths in Florida residents with preexisting liver disease.

Sanitation and water supplies—environmental conditions inside national boundaries—have been the primary focus of public health interventions (and are certainly not meant to be minimized by this analysis). However, it may be that widespread changes in coastal ecology are generating "hot systems" in which mutations (random, perhaps adaptive—bacteriophage, ultraviolet-B light, or chemically initiated) are being selected and amplified under new environmental pressures and then transferred to human populations through the food chain (fish and shellfish). In addition to O139 Bengal, more antibiotic-resistant forms of *V. cholerae* O1, biotype El Tor, have emerged; and in Peru a chlorine-defiant "rugose" variant has surfaced (perhaps related to intermittent disinfection), adding a new mixture of cholera organisms to penetrate poor populations that have little access to potable water.

As threats to marine resources, food safety, and sustainable yields result in direct costs to fishing communities, marine biologists are becoming increasingly concerned for the overall health of marine ecosystems. The new variant of *V. cholerae* intrudes upon planned trials of an oral recombinant vaccine, and although it took the seventh pandemic 30 years to become global, we may expect a more rapid dissemination of O139 Bengal, the agent of an eighth world pandemic. An early warning system—monitoring algal blooms (guided by remote sensing), fish, and shellfish samples for vibrios—is feasible.

CONCLUSIONS

The links between the environment and health may be direct (from toxins to heat waves or cold spells) or indirect (involving intermediate species as vectors and/or reservoirs). At the 1993 Wood Hole conference, participants from the CDC and the World Health Organization, and from universities and institutes in the United States and abroad, concluded that a major impediment to disease monitoring and detection was the fragmentation of epidemiology and scientific disciplines. In response, a new framework is emerging, one that incorporate meteorological mean values (i.e., the climate regime) and anomalies, ecosystem-based findings, molecular epidemiological techniques, *and* surveillance of indicator species (e.g., rodents, insects, and algae) and health outcomes. Integrating surveillance of biological indicators that carry disease—that is, of rapid responders that are therefore sensitive indicators of perturbed environments—is key. It was fortuitous that an ecological station in Sevilleta, NM, was monitoring deer mice, and our knowledge of the marine food web comes from microbiologists, oceanographers, and ichthyologists—groups that do not readily coordinate their findings and data. Geographic information and mapping systems offer a new methodology to integrate systems by overlaying and fusing data sets.

Focusing on critical regions where life-support systems such as water and soil fertility are fragile can also improve monitoring. Land-use changes (deforestation for farming) leading to shifts in rodent species, combined with an influx of nonimmune workers, are apparently related to five emerging arenaviruses in Latin America (Lassa in several nations, Junin in Argentina, Machupo in Bolivia, Guaranito in Venezuela, and Sabiá in Brazil), all of which are associated with hemorrhagic fevers and high case fatality. Many new and resurgent diseases reflect bioclimatic conditions permissive for parasite and pest persistence, and the emergence of hantavirus in a US terrestrial setting, as well as the evolution and spread of cholera in the marine environment, provide illuminating case studies for future health monitoring and environmental management.

Finally, while social, political, and economic factors are not the immediate focus of this paper, they are clearly integral to the condition and management of the environment, for therein lie the driving forces of global change (the cumulative effects of local inputs and transformations) and the inequitable distribution of exposures, vulnerabilities, and access to treatment. Just as the 19th-century confluence of urban epidemics (tuberculosis, cholera, and smallpox) gave rise to modern epidemiology and sanitary reform, so too must the emergence and resurgence of infectious diseases today stimulate interdisciplinary, comparative,

and collaborative epidemiology, as well as a renewed focus on primary prevention—that is, on the forms of development and the fossil fuel–based economies
that drive global change.

The health professions and teaching institutions must reach across scientific
disciplines to study the implications of accelerated environmental change. As
interpreters to the public of the impacts of global change, the medical and
public health professions can assume an influential role in policies that address
our common safety. Finally, risk assessment of anthropogenic activities—from
chemical contaminants to development practices—must include indirect ecological effects, to best ensure that the untoward impacts of our interventions do
not overwhelm the direct effects intended.

7

JUSTICE AND HEALTH CARE

Justice in the allocation of health care is a topic that could easily demand a book of readings on its own. What should be done about the 40 million uninsured in the United States? Should "high-tech" and expensive medical measures be used to extend the life of the very elderly? Should they be used to save very premature infants with dubious prognoses? What would be a fair allocation of organs for donation? Should people whose habits (heavy smoking or drinking) contributed to their need for organ donation be considered on a par with those with healthier lifestyles? How can we control health care spending, and whose responsibility is it to pay for health care? Individuals? Employers? The government? We cannot cover all these important issues in this chapter. What we can do is touch on a few critical issues concerning the future direction of health care in the United States and the prospects for universal access.

It must be acknowledged up front that some people, especially libertarians, do not agree that justice requires that all citizens receive health care. While this is certainly a possible philosophical position, which we discuss below, it is clearly a minority view. For most people, the fact that 40 million Americans lack health insurance contradicts the ideal of "liberty and justice for all." At the same time, the United States has just tried unsuccessfully, yet again, to pass a national health plan. We need to understand the causes for this failure.

On the political front, the American public seems receptive to a scheme for providing universal coverage. The experience with the Clinton plan and the furious storm of opposition it generated from the insurance industry and the Republican Party reveals that the public can be frightened off, at least temporarily. This should not surprise us. The public in democracies is usually reserved in its judgment when vast new schemes for social improvement are offered. The Canadians, for example, passed their national health plan in two stages, between the late 1950s and the late 1960s, and the national electorate was split almost evenly over the issue of a private plan versus a government scheme. The government scheme won in Parliament, and subsequently public support for the Canadian system grew rapidly.[1] Today, despite the difficulties

Canada has undergone—the threat of a secession by Quebec and a very deep recession in this decade, forcing cutbacks in medical spending—support for Medicare (the name of their national plan) remains quite high.

On the question of what went wrong in the United States, almost no expert believes that public opposition was the fundamental barrier to passage of the Clinton plan.[2] Most believe that the opposition of organized interests, primarily small business and the insurance industry (which feared that it might be eliminated by the new plan), helped glue together opposition from Republicans and conservative Democrats.

The Clinton plan accelerated the shift in the United States toward a more competitive health care system and toward managed care, a shift that is in keeping with the promarket balance of political forces that prevail in Washington, D.C. Managed care does this by managing the amount and quality of care received by patients via entry-level doctors and health maintenance organizations (HMOs). Managed care seeks to save money by keeping patients out of hospitals when they don't need it and by putting them in cheaper but equally effective therapies. As an idea it has been around since before World War II. It first got its big push to national attention when President Nixon introduced legislation in the early 1970s to help HMOs spread and to head off a push toward universal health care. And later the idea was altered to include the idea that HMOs would control costs by competing with other HMOs, each offering the same level of comprehensive benefits (with the poor supported by the government).

In the first selection, Amy Gutmann examines the ethical foundations for health care access for all. She considers (and rejects) the libertarian thesis that health care is a preference like any other good and that markets allocate preferences adequately enough. In this view, it is no more the business of government to provide people with health care than it is the business of government to provide people with houses and automobiles. Instead people should be free to spend their income as they choose, whether on health insurance or consumer goods. A market approach to health care is best. As Gutmann points out, some libertarians would support providing more income to the poor to assure more equity in market transactions. But libertarians reject the wholesale application of one system for all as inefficient, as a violation of people's basic right to dispose of their income as they see fit, and as deeply paternalistic. In addition, Richard Epstein, a leading libertarian, argues that universal access is inefficient and wasteful.[3] Viewing health care as a right is not only prohibitively expensive, it rewards the sick and self-indulgent while punishing the healthy and the active. The libertarian view is in the minority in the United States and it is almost nonexistent as a view in other western democracies. In Canada, Germany, France, England, and the Scandinavian countries, health care, like education, is regarded as a public good and is publicly provided for all, although the terms of this public arrangement vary considerably. Moreover, the cost of health care overall is far lower than in the United States. We might add that this approach promotes "hanging together" by the electorate in defense of the common system. Thus a national health plan tends to promote social cohesion around the matter of security against illness and the lack of medical care. Most in these other countries recognize that assuring health care for all is expensive, but they also are well aware that the cost of health care in their countries (Canada, England, France, Germany) is far lower overall than it is in the United States, and public support for continuing these policies remains very high. One of the most important features of the drive to pass a national health insurance plan, and (earlier) to pass Medicare and (even earlier) Social Security, was to strengthen the national community at the expense of the regional and racial fault lines that hobbled the United States in its search for a wider equality.[4]

The Gutmann piece was written long before the failure of the Clinton plan but it still remains a classic argument for a national or universal health care system. A principal feature of her argument is that a one-class health care system, one for the rich, the middle classes and poor alike, promotes a health care system that caters to the needs of the better off as well as the poor, and this will strengthen the overall system level of benefits. Gutmann for practical political reasons acknowledges that a one-class system could not go so far as to forbid the rich from purchasing more health care outside the system, spending out-of-pocket.

Larry Churchill, in our second selection, paints a future in which the market dominates our common life for medicine, and it should raise many questions about the direction of present policies. Churchill suggests that a market-driven system not only undermines principles of justice and the ideal of equality in health care; it also endangers the welfare of patients and weakens trust in physicians. When physicians work for health plans which are not accountable to the electorate, conflicts of interest are inevitable, especially in for-profit plans.

In the third selection, Bradford Gray analyzes the future of trust in physicians in a new era of medical care. A critical question for the future of medicine is whether it will remain a profession in charge of its own destiny. Will physicians who work for HMOs be allowed to set policy for patients in a way consistent with the values of medicine as a profession? Gray argues that trust was already declining for physicians in the traditional fee-for-service settings. Managed care can and should be made to increase the trust patients have for physicians, through codes of ethics, forms of ownership (nonprofit versus profit), and so forth. Gray suggests that it is likely that some form of corporate medicine will be the future of the United States, and the challenge is to marry that future with a medicine that serves the society as well as the corporation. Some will doubt that this can be done.

New threats to the public's health, such as those we discussed in the last chapter, may put a national health plan back on the political agenda. In the last selection for this chapter Phyllis Freeman and Anthony Robbins take up this issue. Freeman and

Robbins argue that public health policy must be a central part of any national health care reform. State departments of health will need to work far more closely with private physicians in forging an effective prevention policy. This cooperation is especially needed if we are to identify new and emergent threats to health, from new hazards in the workplace to new threats from communicable diseases. Epidemic diseases and a whole new host of threats from viral and bacterial pathogens worldwide provide unparalleled opportunities for the spread of infection. These dangers may force us to reconsider a national health plan for reasons of self-protection than out of a concern for justice for all.

NOTES

1. For discussion of this shift in popular opinion in Canada, see Dan Beauchamp, *Health Care Reform and the Battle for the Body Politic* (Philadelphia, PA: Temple University Press, 1996, pp. 43–44).

2. See Haynes Johnson and David S. Broder, *The System: The American Way of Politics at the Breaking Point* (Boston: Little Brown, 1996). Johnson and Broder focus on the difficulties of mobilizing majority support in a badly fragmented political system at the top, plus organized opposition from small business and the insurance industry. See Jacob S. Hacker, *The Road to Nowhere* (Princeton, NJ: Princeton University Press, 1997); Theda Skocpol, *Boomerang: Clinton's Health Security Effort and the Turn Against Government in U.S. Politics* (New York: W.W. Norton, 1996); and Dan Beauchamp, *Health Care Reform and the Battle for the Body Politic. supra.* note 1.

3. Richard Epstein, *Mortal Peril: Our Inalienable Right to Health Care?* (Reading, MA: Addison-Wesley, 1997).

4. Samuel H. Beer, "In Search of a New Public Philosophy," in Anthony King, ed. *The New American Political System.* (Washington, DC: American Enterprise Institute for Public Policy Research, 1978, pp. 5–44).

For and Against Equal Access to Health Care

AMY GUTMANN

There is a fairly widespread consensus among empirical analysts that access to health care in this country has become more equal in the last quarter century. Agreement tends to end here; debate follows as to whether this trend will or should persist. But before debating these questions, we ought to have a clear idea of what equal access to health care means. Since equality of access to health care cannot be defined in a morally neutral way, we must choose a definition that is morally loaded with a set of values. The definition offered here is by no means the only possible one. It has, however, the advantage not only of clarity but also of having embedded within it strong and commonly accepted liberal egalitarian values. The debate is better focused upon arguments for and against a strong *principle* of equal access than disputes over definitions, which tend to hide fundamental value disagreements instead of making them explicit.

An equal access principle, clearly stated and understood, can serve at best as an ideal toward which a society committed to equality of opportunity and equal respect for persons can strive. It does not provide a blueprint for social change, but only a moral standard by which to judge marginal changes in our present institutions of health care.

My purpose here is not only to evaluate the strongest criticisms that are addressed to the principle, ranging from libertarian arguments for more market freedom to arguments supporting a more egalitarian principle of health care. I also propose to examine the sorts of theoretical and practical problems that arise when one tries to defend an egalitarian principle directed at a particular set of institutions within an otherwise inegalitarian society. Since it is extremely unlikely that such a society will be transformed all at once into an egalitarian one, there ought to be room within political and philosophical argument for reasoned consideration and advocacy of "partial" distributive justice, i.e., of principles that are directed only to a particular set of social institutions and

From the *Milbank Memorial Quarterly, Health and Society,* 59 (1981), 542–560. Reprinted by permission of Blackwell Publishers.

whose implementation is not likely to create complete justice even within those institutions.

THE PRINCIPLE DEFINED

A principle of equal access to health care demands that every person who shares the same type and degree of health need must be given an equally effective chance of receiving appropriate treatment of equal quality so long as that treatment is available to anyone. Stated in this way, the equal access principle does not establish whether a society must provide any particular medical treatment or health care benefit to its needy members. I shall suggest later that the level and type of provision can vary within certain reasonable boundaries according to the priorities determined by legitimate democratic procedures. The principle requires that if anyone within a society has an opportunity to receive a service or good that satisfies a health need, then everyone who shares the same type and degree of health need must be given an equally effective chance of receiving that service or good.

Since this is a principle of equal *access*, it does not guarantee equal *results*, although it probably would move our society in that direction. Discriminations in health care are permitted if they are based upon type or degree of health need, willingness of informed adults to be treated, and choices of lifestyle among the population. The equal access principle constrains the distribution of opportunities to receive health care to an egalitarian standard, but it does not determine the total level of health care available or the effects of that care (provided the care is of equal quality) upon the health of the population. Of course, even if equality in health care were defined according to an "equal health" principle, one would still have to admit that a just health care system could not come close to producing an equally healthy population, given the unequal distribution of illness among people and our present medical knowledge.

PRACTICAL IMPLICATIONS

Since the equal access principle requires equality of effective opportunity to receive care, not merely equality of formal legal access, it does not permit discriminations based upon those characteristics of people that we can reasonably assume they did not freely choose. Such characteristics include sex, race, genetic endowment, wealth, and often, place of residence. Even in an ideal society, equally needy persons will not use the same amount or quality of health care. Their preferences and their knowledge will differ as will the skills of the providers who treat them.

A One-Class System

The most striking result of applying the equal access principle in the United States would be the creation of a one-class system of health care. Services and goods that meet health care needs would be equally available to everyone who was equally needy. As a disincentive to overuse, only small fees for service could be charged for health care, provided that charges did not prove a barrier to entry to the poorest people who were needy. A one-class system need not, of course, be a uniform system. Diversity among medical and health care services would be permissible, indeed even desirable, so long as the diversity did not create differential access along nonconsensual lines such as wealth, race, sex, or geographical location.

Equal access also places limits upon the market freedoms of some individuals, especially, but not exclusively, the richest members of society. The principle does not permit the purchase of health care to which other similarly needy people do not have effective access. The extent to which freedom of the rich must be restricted will depend upon the level of public provision for health care and the degree of income inequality. As the level of health care guaranteed to the poor decreases and the degree of income inequality increases, the equal access standard demands greater restrictions upon the market freedom of the rich. Where income and wealth are very unevenly distributed, and where the level of publicly guaranteed access is very low, the rich can use the market to buy access to health care goods unavailable to the poor, thereby undermining the effective equality of opportunity required by an equal access principle.

The restriction upon market freedoms to purchase health care under these circumstances creates a certain discomforting irony: the equal access principle permits (or is at least agnostic with respect to) the free market satisfaction of preferences for nonessential consumer goods. Thus, the rigorous implementation of equal access to health care would prevent rich people from spending their extra income for preferred medical services, if those services were not equally accessible to the poor. It would not prevent their using those same resources to purchase satisfactions in other areas—a Porsche or any other luxurious consumer good. In discussing additional problems created by an attempt to implement a principle of equal access to health care in an otherwise inegalitarian society, I return later to consider whether advocates of equal access can avoid this irony.

Hard Cases

As with all principles, hard cases exist for the equal access principle. Without dwelling upon these cases, it is worth considering how the principle might deal with two hard but fairly common cases: therapeutic experimentation in medicine, and alternative treatments of different quality.

Each year in the United States, many potentially successful therapies are tested. Since their value has not been proved, there may be good reason to limit their use to an appropriate sample of sick experimental subjects. The equal access principle would insist that experimenters choose these subjects at random from a population of relevantly sick consenting adults. A randomized clinical trial could be advertised by public notice, and individuals who are interested might be registered and enrolled on a lottery basis. The only requirement for enrollment would be the health conditions and personal characteristics necessary for proper scientific testing.

How does one apply the principle of equal access when alternative treatments are each functionally adequate but aesthetically or socially quite disparate? Take the hypothetical case of a societal commitment to adequate dentition among adults. Replacement of carious or mobile teeth with dentures may preserve dental function at relatively minor cost. On the other hand, full mouth reconstruction, involving periodontal and endodontal treatment and capping of affected teeth, may be only marginally more effective but substantially more satisfying. The added costs for the preferred treatment are not inconsiderable. The principle would seem to demand that at equal states of dental need there be equal access to the preferred treatment. It is unclear, however, whether the satisfaction of subjective desire is equivalent to fulfillment of objective need.

In cases of alternative treatments, proponents of equal access could turn to another argument for providing access to the same treatments for all. A society that publicly provides the minimal acceptable treatment freely to all, and also permits a private market in more expensive treatments, may result in a two-class system of care. The best providers will service the richest clientele, at the risk of inadequate treatment for the poorest. Approval of a private market in alternative treatments would rest upon the empirical hypothesis that, if the publicly funded level of adequate treatment were high enough, few people would choose to short-circuit the public (i.e., equal access) sector; the small additional free market sector would not threaten to lower the quality of services universally available.

Most cases, like the one of dentistry, are difficult to decide merely on principle. Proponents of equal access must take into account the consequences of alternative policies. But empirical knowledge alone will not decide these issues, and arguments for or against a particular policy can be entertained in a more systematic way once one exposes the values that underlie support for an equal access principle. One can then judge to what extent alternative policies satisfy these values.

SUPPORTING VALUES

Advocates of equal access to health care must demonstrate why health care is different from other consumer goods, unless they are willing to support the more radical principle of equal distribution of all goods. Norman Daniels provides one foundation for distinguishing between health care and other goods. He establishes a category of health care needs whose satisfaction provides an important condition for future opportunity. Like police protection and education, some kinds of health care goods are necessary for pursuing most other goods in life. Any theory of justice committed to equalizing opportunity ought to treat health care as a good deserving of special distributive treatment. Equal access to health care provides a necessary, although certainly not a sufficient, condition for equal opportunity in general.

A precept of egalitarian justice that physical pains of a sufficient degree be treated similarly, regardless of who experiences them, establishes another reason for singling out certain kinds of health care as special goods. Some health conditions cause great pain but are not linked to a serious curtailment of opportunity. The two values are, however, mutually compatible.

A theory of justice that gives priority to the value of equal respect among people might also be used to support a principle of equal access to health care. John Rawls, for example, argues that without self-respect "nothing may seem worth doing, or if some things have value for us, we lack the will to strive for them. . . . Therefore the parties in the original position would wish to avoid at almost any cost the social conditions that undermine self-respect."

Conditions of Self-Respect

It is not easy to determine what social conditions support or undermine self-respect. One might plausibly assume that equalizing opportunity and treating similar pains similarly would be the most essential supports for equal respect within a health care system. And so, in most cases, the value of equal respect provides additional support for equal access to the same health care goods that are warranted by the values of equal opportunity and relief from pain. But at least some kinds of health care treatment not essential to equalizing opportunity or bringing equal relief from pain may be necessary to equalize respect within a society. It is conceivable that much longer waiting time, in physicians' offices or for admission to hospitals, may not affect the long-term health prospects of the poor or of blacks. But such discriminations in waiting times for an essential good probably do adversely affect the self-respect of those who systematically stand at the end of the queue.

Some of the conditions necessary for equal respect are socially relative; we must arrive at a standard of equal respect appropriate to our particular society. Universal suffrage has long been a condition for equal respect; the case for it is independent of the anticipated results of equalizing political power by granting every person one vote. More recently, equal access to health care has similarly become a condition for equal respect in our society. Most of us do not base our self-respect on the way we are treated on airplanes, even though the flight attendants regularly give preferential treatment to those traveling first class. This contrast with suffrage and health care treatment (and education and police protection) no doubt is related to the fact that these goods are much more essential to our security and opportunities in life than is airplane travel. But it is still worth considering that unequal treatment in health care, as in education, may be understood as a sign of unequal respect even where there are no discernible adverse effects on the health or education of those receiving less favored treatment. Even where a dual health care system will not produce inferior medical results for the less privileged, the value of equal respect militates against the perpetuation of such a system in our society.

CHALLENGES

Equality of opportunity, equal efforts to relieve pain, and equal respect are the three central values providing the foundation of support for a principle of equal access to health care. Any theory of justice that gives primacy to these values (as do many liberal and egalitarian theories) will lend prima facie support to a health care system structured along equal access lines.

We are now in a position to consider alternative values and empirical claims that would lead someone to challenge, or reject, a principle of equal access to health care. These challenges also enable us to elaborate further the moral and political implications of the principle.

Proponents of the Market

The most radical and vocal opposition comes from those who support a pure free market principle in health care. A foundation of support for the free market principle is the idea that the relative importance of satisfying different human desires is a purely subjective manner: we can distinguish between one person's desire for good medical care and another person's desire for a good Beaujolais only by the price they are willing to pay for each. If no goods are special because there is no way of ranking desires except by individual processes of choice, then what better way than the unconstrained market to allow us to decide among the smorgasbord of goods society has to offer?

Health care goods and services are likely to be more equally allocated through the market if income and wealth are more equally distributed. Several defenders of the market as a means of allocating goods and services also support a moderate degree of income redistribution on grounds of its diminishing marginal utility, or because they believe that every person has a right to "basic minimum." Neither rationale for redistribution takes us very far toward a principle of equal access to health care. If one retains the basic assumption that human preferences are totally subjective, then the market remains the best way to order human priorities. Only the market appropriately decentralizes decision-making and eliminates all nonconsensual exchanges of goods and services.

Although a minimum income floor under all individuals increases *access* to most goods and services, even at a higher level than that supported by Friedman and others, a guaranteed income will be inadequate to sustain the costs of a catastrophic illness. An exceptionally high guaranteed minimum might result in almost universal insurance coverage at a fairly high level. Supporters of free market allocation do not, however, press for a very high minimum for at least two reasons. They fear its effects on incentives, and they cannot justify a high guaranteed income without admitting that there are many expensive goods that are essential to all persons, and are not just mere consumer preferences.

The first reason for opposing an exceptionally high minimum is probably a good one. A principle approaching equality of income and wealth is likely to have serious disincentive effects on productive work and investment. There are also better reasons for treating health care as a special good, a good that society has an obligation to provide equally to all its members, than there are for equally distributing most consumer goods.

A significant step beyond the pure free market principle is a position that preserves the role of the market in allocating different "packages" of health care according to consumer preferences, but concedes a role for government in supplying every adult with a "voucher" of a certain monetary value redeemable exclusively for health care goods and services. Proponents of health vouchers must assume that there is something special about health care to justify government in taxing its citizens to provide universally for these goods, and not all others. But if health care is a more important good, because it preserves life and expands opportunity, then what is the rationale for effectively limiting the demand a sick but poor person can make upon the health care system? Why should access to health care be dependent upon income or wealth at all?

Opponents of equal access generally imply that more than minimal access will unjustly curtail the freedom of citizens as taxpayers, as consumers, and as providers of health care. Let us consider separately the arguments with regard to the many citizens who are taxpayers and consumers, and the few citizens who are providers of health care.

The Charge of Paternalism

Charles Fried has argued that equal access to health care is a particularly intrusive form of paternalism toward citizens. He claims further that "apart form a rather general commitment to equality and, indeed, to state control of the allocation and distribution of resources, to insist on the right to health care, where that right means a right to equal access, is an anomaly. For as long as our society considers that inequalities of wealth and income are morally acceptable, . . . it is anomalous to carve out a sector like health care and say that *there* equality must reign."

Would an equal access system necessarily be intrusive or paternalistic in its operation? A national health care system simply cannot be said to take away the income entitlement of citizens, since citizens are not entitled to their gross incomes. We can determine our income entitlements only after we deduct from our gross income the amount we owe the state to support the rights of others. To the extent that the rationale of an equal access principle is redistributive, those individuals who otherwise could not afford certain health care services will experience an expansion of their freedom (if we assume an adequate level of social provision). Of course, part of the justification of a national health care system is that it would also guarantee health care coverage to people who could afford adequate health care but who would not be prudent enough to save or to invest in insurance. Even if we accept the common definition of paternalistic actions as those that restrict an individual's liberty so as to further his or her interest, we still have to assess the assertion that this (partial) rationale for an equal access system entails a restriction of individual liberty. Unlike a law banning the sale of cigarettes or forcing people to wear seat belts, the institution of a national health care system forces no one to use it. If a majority of citizens decide that they want to be taxed in order to ensure health care for themselves, the resulting legislation could not be considered paternalistic: "Legislation requiring contributions to some cooperative scheme (such as medical care) . . . is not necessarily paternalistic, so long as its purpose is to give effect to the desires of a democratic majority, rather than simply to coerce a minority who do not want the benefits of the legislation." It is significant in this regard that for the past twenty years the Michigan survey of registered voters has found a consistent and solid majority supporting government measures designed to ensure universal access to medical care.

The charge of paternalism levied against an equal access system is therefore dubious because it is extremely difficult, if not impossible, to isolate the self-protectionist rationale from the redistributive and the democratic rationales. Those who object to a national health care system on the grounds that it is coercing some people for their own good forget that such a system still could be justified as a means to avoid the threat to a one-class system that exempting the rich would create. To condemn such a system as paternalistic would commit us to criticizing all legislation in which a democratic majority decides to protect itself against the wishes of a minority when exemption from the resulting policy would undermine it. Other critics wrongly assume that people have an entitlement to the case equivalent of the medical care to which society grants them a right. People do not have such an entitlement because taxpayers have a right to demand that their tax dollars are spent to satisfy health needs, not to buy luxuries. Indeed, our duty to pay taxes is dependent upon the fact that certain needs of other people must be given priority over our own desires for more commodious living.

Other Restrictions

Nonetheless, two restrictions upon consumer freedom are entailed in an equal access system. One is the restriction imposed by the taxation necessary to provide all citizens, but especially the poorest, with access to health care goods. This restriction does not raise unique or particularly troublesome moral problems so long as one believes that the freedom to retain one's gross income is not an absolute right and that the resulting redistribution of income to the health care sector increases the life chances and thereby the effective freedom of many citizens.

But there is a second restriction of consumer market freedom sanctioned by the equal access principle: the limitation upon freedom to buy health care goods above the level publicly provided. Aside from reasserting the primary values of equality, there is at least one plausible argument for such a restriction. Without restricting the free market in extra health care goods, a society risks having its best medical practitioners drained into the private market sector, thereby decreasing the quality of medical care received by the majority of citizens confined to the publicly funded sector. The lower the level of public provision of health care and the less elastic the supply of physicians, the more problematic (from the perspective of the values underlying equal access) will be an additional market sector in health care.

Without an additional market sector, would the freedom of physicians and other providers to practice wherever and for whomever they choose be unduly restricted? The extent of such restrictions will also vary with the level of public provision and with the diversity of the health care system. Public funds already are crucial to providing many physicians with basic income (through Medicare and Medicaid fees), research opportunities through the National Institutes of Health (NIH), and . . . with hospitals and other institutions in which to practice (through the provisions of the Hill-Burton act). In place of the time and resources now directed to privately purchased add-ons, an equal access system would redirect providers toward meeting previously unserved needs. These types of redirections of supply and redistributions of demand are commonly accepted in other professions that are oriented toward satisfying an important public interest. The legal and teaching professions are analogous in this regard. The equal access principle, strictly interpreted, however, adds another restriction, a limitation upon private practice that supplies health care goods not equally accessible to the entire population of relevantly needy persons. This restriction upon the freedom of providers does not have an analogue in the present practice of law or of education, although the arguments for equal access to the goods of these professions might be similar. And so, one's assessment of the strength of the case for such a restriction is likely to have implications beyond the health care system.

It is hard to see why one ought to prevent people, rich or poor, from spending money upon health care goods while permitting them to spend money on consumer goods that are clearly not essential, and perhaps even detrimental to health. One reason might be the possible systemic effect, mentioned above, that such additional expenditures would deprive the less advantaged of the best physicians. The freedom of providers as well as consumers would have to be restricted in order to curtail this effect. But beyond this empirically contingent argument for restricting any market in health care goods that are not equally accessible to all, the strict limitations upon market freedom in "extra" health care goods are hard to accept if one believes that medical services are at least as worthy items of expense as other consumer goods. One could argue that physicians ought to be free to meet the demand for additional medical goods, especially when that demand is a substitute for demand for less important goods.

This criticism illuminates a more general problem of attempting to equalize access to any good in an otherwise inegalitarian society. The more unequal the distribution of income and wealth within our society, the more likely that the freedom of consumers and providers to buy and sell health care outside the publicly funded sector will result in inequalities that cannot properly be regarded merely as the product of differences in consumer preferences. Therefore, in an inegalitarian society, we must live with a moral tension between granting providers the freedom to leave the publicly funded sector and achieving more equality in the satisfaction of health care needs.

A principle of equal access to health care applied within an otherwise egalitarian society might give little or no reason to restrict the freedom of providers or consumers. One argument often voiced against a publicly funded system that permits a marginal free-market sector is that the government is a less efficient provider of goods than are private parties. But the equal access principle does not require that the government directly provide medical services through, for example, a national health service. Government need only be a regulator of the use and distribution of essential health-care goods and services. This is a role that most people concede to government for many other purposes deemed essential to the welfare of all individuals.

Government regulation may, of course, be more expensive and hence less efficient than government provision of health care services of similar extent and quality. The tradeoff here would be between the additional market choice facilitated by government regulation of private providers and the decreased public cost of government provision. Despite utilitarian claims to the contrary, no simple moral calculus exists that would enable an impartial spectator to determine where the balance of advantage lies. Philosophers ought to cede to a fairly constituted democratic majority the right to decide this issue. What constitutes a fair process of democratic decision-making is an important question of procedural justice that lies beyond the scope of this paper.

Liability for Voluntary Risks?

Another important criticism of the equal access principle cuts across advocacy of the free market and government regulation of health care. Supporters of both views might consistently ask whether it is fair to provide the same level of access for all people, including those who voluntarily adopt bad health habits, and who quite knowingly and willingly take greater-than-average risks with their lives and health. Even if it might be unjust not to provide health care for those people once the need arises, why would it not be fair to force those who choose to drink, smoke, rock climb, and skydive also to bear a greater burden of their ensuing medical costs than that borne by people who deliberately avoid these risky pursuits? An equal access principle seems to neglect the distinction between voluntary and nonvoluntary health risks in its eagerness to ensure that all people have an equal opportunity to receive appropriate health care.

Gerald Dworkin extensively and convincingly argues that it would not be unfair to force individuals to be financially liable for voluntarily undertaken health risks, but only under certain conditional assumptions. These include our ability 1) to determine the relative causal role of voluntary versus nonvoluntary factors in the genesis of illness; 2) to differentiate between purely voluntary behavior and what is nonvoluntary or compulsive; and 3) to distinguish between genetic and nongenetic predispositions to illness. For example, to satisfy the first condition one would have to determine the relative causal role of smoking and environmental pollution in the genesis of lung cancer; to fulfill the second, one must know when smoking (or drinking or obesity) is voluntary and when it is compulsive behavior; and to satisfy the third condition, one must distinguish among those who smoke and get cancer, and those who smoke and do not. In addition, so long as there are no good institutional mechanisms for monitoring certain risky activities or for differentiating between moderate and immoderate users of unhealthy substances, qualifying the equal access principle to take account of voluntary health risks is likely to create more unfairness rather than less. Finally, given great inequalities in income distribution, the poor will be less able to bear the consequences of their risky behavior than will the rich, creating a situation of unfairness at least as serious as the unfairness of equally distributing the burdens of health care costs between those who voluntarily impose risks upon themselves and those who do not. With respect to the health hazards of overeating and obesity, for example, the rich have recourse to expensive programs of weight control unavailable to the poor. Since we have such scanty knowledge of situations when sickness can be attributable to voluntary health risks, criticisms of the equal access principle from this perspective have more weight in principle than they do in practice.

Equal Access to All Health Goods

All criticisms considered so far are directed at the equal access principle from a perspective suggesting that government involvement and public funding of health care would be too great and the role of the market too small in an equal access system. Now let us consider a powerful criticism of the principle for including too little, rather than too much, in the public sector. The criticism can be posed in the form of a challenge: if one crucial reason for supporting a principle of equal access is that health goods are much more essential than many other goods because they provide a basis for equalizing opportunity and relieving substantial pain, then why not require a government to provide equal access to *all* those health goods that would move a society further in the direction of equalizing opportunity and relieving pain for the physically and mentally ill? Without pretending that our society could ever arrive at a condition of absolute equality of health (or therefore strict equality of opportunity), proponents of this principle could still argue that we should move as far as possible in that direction.

In a society in which no tradeoffs had to be made between health care and other goods, equal access to *all* health goods might be the most acceptable principle of equity in health care. Of course, we do not live in such a society. Given the advanced state of our medical and health care technology, and the prevalence of chronic degenerative diseases and mental disorders in our population, a requirement that society provide access to every known health care good would place an enormous drain upon social resources.

Costliness per se is not the main issue. The problem with the principle of equal access to all health goods is that it demands an absolute tradeoff between satisfaction of health care needs and other needs and desires. The simplest argument against this principle is that other needs, such as education, police protection, and legal aid, will be sacrificed to health care, if the principle is enforced. But this argument is too simple. A proponent of equal access to all health goods could consistently establish some priority principle among these goods, all of which satisfy needs derived in large part from a principle of equal opportunity. The weightier counterargument is that, above some less-than-maximum level in the provision of opportunity goods, it seems reasonable for people to value what, for want of a better term, one might call "quality of life" goods: cultural, recreational, noninstrumental educational goods, and even consumer amenities. A society that maximized the satisfaction of needs before it even began to provide access to "quality of life" goods would be a dismal society indeed. Most people do not want to devote their entire lives to being maximally secure and healthy. Why, then, should a society devote all of its resources to satisfying human *needs?*

Democracy and Equal Access

We need to find some principle or procedure by which to draw a line at an appropriate level of access to health care short of what is socially and techno-logically possible, but greater than what an unconstrained market would afford to most people, particularly to the least advantaged. I suspect that no philosoph-ical argument can provide us with a cogent principle by which we can draw a line within the enormous group of goods that can improve health or extend the life prospects of individuals.

This problem of determining a proper level of guaranteed social satisfaction of need is not unique to health care. Something similar can be said about police protection or education in our society. Philosophers can provide reasons why police protection and education are rightly considered basic collective needs and why they should be given priority over individual consumer preferences. But no plausible philosophical principle can tell us what level of police protec-tion or how much education a society ought to provide on an egalitarian basis.

The principle of equal access to health care establishes a criterion of distribu-tion for whatever level of health care a society provides for any of is members. And further philosophical argument might establish some criteria by which to judge when the publicly funded level of health care was so low as to be unfair to the least advantaged, or so high as to create undue restrictions upon the ability of most people to live interesting and fulfilling lives. The remaining question of establishing a precise level of priorities among health care and other goods (at the "margin") is appropriately left to democratic decision-making. The advantage of the democratic process in determining the precise level of health care provision is that citizens have an equal and collective voice in deter-mining a decision that, according to the equal access principle, ought to be mutually binding. Citizens not only reap the benefits; they also share the bur-dens of the decision to expand or limit access to health care.

There is yet another advantage to this procedural method of establishing a fair level of health care provision. If the democratic decision will be binding upon all citizens, as the equal access principle assumes it must be, then one might expect the most advantaged citizens to exercise more political pressure to increase access to health care and hence increase the opportunity of the least advantaged above the level that they could afford in a free market system, or in a system where the rich were not included within the publicly funded health care sector. One finds some evidence to support this hypothesis in comparing the relative immunity from budget cutbacks of the program under universal entitlement of Medicare compared with the income-related Medicaid program. Of course, if costliness to the taxpayer is one's only concern, this added political pressure for health care expenditures is a liability rather than a strength of a one-class system. But from the perspective of equal access, the cost of a two-class system, one privately and one publicly funded, is an inequitable distribution of quantity and quality of care according to wealth, not need. The added nonproductive costs required merely to keep the two classes apart are seldom taken into account. And from the perspective of those supporters of an equal access principle who also want to increase the total level of health care provision, the two-class system threatens to work in the opposite direction, siphoning off the pressure of citizens who have a disproportionate share of political influence. A democratic decision, the results of which are constrained by the principle of equal access, will give a relatively accurate reading of what most people believe to be an adequate level of health care protection. The major disadvantage of the equal access constraint is that the decision of the majority or its representatives binds everyone, even those people who want more than the socially mandated level of health care.

Given the great economic inequalities of our society, it is politically impossible for advocates of equal access to fulfill their task. No democratic legislator could possibly succeed in winning support for a proposal that restricted market freedom as extensively as a strict interpretation of the equal access principle requires. And it probably would be a mistake to insist upon strict philosophical standards: one thereby risks throwing the possibility of greater access to health care for the poor out with the insistence upon curtailing access for the rich.

CONCLUSION

I began by arguing that a principle of equal access to health care was at best an ideal toward which our society might strive. I shall end by qualifying that statement. A sufficiently high level of public provision of health care for all citizens and a sufficiently elastic supply of health care would significantly reduce the threat to universal provision of quality health care of a private market in extra health care goods, just as a very high level of police protection and education reduces the inequalities of opportunity resulting from purchase of private bodyguards or of private school education by the rich.

In the best of all imaginable worlds of egalitarian justice, the equal access principle would be sufficiently supported by other egalitarian social and economic institutions that a market in health care would complement rather than undercut the goals of equal respect and opportunity. But philosophers ought to resist basing their political recommendations solely upon a model of the best of all imaginable worlds.

Market Meditopia: A Glimpse at American Health Care in 2005

LARRY R. CHURCHILL

> *Images of the future are usually only caricatures of the present.*
> *Perhaps this picture of the future of medical care will also prove*
> *to be a caricature. Whether it does depends on choices that Amer-*
> *icans have still to make.*
>
> —Paul Starr
> *The Social Transformation*
> *of American Medicine*

Market forces, unleashed to work their magic after the demise of federal health reform in 1994, continue to dominate the organization and financing of health care. While the number of managed care organizations proliferated in the late 1990s, the smaller and less well-funded companies found it difficult to compete. Many smaller insurance companies sold their health care holdings and returned to their traditional life, fire, and auto insurance products. Shortly after the turn of the century, a handful of very large health care corporations remained and had captured most of the market. These organizations provided comprehensive and integrated health services products, from birthing centers to hospice care.

The key to the success of these corporate winners, in addition to their size, was their skill in risk selection, that is, their ability to avoid persons with complicated and expensive illnesses. Since 30 percent of the population uses more than 90 percent of all health services in any given year, the successful health care corporations succeeded by being sure they had as few of that heavy-utilizing 30 percent as possible.

Early in the twenty-first century, testing for genetic markers for some of the most devastating and costly diseases became sufficiently reliable to be widely used, although effective therapies for most of these diseases were not yet available. Even though the information from genetic tests remains officially confidential, insurers often found a means of access to some of this information, and this enhanced the already quite sophisticated methods by which actuaries predicted which groups would be "undesirable" from a cost perspective. Since genetic markers for diseases are used to exclude persons or treatments under "preexisting condition" clauses, those excluded in this new way became known

From *The Hastings Center Report*, 27 (January, February 1997), 5–6. Copyright ©The Hastings Center. Reproduced by permission of The Hastings Center and the author.

as GEPPEs (genetically predisposed persons). GEPPEs are currently lobbying for recognition and a redress of their grievances under the Americans with Disabilities Act.

The rate of increase in the number of uninsured—roughly one million per year—has continued unabated since 1995, mainly because of small employers dropping health insurance coverage for their employees. Also, in 1998 Medicaid funding for the uninsured was sharply curtailed as the administration and standard-setting for the program was given over entirely to the states. While some states, such as New York and California, continued their programs using roughly the old federal model for benefits, other states, such as Texas and Florida, altered the priorities of their programs dramatically, moving the funding away from poor women and children and placing it in long-term nursing and custodial support for the elderly. An additional ten million persons lost their insurance coverage for health care between 1998 and 2003 because of these Medicaid changes.

The cumulative result was sixty million uninsured persons in the United States, roughly 24 percent of the population, in 2004.

While there have been sporadic movements toward major reform of the health care system, the lobbying power of corporate health care organizations in Washington has never been stronger. Reform movements, led largely by poor and lower middle-class citizens, with disproportionate representation of minorities and females, have had little effect. Corporations have sought to quell the occasional expressions of bad conscience over the exclusion of poor citizens through periodic gestures of medical philanthropy, sometimes on a grand scale. For example, as a grass roots movement for health reform seemed to be gaining steam in 2003, the number of "free" heart transplants for indigent patients rose dramatically, peaking during the fourth quarter. These "Christmas heart" recipients were prominently displayed as "poster patients" in several health care organizations' advertising campaigns about community service in December 2003. Still, most political observers attributed the loss of momentum for reform to the absence of an effective lobbying effort in Washington.

The most recent serious effort at reform occurred in conjunction with the 2004 presidential and congressional elections. At that time, the impetus for reform was fueled in part by the findings of a study done by the Institute of Medicine, and in part by a series in the *New York Times*. The Institute of Medicine study indicated that the health status of Americans had fallen further behind Europeans and Canadians in rates of cancer, coronary artery disease, stroke, infant mortality, and several other measures. Although the reform movement didn't come close to succeeding, it scared the health care establishment enough to lobby Congress for new ways of reporting health statistics. Under the new system, the health indicators of the uninsured are deleted before any official international comparisons are made. This practice of segmenting health statistics was widely hailed as fairer, since it compares insured citizens of one country with insured citizens of another, without the confounding effects of including the medically indigent.

The *New York Times* series appeared in September 2004 and dramatized the plight of Herbert and Jane Spencer. Herbert, 55 and a computer analyst, was made redundant in the "right-sizing and consolidation" of the small firm for which he worked when it was purchased in December 2003. While he did receive some severance benefits, they did not include health insurance. The new year proved to be a disastrous one for the Spencers. Jane was diagnosed with breast cancer in January, requiring a series of surgical and radiation treatments. Herbert had increasing problems with depression, largely due to his wife's illness and his own inability to find employment. Then in May, as Jane was on the rebound from her treatments, she was injured in an automobile accident and spent two weeks in the hospital and several months in rehabilitation. Most of the *Times* series focused on Herbert's frustrating efforts in dealing with the bills for his wife's care, in the midst of being shunted from one health care provider to another in search of effective and affordable psychiatric help for himself. His frustration was underscored by a suicide attempt in late July. By August the Spencers' savings had been exhausted, and they sold their house to pay medical bills.

The *Times* series won a Pulitzer Prize and was later published as a paperback. It also brought the Spencers to the attention of community agencies, and some of the Spencers' problems were dealt with, at least temporarily. Yet the story of the Spencers—the story of impoverishment through medical bills— occupied the national consciousness for only a few weeks. By October the polls indicated that the Spencers had been all but forgotten and political candidates, sensing that this issue had run its course, shifted their campaign speeches away from health care reform issues.

Over the last ten years the consumer rights movement in health care has increased its momentum, largely because of the fears of patients that managed care would mean less quality for them and higher profits for business. Advocacy groups for particular patients, such as Alzheimer patients, AIDS patients, and cystic fibrosis patients, have been particularly vocal and effective in protecting the interests of their constituents. The overall impact of this intensified consumer rights advocacy on the uninsured, however, has been minimal at best. While consumer advocacy groups have been effective for their respective groups, they have not been interested in making common cause with the medically indigent more generally.

While a background concern about the high number of uninsured has persisted, one of the chief dampening factors for political action to correct this problem has been a widely held and deeply seated belief that those without health services are probably less deserving. Personal responsibility for health behaviors has been a constant theme of health educators, professionals, and public figures for several decades. While smoking, beef-eating, and excess alcohol consumption are tolerated among the insured, these practices are frequently cited as a reason for not including the uninsured in a program of care. One watershed event in this lack of sympathy was a speech by the Surgeon General at the turn of the millennium. Her speech linking "moral character" and "health behaviors" was intended to promote good health practices. The result, however, was to correlate personal responsibility and health status so closely that the (uninsured) sick are often seen as reaping the just deserts of their "profligate living."

Health care corporations have made several proposals to provide health services to the uninsured, seeing this large group as another source of business. However, since the uninsured typically are chronically ill, unemployed, or work for modest wages, few of them have sufficient funds to buy into the existing systems of care. Federal and state governments have to date been unwilling or unable to subsidize this care. The continuing high cost of the Medicare program—in spite of reforms to Medicare in 1997, 1999, and 2003—is usually cited as the chief reason for the federal government to stay out of the health care business. Any proposal to raise taxes to benefit the uninsured is considered a political death wish.

The impact of corporate capitalism on health care costs over the past decade has been mixed. Aggressively managed care, under corporate leadership, showed substantial cost reductions during the late 1990s. Careful selection of risks, along with increased co-payments and deductibles, helped to hold down the costs for buyers of services and provided handsome profits for corporations selling health care products. These cost reductions, however, turned out to be short-lived. Skills for rational technological assessment turned out to be less than those for risk selection. As new medical technologies came on line the popular demand for them grew, and the costs of health care began to rise again at a pace that equated cost escalations of the 1970s and 1980s. While the uninsured are using fewer health services than ever before, the services they do use are still provided in the most expensive venues, emergency rooms and intensive care units. For the fiscal year ending October 2005, costs are running at one and one-half times the general inflation rate and consume 21 percent of the gross domestic product.

The phrase "market meditopia" first appeared in an editorial in *The Economist* in the spring of 2005 and has gained wide currency as a shorthand description of the peculiar American proclivity for seeking utopian levels of health through unregulated marketing of medical services. While *The Economist* editorial used this phrase as an ironic indictment of U.S. health policy, American politicians have picked up the phrase as if it were a distinctive American virtue, or a sign of American genius in health policy. Governors in some southern states have begun to campaign for reelection on a platform to extend the reach of market forces even further by eliminating Medicaid completely. As one governor put it, "We have a duty to end the vicious cycle of medical dependence that has enslaved our fellow citizens and sapped their energy for individual health care responsibility." Last week the AMA endorsed market meditopia as essential to protect "the best health care system in the world."

Trust and Trustworthy Care in the Managed Care Era

BRADFORD H. GRAY

Sick people, the physician Eric Cassell observed, are "people who are forced to trust." Trust on the part of patients has long been viewed as fundamental to therapeutic relationships. Patients' willingness to accept medical advice and services has rested on trust in physicians' technical competence and adherence to a fiduciary ethic that held that the physician's responsibility was to put the patient's interests above self-interest. Ethical codes have long encouraged physicians to be trustworthy by discouraging exploitation of patients' vulnerability. Such ethical ideals have been enforced mainly through professional socialization and self-regulation, which are rooted in societal faith in the fiduciary ethic.

The development of third-party payment in fee-for-service medical care also involved trust—between payers and physicians. Payers were not present when services were rendered, and physicians' assessments of patients' needs triggered the flow of dollars from third-party payers to all types of providers. Payers had little choice but to trust those assessments until ways to monitor and assess the appropriateness of services emerged.

Managed care shifts much control over the flow of dollars and patients from physicians to large organizations that have strong economic goals and the power to influence patient care in pursuit of those goals. This combination of purpose and power is a major source of doubts about the trustworthiness of these organizations, particularly because they reduce the power of health professionals who profess adherence to the fiduciary ethic. Thus, even though managed care can reduce the amount of unnecessary and inappropriate care, critics can point to a variety of ways in which managed care might undermine trust, and trustworthiness, in medical care.

Is a decline in trustworthiness an inevitable aspect of managed care, or might new modes of trustworthiness supplant more traditional forms? In this paper I argue that trust in the fiduciary ethic was declining even before the rise of

From *Health Affairs,* 16 (1997), 34–49. Copyright © 1997 The People-to-People Foundation, Inc. All rights reserved. Reprinted by permission.

managed care, that patients' need for trustworthy care is undiminished, and that managed care can operate in ways that merit patients' trust. This trustworthiness may, paradoxically, have its basis in accountability structures that emphasize monitoring and auditing rather than trust in physician autonomy. An important question is whether, and under what circumstances, managed care might make care more trustworthy, not less. To answer that question, I evaluate four alternatives for enhancing the trustworthiness of managed care.

THE EROSION OF TRUST IN FEE-FOR-SERVICE CARE

Critics of managed care often evoke an idealized image of the past, but there is a long history of skepticism about the trustworthiness of doctors, especially under fee-for-service medicine. Early in this century George Bernard Shaw railed against surgeons: "[T]he more appalling the mutilation, the more the mutilator is paid." Voices also have been raised within the profession for more than a century about the pernicious effects of economic conflicts of interest on medicine's performance and public image.

For both patients and payers, trust in the competence and fiduciary ethic of physicians and health care institutions has been strained in recent decades by exploding health care costs, accompanied by much publicity about malpractice crises, fraud and abuse, inexplicable variations in patterns of care and high levels of inappropriate services, and an efflorescence of medical commercialism and conspicuous conflicts of interest. Payers and the attentive public came to understand that services received by patients can be a function of much more than their objective medical needs and that the choice of a physician or hospital can affect care and its outcomes. Professional self-regulatory mechanisms have been widely criticized for ineffectiveness regarding such matters.

Ironically, the fiduciary ethic, as sometimes interpreted by doctors, contributed to payers' desire for alternatives to trust, as when physicians viewed their obligations to patients as including the manipulation of third-party payers' rules to obtain payment for ineligible services. At one time this meant hospitalizing some patients unnecessarily so that services would be covered by their hospital insurance. More recently it has meant "gaming" utilization review systems and payment rules to obtain payment for services deemed by payers to be unnecessary, inappropriate, cosmetic, or experimental. In such ways the fiduciary ethic, thought essential to trust in the doctor/patient relationship, became a source of distrust in the doctor/payer relationship.

Efforts to find alternatives to dependence on trust have developed in recent decades. Patients now routinely seek second opinions, obtain services from "alternative" practitioners, and consume journalistic lists of "the best" physicians and hospitals. More fundamental changes have occurred among purchasers of care, with the embrace of managed care. Cost control is key to the economic success of managed care organizations. Available tools include gatekeepers, practice guidelines and utilization review, and payment methods that discourage the provision of additional services. Health maintenance organizations (HMOs) and preferred provider organizations (PPOs) also can use data on the performance of physicians and other providers to form and manage their networks.

CONTINUING NEED TO PROTECT PATIENTS' INTERESTS

Managed care is a response of purchasers to problems in the doctor/patient/payer nexus. Managed care does not, however, eliminate patients' vulnerability or their need for trustworthy care. An industry of outcomes research, practice guidelines, and utilization review has developed to address the competency aspect of trustworthiness, but the fiduciary aspect has received much less organized attention.

It is apparent, however, that high ethical standards are essential to protecting patients' interests, even in (or perhaps especially in) the era of managed care. For example, the successful operation of utilization management programs relies heavily on physicians' willingness to speak for the patient's interests when threatened by an unsound review decision. A need also exists for adherence to patients' interests within HMOs that use any of the available cost management tools. For example, if physicians were simply to follow their incentives as gatekeepers in individual practice associations (IPAs), major problems would ensue for patients. An orientation toward serving patients' interests among the medical policymakers within managed care organizations also may help to assure that organizations' practice guidelines, medical standards, and review procedures appropriately emphasize patients' needs.

The growth of managed care has itself added sources of doubt regarding the physician's fiduciary ethic as a guardian of the patient's best interests. Managed care has reduced physicians' autonomy in ways that have been widely decried in the profession. Critics charge that the fiduciary ethic is undermined by some managed care methods. They point to conflicts of interest introduced by some compensation arrangements, situations that divide physicians' loyalties, intrusions of external parties into the doctor/patient relationship, and implementation of rules that limit the alternatives that doctors can offer patients.

Physicians' power also has been reduced by their growing dependence on relationships with HMOs and PPOs for a flow of patients, whereas they once depended primarily on satisfactory relationships with existing patients or colleagues. This client or colleague dependency, as Eliot Freidson termed it, may not always have influenced physicians in ways that served patients' best interests, but organization dependency has introduced a powerful new influence into medical care: pressure for physicians to practice in ways that satisfy organizations and their economic interests.

In light of patients' vulnerability, more attention is warranted to the fit between managed care and the fiduciary aspect of medical professionalism. How might continued viability of the fiduciary ethic be assured when the health care system is becoming increasingly price-competitive and dominated by large organizations that have strong economic interests? Sole reliance on the ethical standards of individual physicians seems insufficient, not only because of the loss of confidence in the strength and consistency of such standards within the profession but also because of disparities in power between individual physicians and managed care organizations.

POTENTIAL SOURCES OF TRUST IN MANAGED CARE

Among the ways that the fiduciary ethic might be encouraged in managed care are (1) developing effective ethical standards in the managed care industry, (2) populating the field with mission-oriented nonprofit organizations, (3) increasing physician control within managed care organizations, and (4) using market-oriented solutions involving monitoring, measuring, and public disclosure of the performance of managed care plans.

Ethical Standards

Codes of ethics and statements of ethical ideals are commonplace among professional associations in health care. Their manifest purpose is to provide ethical guidance to members of the profession, although it is uncertain how much and how uniformly behavior is affected. A second purpose is to assure outsiders (potential patients, purchasers, and regulators) that the profession stands for high ethical principles.

The American Medical Association (AMA) has had a code of ethics for 150 years, and its Council on Ethical and Judicial Affairs regularly publishes opinions on ethical issues. Its guidelines on conflicts of interest reflect the fiduciary ethic, holding that "under no circumstances may physicians place their own financial interests above the welfare of their patients" and that "the primary objective of the medical profession is to render service to humanity."

Such an ethical orientation, which is characteristic of professional associations, has not been adopted by organizational providers of health care or their trade associations. Perhaps the closest version is in the American Hospital Association's (AHA's) Patient's Bill of Rights, which dates from the early 1970s. The "rights" imply that hospitals are responsible for treating patients and their privacy respectfully, providing information about treatment, and allowing patients to refuse recommended treatment. The closest the Bill of Rights comes to the fiduciary ethic is in its carefully qualified right to expect a hospital, "within its capacity and policies," to make a "reasonable response" to a patient's request for "appropriate and medically indicated care and services."

Within the managed care industry, statements about ethical responsibilities of providers have been slow to develop and are framed in terms of patients' rights rather than caregivers' obligations. Economic conflicts of interest are not addressed or even acknowledged. Moreover, the language frequently has a contractual flavor and is stated in reciprocal terms, with patients' responsibilities enumerated along with their rights. Of course, since plans are subject to state insurance regulation or federal regulation under the Employee Retirement Income Security Act (ERISA) (or both), their obligations to enrollees are indeed contractual: An open-ended obligation such as the fiduciary ethic is alien to the legalistic relationship between insurers and the insured, in which specificity, precedent, and equity are key considerations.

Changes are occurring regarding managed care organizations' acknowledgment of ethical issues. As recently as late 1994 I was told by the Group Health Association of America (GHAA), the American Managed Care and Review Association (AMCRA), and the American Association of Preferred Provider Organizations (AAPPO) that they had no standards of ethics for member organizations. I received similar responses from such leading nonprofit managed care organizations as Kaiser Permanente, Harvard Community Health Plan, and The HMO Group. Perhaps the youth, rapid evolution, fragmentation, or competitiveness of the managed care industry explains this inattention to ethical ideals. Or perhaps industry leaders and the large purchasers with whom they deal are skeptical about voluntary ethical standards. Or perhaps the industry's priorities have been elsewhere, such as in the development of data systems and other management tools that might protect the interests of patients more effectively than would ethical standards alone.

LATEST DEVELOPMENTS Demand is growing for ethical standards in managed care, with developments on several fronts. In early 1995 the National Health Council (NHC), an association of disease-oriented organizations, not managed care organizations, adopted a set of principles for managed care that were stated in terms of patients' rights and responsibilities. Notably, the number of requests for the document was much greater than anticipated by the NHC, which had to go back to press after 10,000 copies were distributed.

The "Accreditation Standards for Managed Care" that were implemented in 1995 by the National Committee for Quality Assurance (NCQA) cover some pertinent topics, including patients' rights and grievance procedures. To meet accreditation requirements, health plans must adopt their own statement of members' rights and responsibilities that cover matters specified by the NCQA, including access to information, grievance procedures, confidentiality, and so forth. The language is contractual in nature (for example, specifying matters about which enrollees are entitled to information) and contains none of the "best interest of the patient" language that characterizes the fiduciary ethic. . . .

In sum, ethical standards are not well established in the managed care industry and devote little or no attention to the problems addressed by the fiduciary ethic, particularly the conflict-of-interest problem and its resolution in favor of the patient. Moreover, both the limited credibility of associational philosophies and industry accreditation standards as predictors of behavior and the contractual "rights and responsibilities" formulations of the standards that exist suggest that ethical codes within the managed care industry are not a replacement for a fiduciary ethic implemented by physicians with patient care responsibility. Nor are they so intended. Even so, the increasing organizational attention in the managed care field to the problems for which medicine's fiduciary ethic has been a response is a development worth following. . . .

Role of Nonprofits

If medical practice has become organization-dependent, might the ownership form of the organization on which physicians are dependent make a difference? Compatibility between the medical profession and nonprofit health care organizations has been noted in the past by a number of observers. Some have seen it negatively, such as the economists in the 1970s who attributed the predominance of nonprofit hospitals in this country to the power of physicians and the ease with which they could manipulate a nonprofit institution to serve their ends, which were assumed to be economic. However, the link can be viewed more favorably because of an affinity of purposes and moderation of the inevitable tensions between professional prerogatives and organizational requirements. This may seem naïve to persons who are familiar with the conflicts that often typify relationships between medical staffs and hospital administrations. But, at least in ideals, nonprofit health care institutions, like members of the medical profession, are expected to be animated by values other than profit or self-interest.

The nonprofit organizational form and the medical profession's normative emphasis on ethical behavior may serve similar purposes: to facilitate trust and discourage exploitation of vulnerable patients. I have already discussed this with regard to the medical profession, but some parallels with the nonprofit form are worth noting.

Seeking to explain why organizations in certain fields tend to be nonprofit, the legal scholar Henry Hansmann has suggested that the nonprofit organization helps to solve problems of distrust that arise in fields in which purchasers lack the information needed to monitor or evaluate the services provided by sellers. Such purchasers may prefer to deal with nonprofit organizations since they are prohibited from distributing profits and, therefore, have less incentive to exploit their informational advantages vis-à-vis purchasers. Nonprofits thus may play a trust-enhancing role in economic relationships in which informational asymmetries are present. Interestingly, Hansmann questioned the need for the nonprofit form in health care because the interests of vulnerable patients are protected by physicians who adhere to the fiduciary ethic. The possibility that health care organizations could undermine the physician's fiduciary ethic was not considered.

AFFINITY WITH PROFESSIONAL IDEALS The claim of an affinity between medical professionalism and the nonprofit form has plausibility but requires qualification. First, the empirical side of the claim is not well documented. Research a decade ago found some indications that for-profit hospitals were actually more responsive to physicians than were nonprofits, as measured by physicians' presence on boards and their reports of administrative responsiveness. However, this was in the era before diagnosis-related groups (DRGs), when the incentives of profit-oriented hospitals and physicians who believed that "more is better" were aligned.

Other research provides some support for the hypothesized compatibility between the nonprofit form and professional ideals. For-profit hospitals have been more likely than nonprofit hospitals to pressure physicians to act in ways that served the hospital's economic interests—in this case, not to admit Medicaid patients. The incentive systems used by for-profit HMOs have greater influence on physicians than do the incentives of nonprofit HMOs, although the reasons are not wholly clear. There also is some evidence that for-profit HMOs tend to spend less of the premium dollar on medical care than do nonprofits. The values implied by this would presumably be consistent with the values of those who provide patient care. For-profit health plans have headed the list of plans with high levels of complaints and disenrollments among Medicare enrollees, whereas the lowest levels on both measures have been in nonprofits.

This evidence is hardly dispositive of the question of whether there is an affinity between medical professionalism and the nonprofit form, and much more research is needed on ownership forms and physicians' roles in managed care.

SHRINKING SHARE OF HMO MARKET The second problematic aspect of the suggestion that the nonprofit form in managed care might be more trustworthy in a fiduciary sense is that as managed care enrollment has grown over the past fifteen years, the largely nonprofit field has been transformed: More than two-thirds of plans are now for-profit, and a majority of enrollees are in for-profit plans. About a third of nonprofit HMOs converted to for-profit status over the past fifteen years.

(Notably, the current surge of interest in managed care reform is commonly framed in terms of concern about HMOs' profit-oriented behavior.)

Despite their shrinking share of the HMO market, nonprofits provide valuable leadership activities and lessons in organizational performance. For example, of twenty-one HMOs designated as "exceptional quality" by GTE in its *Health Care Consumer Guide* for employees, twenty were nonprofits, as were sixteen of the twenty-one HMOs listed on *U.S. News and World Report's* "Honor Roll" of HMOs with high standards for preventive care. The continued viability of the nonprofit form in managed care merits public policy concern.

POLICY POSSIBILITIES The prevalence of different forms of ownership in managed care has been largely due to governmental policies in the past. Government—as purchaser, regulator, and funder—could do much to encourage the continued availability of nonprofit alternatives in the field. For example, Medicaid managed care has stimulated many nonprofit health centers and hospitals that traditionally have served the poor to move into the world of capitated medical care; they may need both technical assistance and capital if they are to survive. On the regulatory front, flexibility is needed in rules about tax exemptions, speed is needed in response to exemption requests, and greater skepticism might be warranted in response to requests for nonprofit conversions to for-profit status. (On the other hand, it is important that tax exemptions have a meaningful basis, which suggests greater attention to issues of governance and community benefit in managed care.) Finally, insofar as access to capital is driving decisions of existing nonprofits to convert or causing new HMOs to be formed as for-profits rather than nonprofits, government could act to enhance nonprofit plans' access to capital.

Physician Influence Within Managed Care

The oft-stated concern that managed care replaces a fiduciary ethic with an incompatible business ethic implies that managed care might be more trustworthy if the influence of physicians within managed care organizations were enhanced. Physician influence can include complete or shared ownership of a firm, complete or shared ownership of a physician group that contracts with managed care organizations, or a strong voice within managed care organizations.

Intuitions differ regarding whether physician control may enhance managed care organizations' commitment to the fiduciary ethic, and evidence is now sparse. There is some evidence that physicians' influence within managed care organizations may increase, not decrease, the organization's willingness to exert pressure on individual physicians. Thus, my research with Mark Schlesinger and Krista Perreira found that utilization review organizations with high levels of physician control were particularly willing to interfere with practicing physicians' autonomy. This could be compatible with the fiduciary ethic if it enhances appropriateness and quality of services. We also found that review organizations in which physicians had comparatively great influence were more likely to act in an agency capacity toward patients, as indicated by their organization's willingness to intervene (with the patient, hospital, or state authorities) in instances in which problematic care came to light.

Another interesting clue comes from James Robinson and Lawrence Casalino's study of six large medical groups in California that were paid by capitation. These physician-controlled groups had 40 percent lower hospital utilization rates than those in commercial HMOs in California and about half of the national HMO rates for both Medicare and commercial plans. Clearly, simplistic assumptions that physician control of managed care will translate into more extensive services are not correct. How the low rates of hospital use comport with the fiduciary ethic is not clear.

The hypothesis that the fiduciary ethic of the medical profession can be transmitted to managed care organizations via physician control of such organizations is intriguing. It suggests a means for sensitively separating the beneficial and dubious aspects of practitioner autonomy from each other, discouraging nonrational or economically motivated practices while providing the flexibility needed to respond to patients' individual needs. The question is, Does it work that way?

Role of Purchasers and Market Forces

Large purchasers have become very interested in measuring the performance of health plans. Private purchasers took the lead, but interest is growing among governmental purchasers. Important developments include the creation and adoption within the managed care industry not only of accreditation standards and mechanisms but also of standards regarding data that plans should collect and report about services to enrollees. The Health Plan Employer Data and Information Set (HEDIS) is rapidly gaining acceptance as a standardized means for collecting and reporting data on health plan performance.

Increasingly, employers are seeking performance information from HMOs, collecting plan-specific satisfaction data from enrollees, and making this information available to employees. In some instances, the information is published, as with the 1994 and 1995 data on federal employees' satisfaction with more than 200 HMOs in the Federal Employees Health Benefits Program (FEHBP). In other instances, the information is made available to beneficiaries for their use in choosing a health plan. For example, the information given to Xerox employees about the plans from which they may choose includes coverage and costs, whether the plan is accredited by the NCQA, the percentage of primary care physicians who are board-certified, the average waiting time for urgent and emergency care, member satisfaction and the percentage of enrollees who would recommend the plan to family and friends, immunization rates for two-year-olds, the percentage of adults ages forty to sixty-four who have had a cholesterol test in the past five years, the percentage of women ages fifty-two to sixty-four who have had a mammogram in the past two years, the percentage of women ages twenty-one to sixty-four who have had a Pap test in the past three years, and hospital admission rates for asthma patients ages two to nineteen.

Much better monitoring of physician and hospital performance exists in many managed care organizations than ever existed in the traditional fee-for-service system. Anecdotes suggest that when employees are given such information about alternative plans, they tend to move toward efficient, high-quality plans and that HMOs strive to improve performance. . . .

CONCLUSION

Managed care has become a lightning rod for ethical concern. Yet managed care also offers solutions of a sort to ethical problems that existed in the world of unmanaged fee-for-service medicine. Some aspects of managed care—strongly profit oriented plans and powerful physician incentives—seem to exacerbate concerns about ethics and trustworthiness. Greater ethical sensitivity in the managed care industry, preservation or enhancement of a nonprofit sector within the industry, appropriate involvement of physicians, and improvement of monitoring and reporting on the performance of managed care plans might mitigate such concerns.

A system based on trust in the competence and fiduciary ethic of individual physicians is being replaced by a system based on alternatives to trust. Hopes about trustworthiness of physicians' patient care decisions are increasingly being supplemented by evidence. An ideal system would reward physicians who provide excellent care and have high ethical standards. This may be a direction in which managed care is moving, although it is difficult to tell. For the foreseeable future, the new methods of accountability should be viewed as supplements, not alternatives, to trustworthy physicians who adhere to the fiduciary ethic.

The ethical obligations of physicians are more clearly defined than are the obligations of institutions. Building a strong, patient-centered ethic in organizations is one of the great challenges facing managed care. Perhaps the most appropriate starting point is to build institutional settings that allow the fiduciary ethic of health professionals to exist and flourish.

National Health Care Reform Minus Public Health:
A Formula for Failure

PHYLLIS FREEMAN AND ANTHONY ROBBINS

INTRODUCTION

Because renewed energy for health care reform springs from perceptions of risk that center more on economic than on physical vulnerabilities, so too do the remedies. Detailed attention from dozens of consultants to cost containment and to financing universal access to medical services has obscured what should be a decisive distinction between proposals. Do they attend to improving health and reducing disease or only to paying for diagnosis and treatment for those already ill?

Proposals now under serious consideration by the Congress would guarantee Americans payment for doctor visits and hospital services. A great start! But none promises to integrate the medical care system with the public health structure and assure participation of medical care providers in those functions necessary to detect and respond early to health threats. If we accept the pervasive perception that universal access to medical services will address all important health needs, we will miss a magnificent chance to prevent disease—and to hold off unnecessary medical care expenditures. Moreover, if we do not get this right now, the door of political opportunity may not open for a second chance for many years.

Impending health care reform could take advantage of the extensive medical services system, at little additional cost, to accomplish many previously unattainable health goals for the nation, but nothing about the planning process or debate so far makes that outcome seem likely. Repeated references during the debate on health care reform to "access to prevention services" belie a failure to understand the difference between insuring personal health services and assuring public health gains. The distinction is a strategic one. Public health is grounded in the Constitutional authority to protect the health and safety of the entire population. In contrast, medical care is oriented to the needs of the indi-

From the *Journal of Public Health Policy,* 15 (1994), 261–282. Reprinted by permission of the publisher.

285

vidual. Medical services can be preventive, curative or palliative. Good medical care can have a favorable effect on public health even if the services were not offered as features of a population-based strategy. But our nation will never achieve optimal health from our enormous investments in the medical care system without explicitly integrating public health guidance and accountability into the reform of medical care management and finance. Medical care is an element of public health, but the sheer enormity of the medical care system means that it is seen as being separate.

Attention to public health authority has waned. Few professionals remaining in the states or in the Public Health Service can imagine how to marry the tremendous momentum for reform of the medical care industry to a public health strategy designed to achieve gains in public health. Yet each state needs to make use of the expanding federal role in health care reform and of the state's Constitutional police powers to regulate aspects of medical practice that would achieve health benefits for all. The federal health care reform law should make it possible.

Public health reaches far beyond the current popular notion of prevention, which focuses on individual lifestyle rather than on social, economic, and environmental hazards that few individuals can avoid without strong protective legislation and enforcement by the state. Chemical hazards in workplaces, polluted air and water in residential communities, contaminated food in supermarkets and restaurants, and spread of infectious diseases by people, animals and food all pose health risks that can be reduced more efficiently by public health interventions than by medical care. Even when costly medical services can diminish or cure the harm to individuals caused by environmental exposures, other deadly threats remain for which medical care is impotent regardless of how much the individual or society would be willing to spend. . . .

UNIVERSAL SICKNESS INSURANCE POSING AS COMPREHENSIVE HEALTH CARE REFORM

Why has the debate about health care reform neglected public health? Health insurance is a necessity for every American. It buys medical services and avoids personal financial disaster. The ultimate purpose of health care reform as currently debated in the United States is to pay for insurance against the costs of illness. This narrow focus on sickness insurance misses opportunities to improve health, yet it is perfectly tuned to the concerns of the public. . . .

Those who foot the bill for medical care—government, non-government insurers, employers, and citizens—are all engaged in efforts to reduce their financial responsibility and to shift the burden to others. Government tinkers with eligibility rules and benefit limitations for Medicaid to limit spending growth.

Under these pressures Oregon initiated rationing for Medicaid patients, limiting recipients to those medical services the state deemed most cost-effective. No similar limits have been placed on insurance plans for the more affluent. Insurance companies raise premiums, screen out applicants and limit coverage. This reduces workers' ability to change jobs when a "preexisting condition" may be grounds for exclusion from the new employer's group plan—if there is one. Employers in the squeeze are likely to increase each employee's contribution or to cut health benefits from the package. According to a 1991 *New York Times* poll, one-third of those with family incomes below $15,000, and more than one-half of those with incomes above $30,000, had been subjected to this practice within the previous year. . . .

No proposal before the Congress approaches reform from a public health perspective. Yet, if we fail to build into the reformed structure of medical services a way to guarantee those measures that can improve health and dampen the need for medical services, it will be a formula for failure. The costs of unnecessary disease will burden the medical care system, and the health of our people will improve far more slowly.

BEYOND INSURANCE: INCORPORATING BETTER HEALTH INTO REFORM

To achieve the full health potential of the one trillion dollars already spent in the health care sector we need to recognize additional ways to improve health, protect life and make effective use of our medical care resources.

The reformers started down one promising path when they anticipated incorporating in the benefit package a class of personal health services known to have positive impact on the health status of the population. Within this class there are two distinct categories: 1) medical services which are protective for the community as well as for the individual, such as immunizations or treatment for tuberculosis, and 2) those which tend to improve health when provided systematically to all at risk. Screening and treatment for high blood pressure or cancer of the cervix are examples. Reformers talk about reaching optimal coverage for these services through quality control mechanisms, such as "report cards." Today our coverage for pap smears and high blood pressure detection is rarely complete, even in managed care settings. Under health care reform, if the quality control approach works, we are likely to see improved preventive services. But will we see successful control of tuberculosis, toxic exposures, and other public health threats?

In 1983, the Centers for Disease Control was planning a campaign to eliminate tuberculosis. Effective antibiotics were available to render each TB patient noninfectious. All that was needed was a systematic way to screen, treat and monitor several thousand people. Yet without organized and accountable medical services, state tuberculosis programs in health departments had no way to insist that providers of personal health services help. Ten years later the situation is far more grave. Resistant TB organisms are increasingly common, rendering antibiotics ineffective, and the national objective has slipped from elimination to control. If medical practitioners had been engaged in the tuberculosis elimination plan that was proposed in 1983, today our nation might not be searching for over a half billion dollars of new money to control the spreading epidemic of multidrug-resistant tuberculosis which so threatens health care workers and others.

In such programs success in public health terms depends on how public health makes use of the medical care system. Public health authorities should be able to deputize health plans and practitioners, engaging them in managing treatment to protect individuals and the community. Success in the face of challenges to health like tuberculosis remains unlikely under reform. Medical care lacks a tradition of reaching out to patients in need of care who may not seek it. Thus we remain unlikely to provide these people with the therapy to treat themselves and protect the community around them. Society as a whole will suffer little if physicians wait for patients to seek medical care for most problems, but we all pay for missed public health opportunities. Later in this paper we use immunization to illustrate how doctors can become more effective protagonists of public health in a reformed scheme.

Fundamental public health information systems and intervention strategies—the health care analogs of smoke alarms and fire fighting—should be integrated into the health reform bundle. Epidemiology, research and public health information systems are not personal health services. They do not slip easily into an existing niche in medical insurance schemes—the benefit package. But public health systems should be so embedded in reform that they cannot be uncoupled from medical care now or in the future. If cohesion is not assured at the start we will consume our limited resources caring for the equivalent of increasing numbers of smoke and burn victims as preventable problems spread—unnecessarily.

The medical care system can do more than respond with targeted treatment. Medical practitioners can and should strengthen public health capacity by detecting in individuals medical problems which might have been preventable if discovered earlier, and reporting such occurrences to the authorities responsible for controlling further exposures. For example, when a physician discovers that a patient with a neuropathy is suffering from solvent poisoning from his job in a plastics plant, it should be standard practice to report the event and the danger to public health authorities who may be able to protect fellow workers. Similarly for lead poisoning, rat bites, and exposures to environmental toxins, the

medical practitioner must be linked to public health authorities who can intervene at the source as well as directing populations to early treatment.

Reporting of disease is critical for public health, yet there is no reliable
system in place to ensure that doctors will report suspicious cases or that public
health authorities will investigate them in the field and in the laboratory and act
to prevent additional illnesses. Everywhere diseases are under-reported because
physicians do not see themselves as part of a public health system to prevent
disease, except for the patients in their own practice. Too often physicians do
not make the effort to comply with state reporting requirements because in
caring for sick patients they may not see the cumulative consequences of failure
to report—or the benefits of public health interventions.

Practitioners can respond to public health information as well as provide it.
For example, research may reveal that certain chemicals and physical agents
cause cancer, but only many years after initial exposure. For individuals exposed to carcinogens, screening and monitoring may save their lives. Bladder
cancer caused by azo dye exposures in the textile industry, as an example, can
often be cured if detected early. None of the health care reform proposals as yet
incorporates a systematic way to identify, contact and offer early treatment to
all those at risk. No plan yet contemplates making health plans a clinical arm of
the public health departments. At best, plans will be graded for their success in
providing preventive services, such as pap smears, to everyone in the plan for
whom the test is appropriate.

Optimal public health gains will be more difficult to achieve if populations
remain outside the reformed medical care system, that is, if they are not enrolled. From the public health point of view, a policy decision to leave some
individuals outside the health care system does not remove their contribution to
health or disease in the United States. Yet Congress is already debating just
how *universal* health care reform should be, further evidence of inattention to
medical care's role in public health. If the Congress chooses to limit insurance
for health services to some categories of residents, its members should recognize that there is no economic or health justification for withholding payment
and limiting access to those measures which protect the community from the
spread of preventable problems.

The precise list of the services for delivery to populations at risk and to
populations posing risks to others can be argued about and revised over time as
health conditions change and knowledge grows. Similarly, the specific data
needed from providers to bolster epidemiological information systems and research will evolve. But all these activities which unify public health and medical practice into an effective and efficient health care system cannot be grafted
onto reform after organizational, management and financing mechanisms have
been legislated. Instead, the overall design needs to contemplate how to use

enrollment, management and finance components as incentives, checks and balances to improve performance and health. . . .

PUBLIC HEALTH AUTHORITY—A NEGLECTED FOUNDATION FOR REFORM

The need to protect the health of the public will not disappear with health care reform. Public health authority will still exist in the states, even if this topic is neglected in federal health care reform legislation. To protect the public, states should be able to harness the medical care system's highly trained workforce, capable laboratories, linked records system, and billions of contacts with the population.

Authority to regulate human behavior to avoid harm and to enhance health, called the "police power," is contained in Article X of the United States Constitution. The framers included this power among those "not delegated to the United States by the Constitution, nor prohibited by it to the States," thus among those "reserved to the States respectively, or to the people."

States began establishing authority in boards of health more than a century ago, and expanded their activities through state and local health departments. Quarantine of people capable of spreading communicable diseases, searches of housing, restaurants and factories for health hazards, seizures of dangerously mislabeled goods, injunctions to refrain from or engage in certain acts, and licensure of practitioners and of facilities to enforce minimum standards of practice have all been sanctioned by courts as legitimate efforts to protect the public's health.

A measure of federal health regulation began early under the "commerce clause" of the Constitution. Federal interventions in health have expanded in this century. Food and drug laws, and worker, environmental and consumer protections have invoked federal preemption of state authority. Many federal health programs offer grants and financial incentives to the states. The dominant force is financial assistance under the Social Security and Public Health Service Acts to encourage states to expand services for special populations such as children, the poor, the elderly, and migrant workers. . . .

No one asserts that states can protect the public's health without assistance. The tools for improving public health, such as surveillance and information systems, research and development for new diagnostic tests, vaccines and therapies depend on national investment and coordination. Health care reform must assure continued support for the National Institutes of Health, the Centers for Disease Control, the Food and Drug Administration, and programs at the Department of Labor and Environmental Protection Agency created to protect the public health. Yet no health care reform proposal explicitly takes advantage of state public health authority and the federal institutions that support it. Where private medical service providers deliver the bulk of services, public health officials should remember that the states have the Constitutional authority to define the public health and to regulate providers to protect the public health. Where the incentives in the medical care system prove insufficient to protect the public health, states can and should insist on effective and efficient use of resources.

The federal government has resources essential to helping states meet the public health and medical needs of their residents. Federal programs in the Public Health Service should retain and expand their roles in setting health goals for the nation. Federal health care reform legislation should allocate a proportion of medical care funds to states for core public health functions and use the federal guidelines to assure compatible data collection, epidemiological research and reporting systems—and sufficient scope of effort and competence to provide the basis for holding medical practices accountable to public health goals.

Reform legislation should reaffirm the states' Constitutional power to protect the public health, giving them the needed financial and managerial leverage to use the restructured health care system, including its private sector participants, to reach public health objectives. States should translate national health targets into local ones and assist medical practices to improve and contribute to state-wide and national gains. Beyond management systems and rewards, the states will need to use their public health authority to regulate medical practice. When attempting to alter physician behavior, it is "especially important that physicians perceive the proposed changes as beneficial to patients (or at least not harmful)." Thus it will be particularly important for public health regulation to be developed and evaluated in conjunction with the medical care system, rather than imposed from the outside.

States' primary contribution under reform will be public health leadership, technical assistance to medical providers, core public health regulatory systems, and management techniques to squeeze the most health from each medical dollar. Many health departments are unprepared in one of two ways. Some have little experience with regulating medical services, and concentrate regulatory efforts on health hazards in the community. The very idea that such a health department could provide wise guidance and exercise an important measure of control over medical resources may seem incredible. Other departments are principally providers of medical services for the poor and neglect broad-based, strategic public health interventions. These departments seem poorly equipped to exercise regulatory control for the benefit of the whole population. But as poorly equipped as the states may be, they remain the only entities with broad public health authority. National reform architects have neglected to reinforce these powers or to propose any statutory substitute at the federal level.

IMMUNIZATION

To illustrate the risks we face if we bungle health care reform and to suggest the shape of a solution, immunization serves as a useful example. This is a challenge President Clinton is already confronting. The basic public health authority of states can be used to make medical services achieve public health objectives. Failures and subsequent success in the United Kingdom suggest that it will be possible, even before National Health Care Reform is enacted, to know whether the Clinton administration and Congress have recognized the public health element.

Immunization fits perfectly into a reformed medical care system. It is a personal health service, like diagnosis or treatment, but is best understood as a public health strategy to reduce the burden of treatment costs and of disease for society as a whole. If, as our nation designs health care reform, we fail to require that public health interventions like immunization reduce the burden of disease, we will pay for avoidable doctor and hospital visits and escalate the tension around rationing of medical care for the ill.

A fundamental difference separates public health programs prescribed for populations from decisions of individuals to seek treatment. Immunization, for example, generates greatest savings only when it is applied so completely that disease outbreaks are averted altogether. Short of "herd immunity" (a high level of immunity in the population that reduces disease transmission), the unprotected—unvaccinated individuals and those in whom vaccine failed to stimulate immunity—remain vulnerable.

Historical lessons about immunization, starting with Edward Jenner, the inventor of the vaccine against smallpox, should guide reform. Jenner realized that simply administering vaccine to patients seeking medical care would not fulfill his dream of global eradication. Although Jenner understood them intuitively in 1796, two lessons need to be relearned: First, only systematic immunization of entire populations protects society from epidemics. Second, however central the role played by medical practitioners in administering vaccines, an explicit, population-based strategy must exist to assure participation by physicians and immunization of *everyone* who may be at risk. No society has achieved the public health benefit of vaccines simply by waiting for individuals to seek immunization, even where "access" and payment were guaranteed.

In 1979 the U.S. Public Health Service set national goals, asking each state to increase immunization rates for children from 60 to at least 90 percent. A crucial element of the strategy was federal pressure on states to enact and enforce laws requiring full immunization before a child can enter school. The striking operational success of this first systematic program, measured by the number of children fully immunized at school entry, masked a design failure revealed in the 1980s. The initial strategy focused on school age children whose immunization status could be checked on their first day in school. There was no comparable "check point" or enforcement plan for younger children who were not entering school.

About half of preschool children, especially those aged 0–2, remained incompletely immunized. A measles epidemic in 1989–91 brought the error of omission to the front pages of American newspapers. The U.S. Public Health Service acknowledged that a two-year epidemic had resulted in more than 55,000 reported cases of measles, more than 130 measles-related deaths, and 11,000 hospitalizations. President Clinton estimated the hospital costs alone at $20 million for an epidemic that $1 million worth of public health could have prevented. If past experience holds, for every measles death there will be three additional children with permanent brain damage who will continue to add costs to the medical care system throughout their lives. The epidemic was diagnosed as due to failure to immunize preschool children on time.

For immunization monitored at school entry, public health agencies could rely on practitioners and clinics to immunize children identified to need vaccine. Without a tracking and notification system to alert health authorities and families for each immunization visit, there was no population-based accountability for infants and toddlers, as at school entry. In the 1980s diminished federal public health funding, increasing vaccine prices, and increasing demand on public clinics compounded the problem. Even families who sought immunizations for their preschoolers could not always find them.

A reformed medical care system could cure these flaws and assure timely immunization of preschoolers (and adults, too), but only if practitioners are held accountable to a national public health strategy. Everyone must be guaranteed payment for services and a regular place to seek them. Moreover every person should be enrolled in a medical plan or practice which can be held responsible for the results—full and timely immunization of all enrollees. The difference between guaranteed "access" to medical care for those who seek it, and accountability of medical practices to public health authorities to render services that may never be sought by the consumer, is decisive. Bearing the distinction in mind, immunization is not the only public health service which can make use of a reformed medical care system.

When delivery of vaccines is fully integrated into a universal medical care program, public health support will be required as much as ever. We must assure that cases of vaccine-preventable disease are reported to public health authorities so that vaccine failures can be detected and flaws in the delivery system investigated and remedied. Disease surveillance based on competent laboratories will be needed to detect emerging and re-emerging infections. Our capacity to vaccinate with safe and effective vaccines will also depend on government research and development, and regulation. As a public health tool and because they have usually provided less return on investment than pharmaceuticals, vaccines are unlikely to attract sufficient investment without government assistance.

It is not clear that health care reformers understand the difference between clinical and public health laboratories, and no reform proposal acknowledges the difference or incorporates the public health function in its scheme. Public health laboratories perform tests to determine threats to the population even if there will be no diagnostic or therapeutic benefit to the individual from whom a sample is drawn. For example, we now have an effective vaccine for H flu type B, a disease which causes meningitis, predominantly in young children. When the vaccine was introduced in the state of Massachusetts it reduced the incidence of the disease by 70% in the first year. Similar results have occurred wherever the vaccine has been delivered universally.

There is no vaccine for other types of H flu, or for the nontypeable strains which also may cause invasive disease. With increased use of the H flu type B vaccine the relative importance of the other types and nontypeable strains is increasing as public health officials attempt to distinguish disease caused by strains against which there is no vaccine from failures of the vaccine to protect vaccinated children against type B. Similarly it is laboratory testing which allows public health officials to identify outbreaks which can be quelled by immunizing children who may have missed one or all doses of the type B vaccine.

Because there may be no clinical benefit to the individual patient to determine the particular strain, many clinical laboratories do not perform the tests. In the absence of a funded public health laboratory or of public funds to pay a clinical lab for this function, the lab may bill the patient or the patient's insurer, either of whom may refuse to pay the claim because the typing test does not enhance treatment. With increasing emphasis on cost containment, clinical labs are likely to avoid such testing. But most medical care reformers have not appreciated the distinction nor have they made provision to assure that technically competent laboratories handle public health testing—and guarantee remuneration. Public health officials also worry that cost containment-conscious physicians concerned only with their individual patients may not think to order these sorts of tests or to provide samples to their colleagues in public health laboratories. Many states are doing less of this sort of testing as appropriations shrink—or are less equipped to produce reliable results as the technology available in public facilities lags behind the clinical labs.

UNITED KINGDOM EXPERIENCE

Should one doubt that attention to public health strategies is needed when planning health care reform, consider the history of immunization in Britain. Failure of public health authorities to intervene in the National Health Service and of medical practitioners to practice public health subjected Britons to forty years of unnecessary exposure to vaccine-preventable disease.

The British adopted their version of national health care reform in 1947 by establishing the National Health Service. Its designers made the erroneous assumption that universal access to and payment for medical services would suffice. It took forty-four years before they understood the flaw in their original blueprint and were able to correct it. We need not replicate that misjudgment.

Since 1947 basic medical services in England have been provided by general practitioners, salaried by the National Health Service. Since the start every child was on the list of a general practitoner paid and equipped to provide recommended immunizations. The vaccines were available free to doctor and patient which eased the process. Even so, in the 1960s children unimmunized against pertussis fueled the spread of frightening epidemic disease. Whooping cough outbreaks were evident in hospital admission rates. How was this happening with universal, fully paid access to medical services?

The answer was almost too simple: medical practitioners left to their own devices were not very good at public health. Even where they administered vaccines to children whose families sought them at appropriate intervals, physicians did not seek out all those on their lists who came in late or not at all. Doctors saw only the individual child, rarely encountering the broader consequences of missed immunizations. In the absence of data showing that practitioners were giving preventive services principally to patients who sought them, never reaching many who remained at risk, epidemic pertussis erupted before health authorities knew national rates of immunization were too low to maintain herd immunity. Even assigning every child to a doctor had not guaranteed high levels of immunization coverage.

Belatedly the national public health agency (Department of Health) asserted leadership and enlisted the medical care system (National Health Service) in a joint effort to avert further epidemics. In April 1990 the Department set targets and reviews for all levels of operation of the NHS. This time they assured good results.

By 1991 immunization coverage in England rose from a national average of approximately 70 percent to an unprecedented high of 90 percent for children in every age group. . . .

Because success was so impressive, new target levels have been set to raise coverage levels to 95 percent of all children. British public health authorities have made doctors a contributing part of the national immunization effort, and today no one suggests that a separate public health program is required to achieve universal childhood immunization as public health guidance and support has purposefully been integrated into daily medical practice.

Childhood immunization is a powerful example, but other public health objectives can be realized as well—if we articulate the strategy and assign to the medical services delivery system those tasks its medical practitioners can perform most effectively and efficiently. Together, the federal government and the states should build a system in which:

- medical services providers detect, obtain necessary laboratory confirmation, and report cases of disease in a prescribed manner, helping public health inspectors and investigators find and control sources of exposure in the community;
- medical services providers respond promptly with early diagnostic testing and treatment when individuals at high risk (or their characteristics) are identified by public health workers in the community;
- medical services providers reach every member of the population who can benefit individually or when "treatments" are needed to protect others;
- medical services providers know if their interventions are succeeding and if new or different health problems threaten our people.

CONCLUSION

An expanded prescription would require the reformed medical care system to perform certain functions systematically that in the past have been optional for medical practitioners or left to health departments by default. The challenge to reformers is to rebuild the core public health capacity of the states to create a competent national system, and to assure that the medical services that we will pay for under health care reform perform certain functions critical to the health of the public. How can we know that the federal reformers are incorporating every intervention that can improve health and hold off unnecessary expenditures? Do they have a thorough analysis of how medical services will contribute to public health? And if so, does their analysis indicate which of these services require assistance and guidance from public health departments? Have they made sure in each instance to *secure* resources for the public health component as well as for medical services?

This advice is not new, but it is timely. Seventy-five years ago, a warning about inattention to public health agencies was issued to the Medical and Chirugical Faculty of Maryland. It must be heeded today as we reform medical care:

> With the appropriations for health insurance running into millions of dollars annually it goes without saying that legislative bodies will not materially increase the appropriations for their health departments. Owing to this fact, there is a decided probability of sickness insurance acts endangering the very existence of State health departments by absorbing all of the funds available for health work. Our statesmen and lawmakers must, therefore, be careful that proper and ample provisions are made for health machinery in any sickness insurance act.

IV

NEW TECHNOLOGY AND THE PUBLIC'S HEALTH

8

REPRODUCTIVE ISSUES

The right of individuals to decide whether and when and how often to have children has been held to be a basic human right. Procreative liberty[1] can be defended on several grounds. Classic liberals stress the right of individuals to make intimate and private decisions, especially those that reflect religious or spiritual values, without government intervention.[2] In the United States, the Supreme Court has held that a fundamental constitutional right of privacy[3] protects the right of individuals to use birth control and to terminate pregnancies prior to viability.[4] Feminists stress the essential connection between the ability of women to control their fertility and equality.[5] Public health professionals consider access to contraceptives and family planning to be an intrinsic part of women's health care, because of the health risks associated with too many pregnancies and births. Unintended and unwanted pregnancies also result in children who may not be properly cared for. All of these factors contribute to a general recognition of the right of individuals to avoid reproduction, including a right to have access to contraception and abortion. Indeed, many in public health view the legalization of abortion as the greatest advance since penicillin.[6] At the same time, the topic of abortion remains controversial and divisive. Precisely for that reason, it is represented in virtually every textbook on medical ethics, in numerous applied ethics collections, and in several collections devoted solely to abortion.[7] Rather than cover this well-trod ground, we have decided to focus, not on the right to avoid procreation, but rather the right *to have children.* This is the flip side of procreative liberty—the affirmative right to have offspring, and therefore not to be subjected to forced contraception, sterilization, or abortion. Although this too is generally regarded as also part of the right of privacy, nevertheless, from time to time, proposals are made to limit the reproductive freedom of various groups. For example, bills have been introduced to encourage (some would say "force") women on welfare to use Norplant, a long-acting contraceptive. At least one judge made the use of Norplant a condition of probation for a woman who pled guilty to child abuse. Another judge sentenced a couple convicted of sexually molesting the woman's son to ten years in prison, but offered them probation if the woman (not the man!) would consent to a tubal ligation.[8]

All of these proposals have been roundly criticized, on a variety of grounds, not least of which is that they infringe individuals' rights to reproduce. Undoubtedly, such proposals sometimes have punitive and moralistic motives (see Chapter 4), but they also reflect a plausible view that individuals ought, if possible, to refrain from reproducing if they are unable or unwilling adequately to care for children, or if conditions are such that the children would be likely to have lives of extreme suffering or deprivation.[9] The right to procreate is not an absolute right and needs to be balanced in light of both parental and social responsibility. At the same time, proposals to restrict the right to reproduce need to be evaluated in light of the history of forcible sterilization of the "feeble-minded." This sordid chapter in U.S. history is chillingly recounted in the first selection by Philip Reilly. As Reilly points out, some of those who were sterilized were actually not mentally retarded. Many were poor or members of minority groups, or institutionalized for other reasons. Moreover, sterilization programs were often instituted not to protect children from abusive or incompetent parents but out of the belief that some individuals or "races" are inferior and ought not to reproduce. The legacy of eugenics has implications not only for reproduction but also for genetics (covered in Chapter 9).

Over the last few decades, reproductive medicine has made huge strides. Assisted reproductive technologies (ART), from the relatively "low tech" (fertility drugs) to the more "high tech" (*in vitro* fertilization or IVF), enable some infertile individuals to have children they could not have had in the past. New techniques and improvements of existing techniques are being made all the time. At the same time, ART is very expensive, imposes physical and emotional burdens, and has a relatively low success rate, all of which make it unlikely to help more than a small proportion of infertile individuals. Using "the lens of public health," Elizabeth Heitman suggests that a better approach to the problem of infertility includes increased and expanded research on infertility, public education about the effect of sexually transmitted diseases (STDs) on fertility, and increased access to preventive measures against and treatment of STDs.

Some people have wondered why we should be concerned with infertility in a world that is already overpopulated. There is general agreement among experts that overpopulation is a problem, but there is a split in the population field between two different approaches. On one side are those who see overpopulation as the primary problem, because it is thought inevitably to lead to poverty, famine, disease, environmental catastrophe, and social unrest, especially in developing countries. Those who take this approach, which is sometimes labeled "zero population growth," are often willing to impose coercive measures, if necessary, to prevent these disasters.

On the other side are those who advocate a human development approach to population in which reproductive health, improving the status of women, and protecting individual rights are central objectives. This approach holds that allowing individuals to make their own procreative choices and empowering them to carry out these choices is the way to solve the problem of overpopulation. Human development advocates maintain that improving the quality of life of people in poorer countries will lead to population stabilization, as it has in richer countries. Moreover, they point out that coercive policies to limit population often turn out to be ineffective and even counterproductive. Finally, human development advocates do not regard overpopulation as the main problem. They maintain that most resource depletion and environmental damage stems less from population increases in poorer nations than from overconsumption in richer ones. Reducing population by itself will not address these harms.

Further complicating the area of population studies is the complexity of the question of ideal population size, an issue brought out in the selection by Joel E. Cohen. According to Cohen, the question, "How many people can the earth support?" is not a question like, "How old are you?" That is, it does not have a definitive correct answer. How many people at what standard of living? For how long? With what safety net in case of natural disasters? Only after we understand the multitude of issues behind the "deceptively simple" question, "How many people can the earth support?" can we begin to ask which approach to population policy, the "zero population growth" or the human development approach, is most likely to be effective. Readers of this book will also want to ask which approach best reflects a public health perspective.

NOTES

1. "Procreative liberty" is the term John Robertson uses in his book, *Children of Choice: Freedom and the New Reproductive Technologies* (Princeton University Press, 1994), to describe the right to have, or not have, offspring.

2. For a powerful statement of the liberal position, see Ronald Dworkin, *Life's Dominion* (New York: Alfred A. Knopf, 1993).

3. The expression "fundamental constitutional right" is no longer commonly used. Instead, the justices refer to "protected liberty interests." See, for example, *Griswold v. Connecticut,* 381 U.S. 479 (1965); *Roe v. Wade,* 410 U.S. 1134 (1973).

4. See, for example, Susan Sherwin, *No Longer Patient: Feminist Ethics and Health Care* (Philadelphia, PA: Temple University Press, 1992, pp. 99–116); and Rosalind Pollack Petchesky, *Abortion and Woman's Choice: The State, Sexuality, and Reproductive Freedom* (Boston, MA: Northeastern University Press, 1985).

5. Not all public health officials regard abortion as a public health triumph. For some, those who consider abortion to be the killing of innocent children, the legalization of abortion is undoubtedly regarded as a public health catastrophe. Former Surgeon General C. Everett Koop is a notable example. How one regards abortion, then, is not simply a matter of taking a public health perspective but also depends largely on one's views about the moral status of the fetus.

6. See, for example, John D. Arras and Bonnie Steinbock, eds., *Ethical Issues in Modern Medicine,* 5th ed. (Mountain View, California: Mayfield, 1998), and Susan Dwyer and Joel Feinberg, *The Problem of Abortion,* 3rd ed. (Wadsworth, 1997).

7. All of these cases are discussed in my article, "The Concept of Coercion and Long-Term Contraceptives," in Ellen H. Moskowitz and Bruce Jennings, eds. *Coerced Contraception? Moral and Policy Challenges of Long-Acting Birth Control* (Washington, D.C.: Georgetown University Press, 1996, pp. 53–78).

8. For a defense of this view, see, for example, John D. Arras, "AIDS and Reproductive Decisions: Having Children in Fear and Trembling," *Milbank Quarterly* 68, no. 3 (1990), pp. 353–382, and Bonnie Steinbock and Ron McClamrock, "When Is Birth Unfair to the Child?," *Hastings Center Report* 24, No. 6 (1994), pp. 15–21.

9. See Sissela Bok, "Population and Ethics: Expanding the Moral Space," in Gita Sen, Adrienne Germain and Lincoln Chen, eds. *Population Policies Reconsidered* (Cambridge, MA: Harvard University Press, 1994, pp. 15–26).

The Resurgence of Eugenics

Philip R. Reilly

As we have seen, in the first two decades of this century a remarkable number of sterilization laws were enacted, and about thirty-two hundred institutionalized persons were subjected to eugenic sterilization. The bulk of this activity took place from 1909 to 1913, and legislative voting records suggest that the laws had wide support. However, eugenic sterilization programs were actually implemented only in those states in which key persons, such as superintendents of state hospitals, were supportive. Except in California and several Midwestern states, relatively few residents of institutions were sterilized. During World War I, many of the laws were struck down by the courts, and for a time (1918–22), no new sterilization statutes were enacted.

Despite the demise of most of the laws, the number of institutionalized persons who were sterilized each year in the United States continued to rise. This was largely due to the California program. From January 1, 1918, until December 31, 1920, there were 1,150 sterilizations performed upon persons in six California state hospitals for the insane, roughly one for every six persons admitted. About three hundred retarded persons were also sterilized at the Sonoma State Home, an institution with a capacity of twenty-two hundred residents. During those three years, approximately 80 percent of all eugenic sterilizations carried out in the United States were performed in seven institutions in one state.

Despite the quiescence of sterilization programs virtually everywhere except California, the sterilization movement soon made a remarkable comeback. A small number of eugenicists capitalized effectively on the national concern over the dramatic postwar influx of immigrants from Southern and Eastern Europe and growing uneasiness about the northern migration of American blacks. The resurgence of sterilization programs was closely tied to the popular demand to limit immigration. The eugenicists' argument that hordes of immigrants would weaken the American gene pool provided part of the intellectual rationale for

From Chapter 6 in *The Surgical Solution: A History of Involuntary Sterilization in the United States* by Philip Reilly (The Johns Hopkins University Press, 1991). Reprinted by permission of the publisher and the author.

the restrictive Immigration Act of 1924. It is no accident that a second wave of state sterilization laws, targeted at a different threat to the "race," were enacted at the same time.

The issues discussed at the Second International Congress of Eugenics, which met at the American Museum of Natural History in New York City in September 1921, reflect this dual concern. Authorities in genetics, medicine, and eugenics presented 108 papers. Fifty-three reported on laboratory genetics or pedigree studies that documented the inheritance of human traits; 55 addressed the biological and social consequences of marriages between persons of different ethnic backgrounds. As the papers, including those such as "Some Notes on the Negro Problem," "The Problem of Negro-White Intermixture," and "Inter-marriage with the Slave Race" suggest, there was special concern about miscegenation. Nor was that concern limited to eugenic circles. During the first quarter of this century, many states enacted laws that were intended to tighten already existing limits on interracial marriage.

The roots of antimiscegenation law are deeply set in the soil of American history. As early as 1630, only a few years after Negroes were brought to Virginia, the governor's council declared that Hugh Davis, a white man, was to be whipped publicly for "abusing himself to the dishonor of God and shame of Christians by defiling his body in lying with a Negro." In 1662, the state's general antifornication statute was amended to include heavier penalties if the guilty parties had also violated racial boundaries. In tracing Virginia legislative history (which is typical of the South), one finds an unswerving preoccupation with preserving those boundaries. A law enacted in 1787 declared that "every person who shall have one-fourth part or more of Negro blood shall be deemed a mulatto." There the color line held until 1910 when the state legislature, responding to increasing intermarriage between whites and blacks, declared that any person whose ancestry was one-sixteenth Negro was of that race. Many Americans feared that dilution of the ancestral stock by mulattoes and blacks threatened the nation's future. According to one authority, between 1890 and 1910 the "colored" population increased by 81 percent, while the Negro population increased by only 22.7 percent.

In Virginia the legislature responded by passing legislation titled "An Act to Preserve Racial Integrity." The key feature of this law, the most powerful legal obstacle to interracial marriage erected since the Civil War, was to define a "white" person as one "who has no trace whatsoever of any blood other than Caucasian." Officials charged with issuing marriage licenses were ordered not to do so until they had "reasonable assurance that the statements as to color of both man and woman are correct." Existing interracial marriages were declared void regardless of the state in which they had been licensed, and interracial cohabitation was declared a crime. There was one exception to the antimiscegenation policy. The "Pocahontas exception," written in deference to the large number of persons who claimed to be descendants of Pocahontas and John Rolfe, permitted a white to marry "a person with one-sixteenth or less of the blood of an American Indian." At least two other states, Georgia and Alabama, followed Virginia's lead and defined as white only those persons whose genealogy was untainted. . . .

Although many ardent proponents of eugenic sterilization believed that it would reduce the prevalence of crime, most early twentieth-century American criminologists flatly rejected this neo-Lombrosian thesis. For example, in his book, *Criminology* (1918), Maurice Parmelee asserted that Lombroso was "rather ignorant of the modern science of biology, and especially of the theory of heredity." Parmelee argued that what Lombroso had called "atavistic" traits were in reality examples of arrested development caused by an inhospitable environment. He admitted that hereditary factors sometimes figured in criminal conduct, but overall, he saw little value in sterilization as a means of reducing crime.

Six years later, when Edwin Sutherland, a criminologist working at the University of Illinois, published his textbook, the vestiges of Lombrosian thought were sparse indeed. Sutherland wrote that "criminality as such cannot be inherited. If any trait is inherited which predisposes to crime, we do not know what it is. Even in the case of the feeble-minded and insane, it is not clear that their abnormalities are inherited, in the strict sense of the word, in a very large proportion of cases and, in addition, it is not clear that people with such difficulties are more prone to commit crimes than other people." Sutherland concluded that there was "no evidence that criminality would be reduced appreciably" by sterilization laws.

Some contemporary journalists, however, advanced a more titillating view. For example, during 1924 and 1925 French Strother, editor of *World's Work,* a popular tabloid, wrote five articles on the biological basis of crime. These pieces illustrate how eugenics was portrayed for the lay reader. One article, "The Cause of Crime: Defective Brain," was a profile of Harry Olson's work as chief justice of the Chicago Municipal Court. Strother quoted Olson as asserting that "practically all criminals are mentally abnormal." In 1914, convinced that it was time to use scientific methods in the service of crime prevention, Olson had founded the Psychopathic Laboratory. He instructed its director, Dr. William Hickson, a psychometrician, to develop "tests of character" to identify criminals. A decade later Strother reported that Hickson had discovered that dementia praecox (schizophrenia) was the cause of nearly all crimes, a finding that he promised would revolutionize criminology. Hickson's conclusions supplied Judge Olson, a staunch eugenicist, with exactly the mechanistic view of aberrant behavior that he sought. On returning from a tour of European psychology laboratories, Hickson reported to Olson that he had learned a new method of screening for criminal tendencies. He was convinced that nine out of ten criminals were mentally abnormal, and that he could identify more precisely the specific types of defects that led to crime. He suggested to reporters that the Chicago Police should round up the city's one hundred toughest characters and that those found by Psychopathic Laboratory tests to be abnormal should be committed *before* they harmed society.

Another of Strother's articles, "The Cure for Crime," was a strident argument to "stop the breeding of mental defectives" as quickly as possible. A third, which purported to be a primer on heredity, illustrated Mendelian inheritance by discussing the gene for Jewish facial appearance. Analyzing "all possible Jewish-Gentile crosses," Strother advised his readers that "all children of a Jew and a Gentile will look like Gentiles, that if a pure Gentile marries a half-Jew, all the children will look like Gentiles, and that if a half-Jew marries a half-Jew, one child of every four will look like a Jew and the other three will look like Gentiles." Unfortunately, more people probably read Strother's article in one week than read genetics textbooks in an entire year.

The tireless efforts of a few prominent eugenicists like Judge Olson, who oversaw the work of thirty-six other judges, helped to keep prosterilization arguments viable during the years just after defeats in the courts. Olson flatly condemned the view in academic criminology circles that there was no persuasive evidence for the heritability of criminal tendencies. In his 1925 presidential address to the Eugenic Research Association, he asserted: "Crime prevention, finally, is seen to be the weeding out of defective stocks, and it is the first step in the eugenics program."

EUGENICS SOCIETIES

As Americans grew more discontented with the huge influx of immigrants in the postwar years, many people became interested in the problem of racial vigor. In dozens of towns across America, small groups of citizens organized to ponder this and other eugenic questions. Two of these organizations, the American Eugenics Society and the Human Betterment Foundation, attained some prominence. Although it is difficult to assess their impact on sterilization policy, there is no doubt that they published pamphlets, provided speakers, and worked assiduously to keep eugenics proposals, especially sterilization, alive as newsworthy topics.

Although the American Eugenics Society was not incorporated until 1926, it was started shortly after the Second International Congress of Eugenics met in New York City in September 1921. If the First International Eugenics Congress, which had convened in London in 1912, reflected the eugenic thinking in Great Britain, the New York City meeting showed that a group of committed eugenicists had emerged in the United States. Dr. Henry Fairfield Osborn, president of the American Museum of Natural History, was chosen by his American col-leagues as president of the Second International Congress, Madison Grant was elected treasurer, and the tireless Laughlin worked as chairman of the Exhibits Committee. After the congress closed, several prominent Americans, wanting to do more than maintain a committee affiliated with the London-based Interna-tional Commission on Eugenics, formed the Eugenics Society of the United States of America.

By March 1923 this New York-based group, which changed its name to the American Eugenics Society (AES) in 1924, was sufficiently cohesive to be lobbying in Albany against legislation that it felt would have dysgenic effects. With strong support from the New York Charities Aid Association (an organiza-tion abhorred by hard-core eugenicists), two New York legislators had intro-duced a bill providing special educational assistance for "retarded" children (defined as those who were learning at a level that was three or more years below that expected for their age). The Austin-Cole Bill proposed providing state funds to stimulate the schools to hire more teachers to work in special education. A memorandum prepared by Laughlin for the AES about this bill described the proposed program as unequivocally "anti-eugenic," siphoning tax dollars that would be better spent on the gifted. He suggested lobbying to amend the law so that the retarded children could be sterilized. "Otherwise," he feared, "the education of the defective will bolster him or her up to the repro-ductive period and will make it more possible for him or her to become a parent than would be possible if he or she were less well trained." Despite the efforts of the AES, the bill became law.

In the mid-twenties Irving Fisher, a professor of public policy at Yale, was the driving force behind the AES, which then maintained its headquarters in New Haven. Fisher enlisted a zealous but unsophisticated eugenicist named Leon Whitney to be the society's secretary. Whitney, a wealthy farmer and an avid dog breeder, had undergone an almost mystical conversion to eugenics, giving up his comfortable country life to plunge into a new career. In 1928 he published *The Basis of Breeding* (dedicated to Laughlin), a volume intended to educate laypersons about genetics. One key eugenics activity that Whitney ex-tolled in his book was to sponsor "fitter family" contests. These contests fre-quently took place at fairs in the Midwest: judges reviewed human pedigrees to determine the most eugenically positive families, just as the best cattle, chickens, and pigs competed for blue ribbons. He also helped the AES to con-struct a "Eugenics Catechism," a pamphlet of questions and answers about eu-genics, and to launch the publication of a periodical called *Eugenics*. . . .

Gosney first learned of the eugenics movement from a newspaper article that announced the opening of the Eugenics Record Office in Cold Spring Harbor in 1910. He wrote to Charles Davenport to learn more, and his interest soon be-came advocacy. By 1920, Gosney had become convinced that the crucial undertaking in eugenics would be to educate young people about the importance of mate selection. But despite his offers of financial support, he was unable to persuade any university to sponsor his unique educational plan. Thwarted in his first effort, Gosney turned his attention to the study of negative eugenics. He decided to analyze the history of sterilization in California. In 1926 Gosney organized a council of advisers, including Dr. J. H. McBride, a member of the state Commission on Immigration and Housing, and Paul Popenoe, a sociologist who edited the *Journal of Heredity,* to begin a detailed examination of how sterilization of thousands of California's defectives had affected the state. During this period his interest became a conviction, and in 1929 he created the Human Betterment Foundation (HBF), a nonprofit corporation intended to foster eugenics.

From the inception of the California sterilization study Gosney turned to Laughlin for advice. Laughlin provided him with copies of the forms that he used to record and store eugenic data at the ERO and urged him to visit the state hospitals, advice probably given because Laughlin knew the frightening impact that large numbers of poorly housed feeble-minded persons could have on an inexperienced person. A few weeks later Gosney wrote Laughlin that McBride and Popenoe were visiting institutions around the state and that he was gathering the support of physicians and government officials for undertaking a much larger study of sterilization. In reply, Laughlin sent the names and addresses of fifty-two persons whom he knew had been released from California hospitals after being sterilized so that Gosney could conduct a follow-up investigation on the long-term effects of vasectomy.

In March of 1926 Gosney and Laughlin formally agreed to collaborate. From Gosney's perspective, at least, there was ample reason to do so: "It appears to me that there will be great value in having two independent and parallel studies of this topic. The whole project of sterilization is continually under attack, and is certain to be attacked still more vehemently if we proceed with an educational campaign on its behalf. To meet these attacks, we will need all the ammunition available, and it seems unquestionable that a single investigation would be less effective than a double investigation."

By May 1927 Gosney had assembled an impressive list of consultants to the sterilization study. They included David Starr Jordan, chancellor of Stanford University, Lewis Terman, the nation's most prominent psychometrician, and S. J. Holmes, the Berkeley geneticist. Over the next few months the HBF consultants approved eighteen reports on the medical, psychological, economic, and legal dimensions of California's long-running (1909–27) sterilization program. Collectively these reports, all of which were published during the next three years, constituted the first comprehensive "proof" that sterilization was cost-effective and posed no significant medical harm to the institutionalized persons at whom it was aimed. Popenoe, who wrote many of the papers, reassured readers that the data revealed no evidence of discrimination because of race or ethnicity, and that two-thirds of those paroled after sterilization did "reasonably well" outside of the institutions. By 1928 his work was sufficiently well regarded that he was invited to address the annual meeting of the American Bar Association on the topic of sterilization and criminality. *Sterilization for Human Betterment,* published by Gosney and Popenoe in 1929, was the first comprehensive discussion of sterilization aimed at the lay reader. They argued that under a scientifically applied sterilization program, "the number of mentally defective persons in the community could be reduced by perhaps as much as half in three or four generations."

In 1930 the HBF began to conduct an annual survey of state sterilization programs. Like Dr. Sharp before World War I and Harry Laughlin in the 1920s, during the 1930s Edward Gosney and Paul Popenoe were the chief propagandists for and scorekeepers of eugenic sterilization in America. For example, in 1935 the HBF mailed over forty thousand pamphlets containing their sterilization survey results to professors at 436 colleges in every state and several foreign countries. During 1935, Gosney even convinced Harry Chandler, publisher of the *Los Angeles Times,* to run a column, "Social Eugenics," in the paper's Sunday magazine.

By the late 1920s Gosney's name had begun to appear on the letterheads of the various eastern eugenics groups. In 1932 he was invited to speak at the Third International Congress on Eugenics in New York City. He must have regarded this as a signal honor, for despite his age and poor health, he took the long train ride across America. His speech at this last great gathering of eugenicists rejected the belief that segregation or involuntary contraception could effectively limit reproduction by defectives. He was convinced that any technique other than sterilization would result in the births of many more defective persons. The HBF was quite active until Gosney's death in 1942, when it too ceased to exist. . . .

One of the most colorful and zealous (if ineffective) eugenicists of the 1930s was a Kansas City businessman named J. H. Pile. In 1938, extremely concerned by the sharply declining birth rate that the Depression fostered, Pile set up the Eugenic Babies Foundation. It was intended to increase reproduction by women "above the average in intellect" and to deny parenthood to "chronic paupers, confirmed criminals, feeble-minded and insane persons." Pile, who hoped for an endowment of one hundred million dollars, launched a campaign to enlist the United States Chamber of Commerce and the various eugenics societies in his cause. He frequently wrote to the AES. However, Huntington and Osborn eschewed involvement with radical groups, and they decided to "steer clear of Mr. Pile." Pile's utopian fantasy should not, however, be dismissed too quickly, While his proposals were ridiculed in the United States, German officials were initiating *Lebensborn,* a program that involved kidnapping eugenically desirable children from Poland and elsewhere, and setting up special homes where the sturdiest German girls were urged to become pregnant by select German soldiers and bear their "superior" babies.

In 1939 the AES was courted by another would-be eugenic philanthropist. After his graduation from Princeton at the turn of the century, James G. Eddy made a fortune in the lumber industry. He later founded the Institute for Forest Genetics, which contributed substantially to that field and earned the support of the Carnegie Institute. In 1938 Eddy approached Laughlin, offering to support a human heredity clinic that would alert couples to the risk of bearing defective babies. Laughlin carried the plan to the directors of the Carnegie Institute (a mistake, since he was in disfavor), who rejected it as being too removed from basic research. Eddy then asked if the AES would consider operating such a clinic for which he would provide one-half the first year's budget. Although Osborn admired Eddy, he and Huntington agreed that a "marriage reference bureau" was too limited an operation for the AES. Just a few years later the Dight Institute at the University of Minnesota started a similar clinic that was perhaps the nation's first genetic counseling center.

Although the 1930s saw a general shift of emphasis toward programs that enhanced principles of positive eugenics, some groups continued to push for sterilization. The mandate of the Sterilization League of New Jersey . . . which began in Princeton in 1934, was to put "a check on the reproduction of defectives." The president was T. L. Zimmerman, a former judge of the juvenile and Domestic Relations Court in Bergen County. For nearly a decade the league lobbied arduously but unsuccessfully for a sterilization law. Despite repeated legislative defeats at home, the league was a tireless propagandist for eugenic sterilization.

THE SECOND WAVE OF STERILIZATION LAWS

After a peak in 1913, when five new states adopted sterilization laws, legislative activity slowed significantly. From 1918 until the end of 1922, only Washington was added to the ranks, while seven other state laws were invalidated. But in 1923 there was a resurgence of legislative activity, and eugenic sterilization laws were enacted in Oregon, Montana, Delaware, and Michigan. Virginia adopted a sterilization law the following year, and in 1925 the legislative floodgates opened. Nine state legislatures passed bills, and seven were enacted (two were vetoed). Of these Idaho, Utah, Minnesota, and Maine enacted their first eugenic sterilization laws. At the end of 1925, enabling legislation to support sterilization programs was law in seventeen states.

Advocates had learned from the mistakes made in earlier legislative efforts. For example, after carefully analyzing the constitutional infirmities of the early laws, Laughlin drafted a model eugenic sterilization bill that purported to safe-guard the procedural rights of the persons to whom it might be applied, and that satisfied the Equal Protection Clause. The bill required the state eugenicist to conduct surveys to identify persons who were "potential parents of socially inadequate offspring." Such surveys would canvass the entire population, not merely the residents of state institutions, without regard to "personality, sex, age, marital condition, race or possessions." If the state eugenicist determined that an individual was a potential parent of socially inadequate offspring and a candidate for involuntary sterilization, the statute required a hearing, followed automatically by a jury trial and the right of appeal. Although no state enacted the precise text of Laughlin's bill (a draft of which was approved by the American Bar Association Committee on Sterilization), many of its features were incorporated into new bills. The phrase "potential parent of socially inadequate offspring" was widely copied.

What was the attitude of state officials in regard to implementing these new statutes? An unpublished manuscript, entitled "Sterilization of the Unfit Degenerates," which contains the results of a survey of state officials conducted in 1925 by the Rhode Island State Library, sheds some light on this question. For example, the Connecticut state librarian responded that he found no evidence of eugenic sterilizations performed in that state's institutions during the prior ten years.

The executive director of the Delaware Board of Charities, J. Hall Anderson, reported that without benefit of legislation (but with the consent of the families), he had authorized the sterilization of four patients. Anderson strongly advocated a broad sterilization law to cover "cases outside of Institutions," but noted that "in the present state of political opinion it would probably be impossible to get the Legislature to sanction such a drastic measure." This comment was made just when many legislatures were passing compulsory sterilization laws, suggesting that public opinion drew the line firmly at the institution's portals.

Officials in Kansas, a state that adopted a very aggressive sterilization policy in the mid-1920s, worried that the public might be offended by overzealous application of the law. Charles S. Huffman, a member of the Board of Educational, Charitable and Correctional Institutions, noted that "the larger number of protests come from those of the Catholic faith who claim it is against their religious teachings to interfere with nature." Catholic opposition to sterilization became quite active during the mid-1930s. Nevertheless, Kansas was one of the first states whose officials explicitly adopted a policy of sterilizing "most all feeble-minded, institutionalized women patients of the childbearing age."

Just as they had in the past, opponents of involuntary sterilization laws launched a constitutional attack on the flurry of new laws. The battle was joined in two states, Michigan and Virginia. The Michigan law, which contemplated sterilizing "idiots, imbeciles, and the feeble-minded, but not the insane," was not limited to institutionalized persons. Shortly after an order by the Wayne County Probate Court that one Willie Smith should be sterilized by "vasectomy or X-ray," his guardian *ad litem* challenged the law. On June 18, 1925, the Supreme Court of Michigan ruled that the statute was "justified by the findings of Biological Science," and was "a proper and reasonable exercise of the police power of the state." The high court also held that a section of the law that exempted from sterilization wealthy feeble-minded persons who could pay for the care of their children was a violation of the Equal Protection Clause. Nevertheless, the Michigan decision, the first by a state supreme court to uphold a eugenic sterilization law, was a major victory for the pro-sterilization forces.

The constitutional challenge to the Virginia law, which was ultimately decided by the Supreme Court of the United States, had the largest impact on eugenic sterilization programs. Early in 1924 the Virginia legislature, noting that "heredity plays an important part in the transmission of insanity, idiocy, imbecility, epilepsy and crime," overwhelmingly passed an involuntary sterilization bill (the Senate voted 30–0; the House, 75–2). The law, which gave the superintendents of five state institutions the power to petition a special board for permission to sterilize those inmates whom they believed it would benefit, was signed by the governor on March 20, 1924.

On January 23, 1924, an eighteen-year-old woman named Carrie E. Buck, the illegitimate daughter of an allegedly feeble-minded woman named Addie Emmet, who had been adopted by a Charlottesville family at the age of four, was committed to the State Colony for Epileptics and Feeble-Minded. Always a problem child, Carrie, who was said to have a mental age of nine and an I.Q. of about 50, had recently given birth to an illegitimate child who was also allegedly feeble-minded. Fearing that Carrie would bear more children in the State Colony, Dr. A. S. Priddy, the superintendent, petitioned for sterilization. Realizing that the law would eventually be challenged, state officials were eager to make this the test case. In searching for an expert witness, they asked the advice of Judge Olson, who recommended Harry Laughlin. Although he never saw the patient, on the basis of his review of her records Laughlin concluded that Carrie was part of the "shiftless, ignorant and worthless class of anti-social whites of the South." He noted that her sexual immorality was "a typical picture of the low-grade moron," and that the possibility of her feeble-mindedness being due to nonhereditary causes was "exceptionally remote."

On September 10, 1924, the board approved the sterilization of Carrie Buck. A young attorney named R. G. Shelton was appointed as her guardian, and he immediately appealed to the Circuit Court of Amherst County, Virginia. The case was argued on November 18, 1924, and Laughlin's deposition was submitted into evidence. On April 13, 1925, Judge Bennet Gordon upheld the constitutionality of the law and ordered that Carrie be sterilized within ninety days.

The record that the proponents of the law compiled was impressive. Besides the testimony of Laughlin, they secured the support of Dr. J. S. DeJarnett, superintendent of the largest state institution in Indiana, and Dr. Arthur Estabrook, a colleague of Laughlin's at Cold Spring Harbor who specialized in pedigree analysis and who had worked as a eugenics adviser to the state of Indiana. Shelton secured *no* experts to testify on Carrie Buck's behalf. In upholding the decision of the local court, the Virginia Supreme Court of Appeals rejected Carrie's argument that the law violated the Equal Protection Clause of the Constitution. Judge Jesse P. West ruled that the statute constituted a reasonable kind of class legislation that was intended to *benefit* the persons who would be sterilized. The decision was affirmed without dissent.

On February 6, 1926, Carrie Buck appealed to the United States Supreme Court. Although the highest court had refused to hear arguments on the validity of sterilization laws in the past, this time it permitted the appeal, and the case was argued in the autumn. In his brief, Shelton presciently warned that if the law was upheld, "A reign of doctors will be inaugurated and in the name of science new classes will be added, even races may be brought within the scope of such a regulation and the worst forms of tyranny practiced." This is, of course, a capsule summary of Nazi eugenics.

On May 2, 1927, by vote of 8 to 1, the Supreme Court upheld the Virginia involuntary sterilization law. Justice Oliver Wendell Holmes, eighty-six years old at the time, wrote the brief majority opinion. In now famous words, Holmes asserted: "It is better for all the world, if instead of waiting to execute degenerate offspring for crime, or to let them starve for their imbecility, society can prevent those who are manifestly unfit from continuing their kind. The principle that sustains compulsory vaccination is broad enough to cover cutting the Fallopian tubes."

Dismissing the objection that the Virginia statute violated the Equal Protection Clause by treating institutionalized persons differently from those not in institutions as "the last resort of constitutional arguments," Holmes, whose published letters strongly suggest that he was a eugenicist, opened the doors to eugenic sterilization in the United States. Justice Butler, the only dissenter, did not file an opinion. Although the resurgence of sterilization laws had been under way for four years when *Buck v. Bell* was decided, the Supreme Court ruling greatly boosted the pace at which sterilization programs were enacted and implemented. During the next few years the number of states with sterilization laws jumped from seventeen to thirty, and the number of sterilizations performed on institutionalized persons rose substantially. The subsequent fifteen years (1927–42) were a triumphant period for those who embraced hereditarian hopes for social progress.

Infertility As a Public Health Problem: Why Assisted Reproductive Technologies Are Not the Answer

ELIZABETH HEITMAN

Since the late 1970s, remarkable technological developments in the medical treatment of infertility have received tremendous public attention. Almost simultaneously, both the lay and medical press have announced that impaired fertility is a significant health problem in the United States, what some have called an "epidemic of infertility." The lay press commonly cite the alarming statistic that one out of every twelve couples, and as high as one in six in some age groups, is unable to have children. But while the new sub-specialty of reproductive medicine has grown into a multibillion dollar enterprise, the public health dimensions of infertility have received relatively little attention.

In this time of increased interest in preventive and primary care medicine and efforts to develop community priorities for health services, public health perspectives warrant particular consideration. Regrettably, public health's traditional research and strategic agendas in the area of reproduction have left significant gaps in our understanding of the causes, prevention, and treatment of infertility and its implications for health planning, education, and policy. Moreover, public health policies and rhetoric on family planning ironically may appear to support the widespread use of the very sort of high-tech interventions that public health advocates typically consider too costly and ineffective for widespread use.

This article examines the phenomenon of infertility and efforts to address it through the lens of public health. Specifically, it considers how various imprecise and incomplete conceptual definitions skew the epidemiological data on infertility in ways that exaggerate the proportion of infertile couples whom assisted reproductive technologies might help. The article then explores what is known about infertility among segments of the population that have been

From the *Stanford Law & Policy Review,* 6 (1995), 89–102. Copyright © 1995 by the board of Trustees of the Leland Stanford Junior University. Reprinted by permission.

largely overlooked, and why assisted reproductive technologies are not an effective means of addressing their conditions. Finally, this article suggests how new public health policies and community-oriented measures can complement or replace the current emphasis on expensive, high-tech interventions for the treatment of infertility.

THE SCOPE OF PUBLIC HEALTH

Organized community efforts to prevent disease, promote physical and mental health, and address threats to the well-being of communities distinguish public health from clinical medicine. Public health practitioners often express their ethical goals as the protection of the common good and the reduction of health-related inequalities across populations. Public health policies have often concentrated specifically on the poor and others with limited access to medical services. Yet while public health efforts are ultimately intended to benefit individuals, their emphasis on community welfare presupposes that community interests may override individuals' personal interests. This precept can create ethical tension between practitioners and policymakers in public health, who focus on the community as a whole, and those in clinical medicine, who focus on the identified patient.

Perhaps the best known activities of public health are the monitoring of the population's health status and the collection of health statistics. The epidemiological, statistical, and environmental functions of both governmental and nongovernmental public health organizations play a crucial role in health-related research, health planning, and the control of disease at every level of society. Equally important to public health, however, are the less prominent dimensions of health education and community mobilization, the development and evaluation of health policy, and the assessment of health services. A comprehensive approach to infertility must involve each of these disciplines.

EPIDEMIOLOGY AND INFERTILITY

The field of epidemiology measures the distribution, dynamics, and determinants of health and disease in and across populations. These data often provide the basis for disease control, health planning, and health policy formation. Other than studies on environmental and disease-based threats to fertility, public health researchers in reproductive health have typically studied patterns of community fertility, examining population-based birthrates and their determinants rather than the distribution, dynamics, or determinants of the ability to conceive or carry a pregnancy to term. Prior to the development of medical technologies for assisted reproduction, there was virtually no public health literature on infertility.

Definitions, Presuppositions, and Conceptual Issues

Although extensive statistics on worldwide fertility exist, little comprehensive epidemiological data is available on the actual prevalence or causes of infertility. One major reason for this paucity of information on infertility is that, until recently, it has simply not been considered a public health problem. Since the turn of the century, and particularly since the availability of contraceptives, epidemiological efforts and public health concern about reproduction have focused on fertility as a *threat* to the health of women, their children, and society. This response has been particularly directed toward nonwhite and poor women, and women in developing nations. Epidemiologists, health educators, and policymakers have understood the control of fertility to mean its restriction, not its enhancement. Today, the field of public health is dominated by concern for the improvement of women's personal standard of living, and that of their communities, through the stabilization or limitation of reproduction.

Other conceptual considerations also affect the data on infertility in ways that are important for health planning and policy. Differences in the essential terminology used across the literature pose one obstacle to integrating the work of clinical reproductive health specialists and epidemiologists. Classically, the word *fertility* connotes *actual childbearing,* whereas *fecundity* refers to *reproductive ability.* However, *infertility* means *diminished capacity for conception* whereas *infecundity* means the *total inability to reproduce.* Nonetheless, the terms fertility and fecundity are often used as equivalents, and fecundity/infecundity are almost never used in the lay or clinical literature. The phrases *diminished* or *impaired* fecundity and fertility add to the definitional confusion.

In most clinical publications, *infertility* typically refers to a couple's inability to conceive after one or more years of unprotected intercourse, and assumes that neither partner is surgically sterile. This latter distinction may complicate the comparison of clinical reports with broader statistical data, which may include surgical sterilization as one type of infertility. *Primary infertility* refers to the inability to conceive a first child; *secondary infertility* refers to the inability to conceive additional children after one or more live births. Despite these distinctions, the legal, ethical, and sociological literature on infertility has associated almost all forms of involuntary childlessness, including a woman's inability to carry a conceptus to live birth, with infertility. Moreover, despite a growing literature on male infecundity, most of the focus remains on the experiences and treatment of women's infertility. Lay perspectives on the issue may further cloud the terminology; in some cultural contexts, the idea of infertility may also include a woman's failure to bear sons.

An epidemiological issue that is vital to health planning and policy is the appropriate definition of normal, healthy, or appropriate fertility. In 1975, a World Health Organization (WHO) report on the epidemiology of infertility suggested that worldwide a five percent rate of infertility might be a human norm. A clear and consistent definition of fertility is necessary as the baseline for classifying and addressing unhealthy fertility. To date, none exists that can be used in policy to address *both* subfertility and superfertility for *both* populations and individuals.

Part of the problem is the complex biology of fertility. But any definition of healthy or appropriate fertility will also be charged with moral and political implications. Definitions of healthy fertility affect the options of the "unhealthy," and are problematic whether they relate to superfertility or infertility. Many proponents of population control claim that couples and individuals have a right "to decide freely and responsibly on the number and spacing of their children," and have a right of access to family planning information and services to ensure that freedom. This contention suggests that the choice to procreate is the fundamental ethical issue underlying worldwide efforts to control fertility.

However, the rhetoric of reproductive choice and access to medical services seldom includes claims for a right to reproduce, except in terms of freedom from governmental intervention. Although U.S. federal policies require that public facilities providing family planning services also offer basic medical services to assist conception, the treatment of infertility is only rarely mentioned under the umbrella of family planning services. There are also few public infertility clinics in the United States.

For most researchers and policymakers in the field of population control, definitions of "appropriate" fertility are based on the replacement birthrate (2.1 children per woman), population-based average used in national reproductive policy and health education campaigns. As the birthrates in most democratic, industrialized nations have fallen below the replacement rate, this figure has also been linked with such other public health and human rights goals as education and political freedom. However, where specific numerical targets have been applied to individuals, as in the People's Republic of China, public health and human rights advocates have sharply criticized the accompanying governmental interference in personal choice.

Although the concept of replacement has been used to justify a couple's religious or patriotic duty to procreate, it has not been used in policy to support an infertile couple's right to have children. Moreover, the standards of both reproductive choice and replacement affect policy options regarding society's duties to individuals whose fertility has been impaired by the "natural lottery" of disease and disability. In a clinical context, any diagnosis of infertility implies a disease state that, for medical reasons, should be treated. However, even among clinicians there is no consensus on what treatment is adequate or who should pay for such treatment.

In the spring of 1994, the issue of access to infertility treatment at public expense gained considerable attention in New York and Massachusetts when reviews of state-funded health programs revealed that indigent women and men had received drug treatment, surgery, and artificial insemination for infertility under Medicaid. In Massachusetts, the policy debate focused on efforts to reform the welfare program. The dispute was short lived; taxpayer opinion was overwhelmingly against funding. State administrators soon prohibited Medicaid from underwriting such treatment. The public objected most strongly to coverage for the treatment of secondary infertility: 63% of the 260 women receiving fertility drugs in the preceding year already had 1 or more children, and 2 had 8 children each. Critics of the program insisted that the desire to have children was not a medical problem, and that treating infertility at state expense worked against society's interest in preventing the birth of children who would be dependent on public assistance.

In contrast, New York's ongoing debate has focused on the "scandal" of providing specialized treatments when essential primary care services are not available. This broader policy issue of prioritizing medical treatments covered by the state has troubled both public officials and private policy analysts concerned with the just allocation of resources. Recent efforts at health care reform have not adequately addressed the availability of infertility services, perhaps due to the intense debate over access to government-funded abortion. Again, without a clear definition of healthy fertility, neither the scope and meaning of impaired fertility as a public health problem nor the appropriate governmental response can be addressed conclusively.

Defining the "reproductive years," particularly for women, poses another definitional challenge to epidemiology. Definitions of women's reproductive capacity have traditionally been relevant only during the period between menarche (the onset of menses) and menopause, roughly ages fifteen to forty-four. Although a man's reproductive capacity extends throughout his adult life, a man's fertility is effectively limited by his partner's menopause. This distinction has blurred and become politically volatile as in vitro fertilization (IVF) with donor oocytes (female egg) eliminates menopause as the upper age boundary for women's fertility, and the falling age of puberty extends the lower boundary. France has already outlawed the use of IVF with oocyte donation to redress the effects of menopause. French legislators claimed that the natural course of a woman's reproductive life should not be artificially extended. Women's rights advocates and infertility researchers have argued, however, that women should have the option to bear children for as long as they wish, both because of today's longer life expectancy and more active old age, and as a matter of gender equity.

A final consideration involves defining the population for purposes of conducting reproductive health studies. This is perhaps the most serious challenge for public health research on infertility. A number of public health investigators have observed that the recent epidemiological interest in infertility has been due less to a concern about the condition as a public health problem than to the marked increase in infertility consultations that began in 1972. In the United States and elsewhere in the industrialized world, the causes of infertility have been measured primarily by clinicians and epidemiologists affiliated with infertility clinics. As a result, the research population has consisted almost exclusively of those people already seeking medical diagnosis and treatment for childlessness, and the needs and interests of these individuals have shaped the collection of demographic data on infertility.

Reliance on projections from patient data is partly due to methodological constraints, as infertility is a medical diagnosis that can be established only after a thorough medical evaluation. However, this data cannot reflect the more general concerns of community-based perspectives on reproductive health or disease prevention and control. Because most couples seeking high-tech treatment for infertility have been affluent whites, published studies typically do not reflect the traditional public health concern for under-served and at-risk populations. Experts have questioned the validity of inferring population-based infertility rates from the experiences of a narrow spectrum of clinic patients. Nonetheless, little has been done to elaborate the differences between the experiences and needs of this group and those of the public at large. Such clarification is essential to making future epidemiological research on infertility widely applicable.

The Population-Based Data

In 1976, the Center for Health Statistics conducted the National Survey of Family Growth (NSFG), the first direct, population-based study of infertility carried out in the United States. The study was repeated in 1982 and 1988. The 1982 NSFG surveyed 7,969 women between the ages of 15 and 44 regarding their reproductive history. This study has been the cornerstone of the U.S. literature on the epidemiology of infertility. Its results form the primary basis of the 1988 report on infertility by the Congressional Office of Technology Assessment (OTA), probably the most widely cited publication in the field. Advance data from the 1988 NSFG have been available since late 1990, but the survey's results are not yet reported in full.

Using personal interviews, the 1982 NSFG examined the fecundity, use of contraception, dates and outcomes of any pregnancies, marriages, use of family planning and infertility services, and demographics of a national sample of women between fifteen and forty-four years old. From this survey, researchers estimated that nationally approximately 4.5 million, or 8.4% of the 53.6 million married women of childbearing age had an impaired ability to have children. Approximately half of these women, 1.9 million, had no children; 2.6 million had 1 or more previous births. When these figures included those surgically sterilized, infecund couples constituted 13.9% of the study's population.

The 1988 interviews with 8,450 women echo the 1982 figures. In 1988, the NSFG projected that 4.9 million women, 15 to 44 years of age, or 8.4% of the 57.9 million married women of childbearing age nationwide, had impaired fecundity. Of this total, 2.2 million were classified as having primary infertility and 2.7 million as having secondary infertility. While a specific figure excluding surgically sterilized couples is not yet available, commentaries accompanying the data suggest that the 1982 rate of 13 to 14% remains applicable because there was no significant change in the rates of impaired fecundity in any category.

Claims about an epidemic of infertility first arose from the 1982 NSFG's finding that rates of primary infertility had doubled since the National Fertility Study in 1965. In reality, the overall infertility rate for couples had remained relatively constant, growing only 0.6% from 13.3% in 1966 to 13.9% in 1982. However, rates for women in some age groups had increased. In particular, the percentage of infertile women between ages 35 to 39 rose from 18.4% to 24.6%, and the rate among women ages 20 to 24 more than doubled, from 3.6% in 1965 to 10.6% in 1982. Epidemiologists have pointed out repeatedly that the rise in the number of childless women over age thirty-five is not surprising in light of the large increase in the population of women over age thirty-five during the period, coupled with the "baby boom" generation's postponement of childbearing. However, the enormous publicity surrounding the treatment of infertility among women over thirty-five and the ethical and legal controversy over IVF and commercial surrogacy created the popular perception that infertility had increased dramatically across the board.

Despite the assurances of epidemiologists that "there is no epidemic" of infertility, NSFG data suggest several areas in which public health problems do exist. First, there are significant disparities in the rates of infertility among women of different demographic backgrounds. Second, the reasons for the prevalence of impaired fecundity among young women is unclear, and what is known is not fully explained by changes in the size of the cohort. And third, the apparent stability of rates of impaired fecundity generally, despite the greater availability and use of a variety of treatments for infertility, calls into question both the effectiveness of these technologies and their role in infertility policy.

ETHNIC AND SOCIOECONOMIC DIFFERENCES IN INFERTILITY The 1982 NSFG, providing the most recent data organized by race and socioeconomic group, reported the prevalence of infertility among black couples (excluding the surgically sterile) across women's age groups to be roughly twenty-one percent. This figure is 1.5 times greater than the rate of 13% reported among white couples. The most recent data available also suggest that women with less than a high school education (a standard measure of lower socioeconomic status) are more likely to be part of an infertile couple than are their more educated counterparts.

The causes of the higher rate of infertility among blacks are not known. A number of researchers have suggested that there may be an important correlation with black women's higher reported incidence of pelvic inflammatory disease (PID), a leading cause of infertility worldwide. The 1982 NSFG found that black women were about twice as likely to have been treated for PID as were white women, and that both whites and blacks were more likely to have been treated than Hispanic women. Although the percentage of women treated for PID did not vary statistically with income, women with only high school educations were more likely than college-educated women to have been treated. These data may also seriously underestimate the effects of PID on the fertility of black women, because a considerable proportion of women with PID do not seek treatment.

The documented prevalence of infertility among black couples suggests that black women should constitute a considerable proportion of those seeking infertility services. However, the opposite is true: infertile nonwhite women appear to seek reproductive services much less often than their white counterparts. Only thirty percent of both black and Hispanic women reporting impaired fecundity in the 1988 NSFG, as compared with forty-seven percent of white women, had sought some form of infertility service, including simple medical advice on becoming pregnant.

The high percentage of infertility among black women that is attributed to PID also suggests that these women might be candidates for surgery to repair blocked fallopian tubes or for IVF. Nonetheless, only 12.8% of black women in the NSFG had sought specialized infertility services (including ovulatory drugs, artificial insemination, surgery or other intervention for blocked fallopian tubes, or IVF), compared with 17% of Hispanics and 27.2% of whites. Socioeconomic status also plays a role, as only 8% of poor women (0 to 149% of poverty level) had sought specialized fertility services, compared with 32% of affluent women (400 + % of poverty level).

Insurance coverage, not discussed in the NSFG, impacts heavily on access to specialized reproductive services. Many people with excellent health insurance may discover that their policies exclude treatment for infertility beyond a diagnostic work-up or perhaps surgical intervention to repair damaged organs. While at least eight states now require insurance companies to cover or offer coverage for IVF as part of any policy that includes pregnancy-related services, many basic health insurance policies do not always cover pregnancy. Doctors who know of a couple's financial constraints and limited insurance coverage may not refer them to fertility clinics. Moreover, both private clinics and state-funded medical school clinics typically have eligibility criteria for prospective IVF couples that include such socioeconomic factors as a "stable" marriage, sufficient education to comply with treatment regimens, and the financial resources to provide "adequately" for a child. Each of these factors may weigh against the poor, as well as against nonwhite couples whom clinic personnel may assume to be more financially at risk.

Even if treatment for infertility were readily accessible to poor and nonwhite couples, their use of such services might still depend on the extent to which they perceive infertility to be a medical problem. The belief that pregnancy is not a medical condition is considered a significant barrier to the use of prenatal services by poor, black, and Hispanic women. These women receive significantly less prenatal care compared to middle-class whites. Even less is known about the psychosocial experiences of infertile nonwhite and poor women than is known about their rates of impaired fertility. Discovering couples' motives for seeking infertility services has dominated the question of how demographic variables affect perceptions of infertility and responses to it.

Many middle-class white women experience infertility as a frustrating foreclosure of choice. They seek to regain personal control over their lives and bodies through medical intervention. By contrast, many poor and nonwhite women who have endured other hardships and who consequently may not focus on issues of personal control, may experience infertility more in terms of general adversity. If infertility is one in a series of negative, seemingly irreversible events in a woman's life, she may be more likely to attribute it to fate or God's will than seek to address it through science. Women with such beliefs are less likely to seek medical treatment irrespective of their rates of infertility.

IMPAIRED FERTILITY AMONG YOUNG ADULTS AND TEENAGERS The prevalence of infertility among young women is not as well documented as that of women over age twenty-five. Nonetheless, the available data suggest that impaired fecundity among women ages fifteen to twenty-four is a considerable problem. The 1982 NSFG reported that between 1965 and 1982 the rate of infertility (excluding surgical sterilization) among married women ages 15 to 19 rose from 0.06% to 2.1%, and from 3.6% to 10.6% for women ages twenty to twenty-four. Unfortunately, the NSFG's focus on married women and changes in the age categories make population wide inferences difficult.

The most recent NSFG found that the rate of impaired fecundity among married women ages 15 to 24 dropped from 8.8% in 1982 to 7.6% in 1988. However, because the 1988 NSFG does not use the same age-groups as the 1982 report, it is difficult to interpret the prevalence of infertility among women twenty to twenty-four, whose infertility rates had increased so dramatically in the previous cycle. Moreover, by focusing exclusively on married women, the

NSFG does not address the fecundity of the large numbers of unmarried, sexually active women in this age-group. Particularly among young black women, a greater proportion of whom experience motherhood without marriage, impaired fertility may be a real concern.

Much of the increase in infertility among young women has been attributed to an increased incidence of chlamydia and gonorrhea, sexually transmitted diseases (STDs) which can lead to PID and occlusion of the fallopian tubes. The rates of sexually transmitted diseases have increased across all age and demographic groups. This increase appears to be especially significant for black adolescents and young adults. These groups typically have limited access to the medical care that can prevent the serious health consequences of STDs. Rising infertility rates among young black women appear to be one of the most serious effects of PID resulting from untreated STDs.

THE EFFECTIVENESS AND COSTS OF REPRODUCTIVE TECHNOLOGIES The lack of change in the prevalence of infecundity and infertility reported in the United States over the past two decades raises a serious challenge to the role of clinical infertility treatment in reproductive health policy. Most specialized infertility treatments (ovulation-inducing drugs, artificial insemination, tubal surgery, and IVF) attempt to redress childlessness rather than to cure biological infertility per se. If, as the data suggest, assisted reproductive technologies have had little effect on rates of infertility or on the differentials among subgroups, it is difficult to justify their apparent primacy among interventions against infertility. It is even harder to rationalize any future widespread application at public expense.

The effectiveness of reproductive technologies depends on whether their effects are measured in terms of live births or improved natural procreative capacity. Couples who successfully conceive and deliver a child using assisted reproductive techniques may still be considered infertile for epidemiological purposes if they remain unable to procreate without medical assistance. If the policy question is how best to resolve childlessness among the infertile rather than how best to address its biological causes, the answers may differ greatly.

As is typical of most high-tech medical interventions in the United States, the major infertility treatments were not well evaluated before they were adopted into widespread practice. In the past few years, however, clinical studies and technology assessments have suggested that even measured in terms of individual births following infertility treatment, the demonstrated effectiveness of specialized techniques has not been high. For example, using the delivery of a live infant as the measure of successful treatment, researchers report that the most effective use of IVF (to treat tubal blockage) has a marginal success rate of only 10 to 15 live births per 100 women over as many as 6 cycles. The reported effectiveness of IVF for the treatment of low sperm count, endometriosis, and advanced maternal age has varied across clinical studies. While some clinics claim success rates of fifteen to twenty percent, the comprehensive analysis performed by the Canadian Royal Commission on New Reproductive Technologies concluded that there is no clear indication of IVF's effectiveness for these conditions.

Beyond the issue of effectiveness, the costs and potential unwanted side effects of assisted reproductive technologies raise further questions about their widespread application and their potential coverage by public health policies. Three recent evaluations of the direct charges and indirect economic consequences of infertility treatment concluded that the costs of induced ovulation, tubal surgery, and IVF are too great to ignore in the formation of public policy.

Although the charge for a single treatment cycle may be as low as a few hundred dollars for fertility drugs and several thousand dollars for IVF, the cumulative cost for a successful delivery after such interventions is dramatically higher. In 1991, the average hospital delivery charge for mother and infant in one Boston teaching hospital was slightly under $10,000. Although total hospital charges do not reflect total costs, this figure is profoundly less than the costs of a live birth after tubal surgery, projected at $85,000. Similarly, the costs of a live delivery range from $50,000 to $72,727 when IVF is used for tubal occlusion and from $160,000 to $800,000 when IVF is used to overcome the combination of male-factor infertility and advanced maternal age. The average range for IVF generally is $66,667 to $114,286. Moreover, the eighty-five to ninety percent of couples who do not achieve pregnancy or live birth despite multiple interventions may incur the bulk of these costs as they undergo treatment.

One element often overlooked in the greater cost of delivery associated with assisted reproductive technologies is the cost of multiple-gestation pregnancies, which may be ten to thirty times more likely with the use of ovulation-inducing drugs and the implantation of more than one embryo. The growing use of infertility treatments nationwide has been associated with a marked rise in the number of multiple-gestation pregnancies and an attendant incidence of related complications and costs for mothers and babies. Counting only the hospital charges for delivery and subsequent care of mother and infant, studies have estimated the cost per baby of twins at $18,974 and of triplets at $36,588.

Assisted reproductive technologies also carry significant non-economic costs. The social costs of higher morbidity and mortality among infants from multiple-gestation pregnancies are occasionally compounded by the tragic need for "selective reduction," the abortion of one or more fetuses when multiple gestation itself threatens the lives of the woman and/or all of her would-be progeny. Moreover, there is growing evidence that ovulation-inducing drugs may be linked to an increased risk of ovarian cancer, especially for those women who ultimately never conceive.

Even when the physical costs are few, the psychological consequences of infertility treatment may be quite burdensome. Many commentators have observed that the use of reproductive technologies often involves a tragic medicalization of women's (and men's) experiences of procreation, and creates false hopes for biological parenthood. Particularly for those couples who never conceive, the resulting anxiety, confusion, and shame of failure can be devastating.

Infertile couples reportedly willing to try and to pay "almost anything" to create their own baby are not unlike many chronically ill Americans searching for a cure. Their choice to pursue high-cost and marginally effective treatment at their own expense is an essential freedom afforded by the private health care system in the United States. However, the public health policy goal of reducing health-related inequalities across the population does not require that society underwrite the universal pursuit of low-probability outcomes.

While standards of appropriate intervention and coverage have been more difficult to establish in the United States than in countries with nationalized health care, reform of the United States' system will depend on the establishment of such standards and the demonstrated effectiveness of specific interventions. The challenge for policymakers is to evaluate the benefits of biological parenthood, to weigh the costs and effectiveness of intervention against those benefits, and to assess the results with respect to essential health services. It was in this context that the Clinton administration excluded IVF from its standard health insurance package and the Canadian province of Ontario restricted IVF coverage to use for bilateral tubal blockage.

In the absence of widespread insurance or governmental coverage of specialized reproductive services, those couples who cannot afford to pay for treatment may never gain access to the technologies. Governmental decisions that simply limit the availability of these technologies would perpetuate not only the current inequity in access to specialized procedures but also the narrow clinical view of infertility as a disease that demands a high-tech cure. It is essential that comprehensive health policy on infertility also incorporate a preventive element. By promoting research and education on the *causes* of infertility, and providing programs to modify or prevent behaviors that increase infertility-causing disease, the need for infertility treatment could be reduced and the medical services provided more effectively.

RECOMMENDATIONS FOR POLICY AND RESEARCH

Increased and expanded research on infertility is essential if this complex problem is to be resolved. The lack of comprehensive epidemiological data on the prevalence and causes of infertility compromises both the value of what is known and the manner in which that knowledge is used to form policy. In 1988, the OTA suggested that the federal government improve the collection of data on infertility by expanding the NSFG's sample and the frequency of follow-up surveys. Populationwide statistics on infertility are still badly needed to form public policy, because the absence of data limits the political voice of groups whose problems affect all of society. Future demographic studies must be crafted carefully because their design can influence not only the interpretation of issues, but also the identification of key players and the definition of their roles and needs for many years.

The usefulness of future research will also depend on the standardization of definitions and methods in the epidemiology of infertility. For example, the definition of groups included in an expanded study of infertility must consider both the statistical and political meaning of "significant population." To maximize the applicability of data to both medical and public health intervention, classification should consider:

- strictly biological/genetic factors that appear to be important for fertility and its impairment;
- socio-cultural beliefs and practices, such as late marriage or the acceptance of adolescent parenthood, that may have important biological consequences for fertility; and
- socio-cultural beliefs and practices that affect the perception of infertility and the use of medical services.

Each of these factors must also be examined with regard to their relationship to race, ethnicity, and socioeconomic status.

Importantly, additional epidemiological research is also needed to study the relationship between the spread of sexually transmitted diseases and the incidence of infertility. One of the OTA's first recommendations on addressing infertility was that Congress establish a national data collection system to study chlamydia and PID. To date, no such database exists, and we may in fact have a less clear picture of the prevalence and consequences of STDs than we had before the OTA report. Because infertility caused by PID appears to disproportionately affect poor and nonwhite women, and because such infertility may be perceived as the result of sexual behavior that some would consider immoral, this research has not had the moral appeal of providing treatment for the "innocent" and "responsible" women whose infertility stems from other causes. Yet without such data it is difficult to separate the preventable from the unpreventable causes of infertility.

Together with increased and re-focused research into the epidemiology of infertility, changes in policy are also essential. As discussed earlier, the prevention of infertility has received very little attention in either practice or in policy. The general emphasis on treatment over prevention is a noted consequence of Americans' desire for a technological "quick fix" to problems. This search for immediate solutions is coupled with an unwillingness to invest in less tangible, future effects of prevention where only statistical persons are at risk. This emphasis is illustrated by the reality that less than one percent of the nation's aggregate health expenditures are spent on preventive public health activities, despite their typically greater effectiveness and lower cost. Where treatment is difficult, expensive, or largely ineffective, however, the importance of prevention grows. Infertility is a classic example demonstrating why the need for prevention is central to comprehensive health policy.

In 1993 the Canadian Royal Commission on New Reproductive Technologies confronted these issues and recommended the establishment of a centralized, integrated, national preventive strategy to address infertility. While the differences in the U.S. health care system make centralized oversight unlikely, an integrated strategy on prevention is still necessary. Efforts to prevent infertility should take place at four levels:

- education
- access to preventive health services
- access to treatment for STDs
- ongoing evaluation and research of the successful approaches to reduce the risk and incidence of infertility.

Education

Although public education about sexually related matters continues to be a politically volatile topic, the OTA's primary recommendation for Congressional involvement in the prevention of infertility was to increase the public's understanding of PID and the STDs that cause it. Community clinic-based educational campaigns on sexual and reproductive health may be particularly valuable among populations where childbearing is central to a woman's identity. However, such programs should also actively target men as potential carriers of infertility-causing STDs. In addition to their current emphasis on the prevention of HIV and unwanted pregnancy using barrier contraceptives, these educational programs should stress that barrier methods have the additional advantage of protecting future fertility. This approach is consistent with campaigns that present birth control as a means of increasing a woman's reproductive choices, as barrier contraceptives protect the choice to bear children in the future.

Across the country, the principal site for public health education is the school. Health education classes typically include material on sexuality, reproduction, and sexually transmitted diseases, including HIV. Although the timing of school-based sex education varies tremendously among communities, experts advocate educational programs beginning in elementary school as part of a comprehensive strategy to reduce the incidence of teen pregnancy, STDs, and HIV. This approach may help to reduce infertility among young women, as the increased rate of sexual activity among preteens suggests that education in middle school may occur too late to prevent some PID-related infections.

However, in spite of the intellectual appeal of educational efforts, there is controversy over the effectiveness of sex education in the schools because there has been no demonstrated decrease in teen pregnancy or STDs in communities with even the most comprehensive programs. At the same time programs that teach only abstinence do not seem to have any significant effect either. Experience with integrated community approaches to sex education suggests that multilateral efforts may be more successful. Providing a combination of factual knowledge about sexual issues, help in developing interpersonal and decision-making skills, and social support for responsible behavior has been shown to reduce the incidence of teen parenthood. Especially in communities where adolescent parenthood is accepted, such educational programs may make a convincing case for both abstinence and "safe sex" by stressing that unprotected intercourse *threatens* one's future ability to have children. Such a unified approach may be the key to an effective educational strategy targeting preventable infertility.

Increased Access to Preventive Health Services

Beyond education, increased access to preventive measures against PID-induced infertility, particularly the greater availability of barrier contraceptives, is an essential aspect of a comprehensive public health campaign. For adult patients of public family planning clinics, the emphasis on birth control and assumptions about women's willingness or ability to use more active forms of contraception have led to an increased use of Norplant (time released contraceptive placed in the arm for up to five years) and Depo-Provera (hormone shot contraceptive lasting three months) over both the Pill and diaphragms. But with any of these types of contraception, women must be encouraged to also use a barrier method to protect against both conception and STDs. The "female condom," intended to give women the power to protect themselves against both pregnancy and STDs, has met with little acceptance. The use of traditional condoms with other forms of contraception may be abandoned unless women have equally easy access to both. Similarly, STD clinics, which treat primarily male patients, should provide condoms cheaply or free of charge as part of their treatment. In doing so, clinics should also emphasize the protection of fertility to add weight to current warnings about HIV and the personal benefits of using condoms.

Efforts to distribute condoms in public schools have prompted heated criticism from religious authorities and conservative political activists who claim that the easy availability of contraceptives is a tacit approval of adolescent sexual activity. Nonetheless, educational programs that teach adolescents the social and developmental skills necessary to postpone sexual activity, and programs to protect young people from STDs and their consequences, must acknowledge the early age at which many adolescents already engage in sexual intercourse. The practice of making condoms available would recognize and confront this reality.

Access to Treatment for STDs

Access to diagnosis and treatment of infertility-causing STDs is both essential to any personal health care package and integral to any meaningful public health system. Attention to the diagnosis and effective treatment of STDs can significantly reduce the incidence of infertility from PID and the potential demand for reproductive services. Typically, treatment consists of low-tech antibiotics which are simple and inexpensive to administer. Contact tracing of persons infected with chlamydia and gonorrhea, a traditional dimension of public health efforts to track and control the spread of STDs, may also play an important role in advancing this treatment strategy.

Ongoing Evaluation and Research

Measuring the effects of prevention and identifying the relevant variables is a complex process that may make the success of preventive health campaigns difficult to ascertain in the short term. Population-based research on the prevention of infertility will require policymakers' patience to view successes in the long-term. A long-range outlook is necessary if the educational and treatment programs under study are to remain in place until their goals, methods, and outcomes can be evaluated.

Whether focused on school-based, clinic-based, or community-based education, health educators need to determine which strategies work for specific populations and why. In particular, more research is needed into the often-acknowledged gap between awareness of health risks and associated behavior. Studies examining the effectiveness of condom distribution among various populations from various sites are needed to establish which variables affect the actual use of condoms once they have been made available. Research into the prevention of HIV also affords an important opportunity to evaluate measures to control the STDs that affect fertility. Finally, evaluation of treatment programs for STDs must explore whether emphasis on the treatment of men, whose symptoms appear earlier and more markedly, can improve the prevention of infertility among women. Such an integrated research agenda can enhance policy for the treatment of infertility in several ways by indicating the areas in which preventive strategies do not work and thus where medical efforts to understand the causes of infertility must be redoubled. This knowledge can then illuminate those situations in which prevention is indeed the key to eliminating infertility.

How Many People Can the Earth Support?

JOEL E. COHEN

On April 25, 1679, in Delft, Holland, the inventor of the microscope, Antoni van Leeuwenhoek, wrote down what may be the first estimate of the maximum number of people the earth can support. If all the habitable land in the world had the same population density as Holland (at that time about 120 people for every square kilometer), he calculated, the earth could support at most 13.4 billion people—far fewer than the number of spermatozoans his lenses had revealed in the milt of a cod.

In subsequent centuries, van Leeuwenhoek's estimate has been followed by dozens of similar calculations. Around 1695 a Londoner named Gregory King estimated that the earth's "Land If fully Peopled would sustain" at most 12.5 billion people. In 1765 a German regimental pastor, Johann Peter Süssmilch, compared his own figure (13.9 billion) with the estimates of van Leeuwenhoek, the French military engineer Sébastien Le Prestre de Vauban (5.5 billion) and the English writer and cartographer Thomas Templeman (11.5 billion).

In recent decades estimates of maximum population have appeared thicker and faster than ever before. Under the rubric of "carrying capacity" they crop up routinely in environmental debates, in United Nations reports and in papers by scholars or academic politicians trained in ecology, economics, sociology, geography, soil science or agronomy, among other disciplines. Demographers, however, have been strangely silent. Of the more than 200 symposiums held at the 1992 and 1993 annual meetings of the Population Association of America, not one session dealt with estimating or defining human carrying capacity for any region of the earth. Instead, professional demographers tend to focus on the composition and growth of populations, restricting their predictions to the near term—generally a few decades into the future—and framing them in conditional terms: *If* rates of birth, death and migration (by age, sex, location, marital status and so on) are such-and-such, *then* population size and distribution will be so-and-so.

Such conditional predictions, or forecasts, can be powerful tools. Projections by the U.N. show dramatically that *if* human populations continued to grow at 1990 rates in each major region of the world, *then* the population would increase more than 130-fold in 160 years, from about 5.3 billion in 1990 to about 694 billion in 2150. Those figures are extremely sensitive to the future level of average fertility. If, hypothetically, from 1990 onward the average couple gradually approached a level of fertility just one-tenth of a child more than required to replace themselves, world population would grow from 5.3 billion in 1990 to 12.5 billion in 2050 and 20.8 billion in 2150. In contrast, if (again hypothetically) starting in 1990 and ever after couples bore exactly the number of children needed to replace themselves, world population would grow from 5.3 billion in 1990 to 7.7 billion in 2050 and would level off at around 8.4 billion by 2150.

The clear message is that people cannot forever continue to have, on average, more children than are required to replace themselves. That is not an ideological slogan; it is a hard fact. Conventional agriculture cannot grow enough food for 694 billion people; not enough water falls from the skies. The finiteness of the earth guarantees that ceilings on human numbers do exist.

Where are those ceilings? Some people believe that any limit to human numbers is so remote that its existence is irrelevant to present concerns. Others declare that the human population has already exceeded what the earth can support in the long run (how long is usually left unspecified). Still others concede that short-term limits may exist, but they argue that technologies, institutions and values will adapt in unpredictable ways to push ceilings progressively higher so that they recede forever. The differences of opinion are buttressed by vast disparities in calculation. In the past century, experts of various stripes have made estimates of human carrying capacity ranging from less than a billion to more than 1,000 billion. Who, if anybody, is right?

For several years I have been trying to understand the question, "How many people can the earth support?" and the answers to it. In the process I came to question the question. "How many people can the earth support?" is not a question in the same sense as "How old are you?"; it cannot be answered by a number or even by a range of numbers. The earth's capacity to support people is determined partly by processes that the social and natural sciences have yet to understand, partly by choices that we and our descendants have yet to make.

In most of its scientific senses, *carrying capacity* refers to a population of wild animals within a particular ecosystem. One widely used ecology textbook defines it as follows: "Number of individuals in a population that the resources of a habitat can support; the asymptote, or plateau, of the logistic and other sigmoid equations for population growth." Even within ecology, the concept of carrying capacity has important limitations. It applies best under stable conditions and over relatively short spans of time. In the real world, climates and habitats fluctuate and change; animals adapt to their conditions and eventually evolve into new species. With each change, the carrying capacity changes, too.

When applied to human beings, the concept becomes vastly more volatile. I have collected twenty-six definitions of human carrying capacity, all published since 1975. Most of them agree on a few basic points—for instance, that the concept refers to the number of people who can be supported for some period (usually not stated) in some mode of life considered plausible or desirable. Most of the definitions recognize that ecological concepts of carrying capacity must be extended to allow for the role of technology. Most also agree that culturally and individually variable standards of living, including standards of environmental quality, set limits on population size well before the physical requirements for sheer subsistence start to become an issue.

In other respects, however, the definitions vary widely or even contradict one another. How long must a population be sustainable? Does it make sense to speak of local or regional carrying capacity—or do trade and the need for inputs from outside any specified region imply that only a global scale will do? More fundamental, how constraining are constraints? Some definitions deny the existence of any finite carrying capacity altogether, holding that human ingenuity will win out over any natural barriers; others acknowledge that the limits are real but recognize that human choices, now and in the future, will largely decide where those limits fall.

In my opinion, that last point—the interplay of natural constraints and human choices—is the key to making sense of human carrying capacity. The deceptively simple question "How many people can the earth support?" hides a host of thorny issues.

HOW MANY PEOPLE AT WHAT AVERAGE LEVEL OF MATERIAL WELL-BEING?

The human carrying capacity of the earth will obviously depend on the typical material level at which people choose to live. Material well-being includes food (people choose variety and palatability, beyond the constraints imposed by physiological requirements); fiber (people choose cotton, wool or synthetic fibers for clothing, wood pulp or rag for paper); water (tap water or Perrier or the nearest river or mud hole for drinking, washing, cooking and watering your lawn, if you have one); housing (Auschwitz barracks, two men to a plank, or Thomas Jefferson's Monticello); manufactured goods; waste removal (for human, agricultural and industrial wastes); natural-hazard protection (against floods, storms, volcanoes and earthquakes); health (prevention, cure and care); and the entire range of amenities such as education, travel, social groups, solitude, the arts, religion and communion with nature. Not all of those features are captured well by standard economic measures.

HOW MANY PEOPLE WITH WHAT DISTRIBUTION OF MATERIAL WELL-BEING?

An ecologist, an economist and a statistician went bow hunting in the woods and spied a deer. The ecologist shot first, and his arrow landed five meters to the left of the deer. The economist shot next, and her arrow landed five meters to the right of the deer. The statistician looked at both arrows, looked at the deer, and jumped up and down shouting: "We got it! We got it!"

Estimates of human carrying capacity rarely take into account the scatter or distribution of material well-being throughout a population. Yet paying attention to average well-being while ignoring the distribution of well-being is like using an average arrow to kill a deer. People who live in extreme poverty may not know or care that the global average is satisfactory, and the press of present needs may keep them from taking a long-term view. For example, thanks to genetic engineering, any country with a few Ph.D.s in molecular plant biology and a modestly equipped laboratory can insert the genes to create stronger, more disease-resistant, higher-yielding plants. If every region has the scientific and technical resources to improve its own crop plants, the earth can support more people than it can if some regions are too poor to help themselves.

HOW MANY PEOPLE WITH WHAT TECHNOLOGY?

The complexities of technological choices often disappear in heated exchanges between environmental pessimists and technological optimists:

Ecologist: When a natural resource is being consumed faster than it is being replenished or recycled, an asset is being depleted, to the potential harm of future generations.

Technologist: If new knowledge and technology can produce an equivalent or superior alternative, then future generations may turn out to be better off.

Taxpayer: Which natural resources can be replaced by technology yet to be invented, and which cannot? Will there be enough time to develop new technology and put it to work on the required scale? Could we avoid future problems, pain and suffering by making other choices now about technology or ways of living? *[No answer from ecologist or technologist.]*

The key to the argument is time. As Richard E. Benedick, an officer of the U.S. Department of State who has also served with the World Wildlife Fund, worried:

While it is true that technology has generally been able to come up with solutions to human dilemmas, there is no guarantee that ingenuity will always rise to the task. Policymakers must contend with a nagging thought: what if it does not, or what if it is too late?

HOW MANY PEOPLE WITH WHAT DOMESTIC AND INTERNATIONAL POLITICAL INSTITUTIONS?

Political organization and effectiveness affect human carrying capacity. For example, the United Nations Development Program estimated that developing countries could mobilize for development as much as $50 billion a year (an amount comparable to all official development assistance) if they reduced military expenditures, privatized public enterprises, eliminated corruption, made development priorities economically more rational and improved national governance. Conversely, population size, distribution and composition affect political organization and effectiveness.

How will political institutions and civic participation evolve with increasing numbers of people? As numbers increase, what will happen to people's ability to participate effectively in the political system?

What standards of personal liberty will people choose?

How will people bring about political change within existing nations? By elections and referendums, or by revolution, insurrection and civil war? How will people choose to settle differences between nations, for instance, over disputed borders, shared water resources or common fisheries? War consumes human and physical resources. Negotiation consumes patience and often requires compromise. The two options impose different constraints on human carrying capacity.

HOW MANY PEOPLE WITH WHAT DOMESTIC AND INTERNATIONAL ECONOMIC ARRANGEMENTS?

What levels of physical and human capital are assumed? Tractors, lathes, computers, better health and better education all make workers in rich countries far more productive than those in poor countries. Wealthier workers make more wealth and can support more people.

What regional and international trade in finished goods and mobility in productive assets are permitted or encouraged? How will work be organized? The invention of the factory organized production to minimize idleness in the use of labor, tools and machines. What new ways of organizing work should be assumed to estimate the future human carrying capacity?

HOW MANY PEOPLE WITH WHAT DOMESTIC AND INTERNATIONAL DEMOGRAPHIC ARRANGEMENTS?

Almost every aspect of demography (birth, death age structure, migration, marriage, and family structure) is subject to human choices that will influence the earth's human carrying capacity.

A stationary global population will have to choose between a long average length of life and a high birthrate. It must also choose between a single average birthrate for all regions, on the one hand, and a demographic specialization of labor on the other (in which some areas have fertility above their replacement level, whereas other areas have fertility below their replacement level).

Patterns of marriage and household formation will also influence human carrying capacity. For example, the public resources that have to be devoted to the care of the young and the aged depend on the roles played by families. In China national law requires families to care for and support their elderly members; in the United States each elderly person and the state are largely responsible for supporting that elderly person.

HOW MANY PEOPLE IN WHAT PHYSICAL, CHEMICAL AND BIOLOGICAL ENVIRONMENTS?

What physical, chemical and biological environments will people choose for themselves and for their children? Much of the heat in the public argument over current environmental problems arises because the consequences of present and projected choices and changes are uncertain. Will global warming cause great problems, or would a global limitation on fossil-fuel consumption cause greater problems? Will toxic or nuclear wastes or ordinary sewage sludge dumped into the deep ocean come back to haunt future generations when deep currents well up in biologically productive offshore zones, or would the long-term effects of disposing of those wastes on land be worse? The choice of particular alternatives could materially affect human carrying capacity.

HOW MANY PEOPLE WITH WHAT VARIABILITY OR STABILITY?

How many people the earth can support depends on how steadily you want the earth to support that population. If you are willing to let the human population rise and fall, depending on annual crops, decadal weather patterns and long-term shifts in climate, the average population with ups and downs would include the peaks of population size, whereas the guaranteed level would have to be adjusted to the level of the lowest valley. Similar reasoning applies to variability or stability in the level of well-being; the quality of the physical, chemical and biological environments; and many other dimensions of choice.

HOW MANY PEOPLE WITH WHAT RISK OR ROBUSTNESS?

How many people the earth can support depends on how controllable you want the well-being of the population to be. One possible strategy would be to maximize numbers at some given level of well-being, ignoring the risk of natural or human disaster. Another would be to accept a smaller population size in return for increased control over random events. For example, if you settle in a previously uninhabited hazardous zone (such as the flood plain of the Mississippi River or the hurricane-prone coast of the southeastern U.S.), you demand a higher carrying capacity of the hazardous zone, but you must accept a higher risk of catastrophe. When farmers do not give fields a fallow period, they extract a higher carrying capacity along with a higher risk that the soil will lose its fertility (as agronomists at the International Rice Research Institute in the Philippines discovered to their surprise).

HOW MANY PEOPLE FOR HOW LONG?

Human carrying capacity depends strongly on the time horizon people choose for planning. The population that the earth can support at a given level of well-being for twenty years may differ substantially from the population that can be supported for 100 or 1,000 years.

The time horizon is crucial in energy analysis. How fast oil stocks are being consumed matters little if one cares only about the next five years. In the long term, technology can change the definition of resources, converting what was useless rock to a valuable resource; hence no one can say whether industrial society is sustainable for 500 years.

Some definitions of human carrying capacity refer to the size of a population that can be supported indefinitely. Such definitions are operationally meaningless. There is no way of knowing what human population size can be supported indefinitely (other than zero population, since the sun is expected to burn out in a few billion years, and the human species almost certainly will be extinct long before then). The concept of indefinite sustainability is a phantasm, a diversion from the difficult problems of today and the coming century.

HOW MANY PEOPLE WITH WHAT FASHIONS, TASTES AND VALUES?

How many people the earth can support depends on what people want from life. Many choices that appear to be economic depend heavily on individual and cultural values. Should industrial societies use the available supplies of fossil fuels in households for heating and for personal transportation, or outside of households to produce other goods and services? Do people prefer a high average wage and low employment or a low average wage and high employment (if they must choose)?

Should industrial economics seek now to develop renewable energy sources, or should they keep burning fossil fuels and leave the transition to future generations? Should women work outside their homes? Should economic analyses continue to discount future income and costs, or should they strive to even the balance between the people now living and their unborn descendants?

I am frequently asked whether organized religion, particularly Roman Catholicism, is a serious obstacle to the decline of fertility. Certainly in some countries, church policies have hindered couples' access to contraception and have posed obstacles to family planning programs. In practice, however, factors other than religion seem to be decisive in setting average levels of fertility for Roman Catholics. In 1992 two Catholic countries, Spain and Italy, were tied for the second- and third-lowest fertility rates in the world. In largely Catholic Latin America, fertility has been falling rapidly, with modern contraceptive methods playing a major role. In most of the U.S. the fertility of Catholics has gradually converged with that of Protestants, and polls show that nearly four-fifths of Catholics think that couples should make up their own minds about family planning and abortion.

Even within the church hierarchy, Catholicism shelters a diversity of views. On June 15, 1994, the Italian bishops' conference issued a report stating that falling mortality and improved medical care "have made it unthinkable to sustain indefinitely a birthrate that notably exceeds the level of two children per couple." Moreover, by promoting literacy for adults, education for children and the survival of infants in developing countries, the church has helped bring about some of the social preconditions for fertility decline.

On the whole the evidence seems to me to support the view of the ecologist William W. Murdoch of the University of California, Santa Barbara: "Religious beliefs have only small, although sometimes significant, effects on family size. Even these effects tend to disappear with rising levels of well-being and education."

In short, the question "How many people can the earth support?" has no single numerical answer, now or ever. Human choices about the earth's human carrying capacity are constrained by facts of nature and may have unpredictable consequences. As a result, estimates of human carrying capacity cannot aspire to be more than conditional and probable: if future choices are thus-and-so, then the human carrying capacity is likely to be so-and-so. They cannot predict the constraints or possibilities that lie in the future; their true worth may lie in their role as a goad to conscience and a guide to action in the here and now.

The following beautiful quotation from *Principles of Political Economy*, by the English philosopher John Stuart Mill, sketches the kind of shift in values such action might entail. When it was written, in 1848, the world's population was less than one-fifth its present size.

> There is room in the world, no doubt, and even in old countries, for a great increase of population, supposing the arts of life to go on improving, and capital to increase. But even if innocuous, I confess I see very little reason for desiring it. The density of population necessary to enable mankind to obtain, in the greatest degree, all the advantages both of cooperation and of social intercourse, has, in all the most populous countries, been obtained. A population may be too crowded, though all be amply supplied with food and raiment. It is not good for man to be kept perforce at all times in the presence of his species. A world from which solitude is extirpated, is a very poor ideal. . . . Nor is there much satisfaction in contemplating the world with nothing left to the spontaneous activity of nature; with every rood of land brought into cultivation, which is capable of growing food for human beings; every flowery waste or natural pasture ploughed up, all quadrupeds or birds which are not domesticated for man's use exterminated as his rivals for food, every hedgerow or superfluous tree rooted out, and scarcely a place left where a wild shrub or flower could grow without being eradicated as a weed in the name of improved agriculture. If the earth must lose that great portion of its pleasantness which it owes to things that the unlimited increase of wealth and population would extirpate from it, for the mere purpose of enabling it to support a larger but not a better or a happier population, I sincerely hope, for the sake of posterity, that they will content to be stationary, long before necessity compels them to it.
>
> It is scarcely necessary to remark that a stationary condition of capital and population implies no stationary state of human improvement. There would be as much scope as ever for all kinds of mental culture, and moral and social progress; as much room for improving the Art of Living, and much more likelihood of its being improved, when minds ceased to be engrossed by the art of getting on. Even the industrial arts might be as earnestly and as successfully cultivated, with this sole difference, that instead of serving no purpose but the increase of wealth, industrial improvements would produce their legitimate effect, that of abridging labour. . . . Only when, in addition to just institutions, the increase of mankind shall be under the deliberate guidance of judicious foresight, can the conquests made from the powers of nature by the intellect and energy of scientific discoverers, become the common property of the species, and the means of improving it and elevating the universal lot.

9

GENETIC SCREENING, TESTING, AND THERAPY

Perhaps no other field in health care has advanced as rapidly in the last few years as genetics. Rapid breakthroughs in genetic research, a $3 billion federal Human Genome Project that will map and sequence the genetic makeup of humans, and advances in molecular biology are all contributing to this genetic revolution. According to one commentator, "Conservative estimates are that some 50,000 gene markers will be developed as a result of molecular biology and translated into easy-to-employ biochemical assays, genetic tests, new drugs, and genetic therapies."[1]

Genetic screening can be done to identify those who have, or are likely to develop, a disease, although they are as yet asymptomatic, or it can be done to identify carriers, that is, those who will not develop the disease but who could pass it to offspring. Screening can be done on an entire population, or it can be targeted to some subset, such as an ethnic group at high risk for a particular disease. The most pervasive form of screening currently practiced is neonatal screening, for example, for phenylketonuria (PKU), a metabolic disorder which causes severe mental retardation if not treated with a special, and extremely restrictive, diet. Prenatal screening can identify fetuses with hereditary conditions, which may lead to treatment after or even before birth. Most commonly, however, the detection of genetic disease in fetuses results in abortion.

The genetic defects which cause many single-gene disorders, such as Huntington disease (HD) and cystic fibrosis (CF), have already been discovered, and screening tests have been developed. However, diseases caused by the malfunction of a single gene are relatively rare. The most prevalent diseases—and thus the ones most important from a public health perspective—result from a complex interaction of genetic and environmental factors. Screening for multifactorial diseases, such as breast and ovarian cancer, prostate cancer, coronary artery disease, diabetes, hypertension, Alzheimer's disease, and some forms of mental illness, may be on the horizon.

Genetic testing can contribute to the prevention or reduction of disease. For example, genetic testing of presymptomatic individuals enables them to benefit from early intervention (if it is available). Prenatal genetic testing can help at-risk couples avoid the birth of a seriously ill baby. However, genetic testing could also result in stigmatization and discrimination. For example, information about a person's genetic predisposition to disease might be used by insurance companies to deny coverage or increase premiums. A number of states have passed laws that prohibit insurance companies from doing this.[2]

Another problem with genetic testing is that there are literally thousands of inherited conditions: how should society, insurers, the medical profession, and drug companies decide which tests should be developed and offered? As more and more markers for genetic diseases are discovered, there is increased pressure for genetic testing, due in part to the emergence of a biotechnology industry with a financial interest in testing. Unless it is done appropriately, genetic screening may not yield useful information or improve the public's health. Elias and Annas comment:

> The optimal genetic screening program would only be initiated after adequate public education, with community support and involvement in the program; those screened would be informed of the purpose of the screening and give consent; confidentiality would be maintained; results would be conveyed through nondirective counseling; screening tests would be inexpensive, simple, and accurate; there would be sufficient qualified personnel and laboratory facilities for required follow-up; and the program would provide means of self-assessment.[3]

A good example of a successful population screening program is screening in the Jewish community for Tay-Sachs disease (TSD). The devastating nature of the disease, combined with the lack of a therapy or cure, made it a good candidate for prenatal and carrier screening. Since testing for Tay-Sachs began in the 1970s, there has been a greater than 90% reduction in the incidence of the disease in the Jewish population in the United States and Canada.

However, screening for genetic disease has not always been beneficial, and sometimes has caused great harm. The story of sickle cell disease is a case in point. Law professor Patricia King writes:

> Sickle cell screening programs were often mandated by state legislatures, in contrast to voluntary screening programs for Tay-Sachs disease, which primarily affects Jews. Only after the passage of the National Sickle Cell Anemia Control Act in 1972, which required that federal funds be used in voluntary programs, was the movement toward mandatory laws halted. These programs developed in an ad hoc fashion with disastrous consequences for the African-American community. Inadequate provisions for confidentiality led to stigmatization and discrimination in employment and insurance. As a result of inadequate education and counseling, the difference between sickle cell trait and sickle cell disease was poorly understood by those affected and the general community.[4]

Other problems in mass screening stem from the reliability of the test and the dual problems of false negatives and false positives. Consider newborn screening for PKU, mandated by most states. As Norman Fost points out in the first selection in this chapter, the Guthrie test identified some children with a variation of abnormal phenylalanine metabolism as having PKU when they were not in fact at risk for retardation. Moreover, since the severely restrictive PKU diet itself can cause brain damage, the mass screening program caused some children who would have been of normal intelligence to become retarded.

Abby Lippman discusses another problem raised by prenatal genetic testing, namely, that it "prevents" genetic disease by eliminating fetuses who have certain genetic traits. "Prenatal diagnosis," she writes, "presupposes that certain fetal conditions are intrinsically not bearable." While this is undoubtedly true of the severest diseases, like Tay-Sachs, it is not the case for some of the most common conditions for which prenatal diagnosis is performed, such as Down syndrome, spina bifida, or cystic fibrosis. Individuals living with these conditions may object to prenatal testing because they think it suggests that they should never have come into existence, that their lives are not worth living. Many in the disability community argue that resources would be better spent on making society more accommodating of those with disabilities rather than on screening programs aimed at preventing the births of people likely to be disabled.

Some feminists also object to prenatal testing because they do not believe that it has improved the lot of women or enhanced their choices. Instead, the routinization of prenatal testing makes the "decision" to be tested, and to abort if the fetus is affected, a foregone conclusion. As Lippman notes, "Society does not truly accept children with disabilities or provide assistance for their nurturance. Thus, a woman may see no realistic alternative to diagnosing and aborting a fetus likely to be affected." Lippman does not totally reject prenatal testing, but she does advocate a closer look at the assumptions that motivate it.

Another aspect of the "dark side of genetic screening" is the potential it has to be used not only to prevent serious disease, but to select against relatively minor medical conditions, such as near-sightedness or hay fever. Will there be pressure on prospective parents to have a "perfect baby"? Genetic screening might also be used to prevent the births of people with nonmedical conditions, such as homosexual orientation, which some scientists think has a significant genetic component. Should such tests be developed and made available to people who want them? Some argue that this would be an inappropriate use of technology, one that would contribute to prejudice and discrimination against homosexuals.[5] A related fear is that prenatal testing and genetic engineering might be used, not for the prevention of disease, but for enhancement: to create children who are stronger, smarter, taller, or better looking. Many consider this to be a "new eugenics" and almost as scary as the old eugenics.

The last selection, by LeRoy Walters and Julie Gage Palmer, comes from their book, *The Ethics of Human Gene Therapy*. (Readers interested in understanding the science of genetic disease and how gene therapy works are advised to consult this excellent book.) Gene therapy attempts to treat diseases that result from errors in the structure or function of genes by adding new genes to cells or by substituting new genes for original malfunctioning genes. Sickle cell anemia, cystic fibrosis, rheumatoid arthritis, familial hypercholesterolemia, coronary artery disease, various cancers, and AIDS are among the diseases that might someday be successfully treated with gene therapy. Gene therapy in humans has so far been limited to somatic cell gene therapy. Because somatic cell gene therapy affects only nonreproductive cells, none of the genetic changes produced by somatic cell gene therapy will be passed on to the patient's children. At present, somatic cell gene therapy is still in the experimental stage. While the prospects hold great promise, it remains true that "no approach has definitely improved the health of a single one of the more than 2,000 patients who have enrolled in gene therapy trials worldwide."[6] Nevertheless, somatic cell gene therapy is accepted in principle as no more problematic than any other experimental therapy.

Germ-line gene therapy involves a therapeutic genetic alteration in germ-line or reproductive cells, and is usually done on zygotes or preimplantation embryos. It has several advantages over somatic cell gene therapy. First, in the treatment of genetic diseases, such as CF, which affect many different organs, somatic cell therapy might require several different procedures to accomplish delivery to the various cell types involved. By contrast, germ-line gene therapy would allow the addition of a properly functioning gene to all of the affected cell types in one fell swoop.[7] Second, because germ-line gene therapy would be performed at the earliest stages in human development, it could prevent damage that might occur during fetal development. Third, because germ-line gene therapy alters reproductive cells, any changes would be transmitted to the patient's offspring, if any. Thus, germ-line therapy offers the attractive possibility of reducing the incidence of certain inherited diseases, such as CF, in the human gene pool.

At the same time, the ability to introduce permanent changes into the genome is regarded by many people as making germ-line gene interventions ethically unacceptable. In addition to fear of unalterable mistakes being introduced into the gene pool, critics are concerned about the potential for abuse of the technology to enhance healthy individuals. Such concern, in part, informed a bioethics convention produced by the Council of Europe in 1997 that gathered signatures from twenty-two European states. This convention says that genetic manipulation may be undertaken for purposes of prevention, diagnosis or therapy—but only if it does not aim to introduce a permanent modification in the genome.[8]

Walters and Palmer consider the arguments for and against germ-line gene

therapy and conclude that voluntary programs are ethically acceptable in principle. They note that in order to accomplish the permanent elimination of genes
that cause disease, germ-line gene therapy would have to be given not only to
individuals who suffer from the disease but to healthy carriers of defective
genes as well. In their book, Walters and Palmer concede that screening and
treating healthy carriers would be an "ambitious public-health program" but
maintain that it is "not an entirely unrealistic prospect," noting that programs of
a similar scale have been carried out to counteract infectious disease such as
tuberculosis and small pox.[9] We leave it to the reader to decide whether germ-
line gene therapy ought to be permanently and universally banned, or wel-
comed as the next contribution to public health.

NOTES

1. Philip J. Boyle, "Shaping Priorities in Genetic Medicine," Special Supplement,
Hastings Center Report 25, no. 3 (1995), p. S2.
2. Robert Pear, "States Pass Laws to Regulate Uses of Genetic Testing," *New York
Times,* October 18, 1997, A1.
3. Sherman Elias and George J. Annas, *Reproductive Genetics and the Law* (Chicago:
Yearbook Medical, 1987, p. 54).
4. Patricia A. King, "The Past as Prologue: Race, Class, and Gene Discrimination," in
George J. Annas and Sherman Elias, eds. *Gene Mapping: Using Law and Ethics as
Guides* (New York: Oxford University Press, 1992, p. 99).
5. Udo Schuklenk, Edward Stein, Jacinta Kerin, and William Byne, "The Ethics of
Genetic Research on Sexual Orientation," *Hastings Center Report* 27, no. 4 (1997), pp.
6–13.
6. Theodore Friedmann, "Overcoming the Obstacles to Gene Therapy," *Scientific
American* (1997), p. 96.
7. LeRoy Walters and Julie Gage Palmer, *The Ethics of Human Gene Therapy* (New
York: Oxford University Press, 1997, p. 62).
8. Meredith Wadman, "European States Outlaw Permanent Changes," *Nature* (1998),
http://www.nature.com/Nature2.
9. Walters and Palmer, *supra* note 7, p. 63.

Ethical Implications of Screening Asymptomatic Individuals

NORMAN FOST

There is nothing new about screening asymptomatic individuals. It has become more common as health supervision and prevention have become a larger part of medical practice. Individual patients are routinely screened for hypertension, diabetes, and urinary tract infection. Mass screening of school children for intelligence, visual problems, and scoliosis are familiar activities.

Nor is genetic screening new. Mass screening of newborns for phenylketonuria (PKU) began decades ago, and has long been supplemented by tests for other genetic disorders such as maple syrup urine disease, and more recently, hemoglobinopathies. Adults have long been screened for sickle cell disease or trait.

What is new is the rapid growth of laboratory tests for genetic disorders. Molecular biology and the Human Genome Project are increasing the ability to identify genetic disorders and predisposition to disease at a dizzying pace, and each disorder and test has its own unique complexities. The discovery of the gene for cystic fibrosis was a remarkable achievement but not surprising. What was surprising was the discovery that there was not one mutation but hundreds, raising a variety of unanticipated scientific questions and complicating familiar ethical and legal questions about population screening.

Much has been made of the distinction between *screening* and *testing*. The former, as defined by Holtzman in this volume, generally refers to a program aimed at a defined population, often under public auspices. The latter generally refers to a procedure performed on an individual in a doctor-patient relationship. I do not find this distinction a particularly useful one in considering the ethical issues. All screening programs involve performing a test on individuals. If the program is voluntary, then at least minimal standards for consent are implied and the issues overlap substantially with what is called testing. Conversely, some forms of testing are so widespread as to constitute a standard of

From *FASEB Journal*, 6 (1992), 2813–2817. Reprinted by permission of the publisher and the author.

practice and have become de facto screening programs. The central question is what ethical principles and policies should guide proposals to perform a test on an asymptomatic individual or population of individuals.

The principles that should guide genetic screening have been identified with broad consensus for nearly 20 years. Studies and reports from the National Academy of Sciences Institute of Medicine, the President's Commission for the Study of Ethical Problems in Medicine and Biomedical and Behavioral Research, and the Hastings Center are remarkably homogeneous in their conclusions and recommendations. More recently, considerations of presymptomatic screening programs for specific disorders, such as cystic fibrosis and HIV infection, have rediscovered the same principles. The participants in these committees and reports typically include scientists, clinicans, lawyers and ethicists, advocates, and skeptics. Two factors are constant: agreement on the principles that should guide screening and the recurrent appearance of screening programs that ignore these principles.

A BRIEF HISTORY OF GENETIC SCREENING: TWO CASE STUDIES

Mass population screening for genetic disorders in asymptomatic individuals has been conducted for four purposes: presymptomatic detection of disorders for which effective *treatment* is thought to be available; *reproductive counseling,* particularly when effective treatment is not available; *research,* including studies of prevalence or natural history, or to recruit individuals into experimental treatment studies; and *inclusion or exclusion,* particularly for decisions regarding insurance employment. Two case studies will be reviewed to illustrate the ethical problems that arise.

Screening for Treatment: Phenylketonuria

The basic biochemistry of this rare inborn error of metabolism has been understood for more than 60 years. By 1960 it was clear that early detection and institution of a diet restricted in phenylalanine could ameliorate and possibly prevent the severe brain damage that developed in nearly all affected children. The development of the Guthrie test made it possible to screen all newborns cheaply and efficiently, and the development of an inexpensive and palatable milk created the opportunity to make PKU a model for preventing mental retardation. Aided by the leadership of a president passionately concerned about retardation—John F. Kennedy—state statutes were passed mandating newborn screening and referral to treatment centers.

In its early days, there was imperfect knowledge about the many variations of abnormal phenylalanine metabolism and about use of the diet. As a result, some children with variants of hyperphenylalaninemia who were not at risk for retardation were started on the diet. Because severe restriction of this essential amino acid could cause brain damage as surely as could excess, some children were made retarded by the program, and a smaller number died from complications of severe malnutrition. Despite a plea from the American Academy of Pediatrics Committee on Nutrition that mandatory screening be stopped, the program continued and expanded.

Later advances in the understanding of phenylalanine metabolism clarified the indications for treatment and its appropriate limits, but another complication appeared. The survival of women with PKU to reproductive age created a cohort of potential mothers at risk for causing even more extensive damage to potentially normal infants. High serum phenylalanine is one of the most potent teratogens known, causing retardation or structural malformations in 90% of exposed fetuses. As most affected fetuses would not be at risk for PKU, and because one affected mother could give birth to many damaged children, the net potential effect of the newborn screening and treatment program could be an increase in severely damaged children. Such damage can theoretically be prevented if mothers at risk maintained normal serum phenylalanine throughout pregnancy, but such a diet is onerous and must be initiated soon after conception.

In summary, several lessons were learned from the PKU program that should be expected in any screening program whose primary purpose is presymptomatic treatment.

1. *Genetic disorders, like all diseases, are heterogeneous.* There is probably no single-gene disorder, in the sense that phenotype will be determined by a single gene. This is certainly the case when the screening test is a gene product, rather than the gene itself, as such products may be controlled by a number of genes. The disease may be caused by many mutations, as in cystic fibrosis, with widely varying clinical manifestations. Even when there is a single mutation, as in sickle cell disease, the clinical course may be variable, affected by other genes and environmental factors, so that not all individuals will have a similar need for treatment and may not respond similarly to treatment. Treatment that may be lifesaving for some individuals may be unnecessary for others, so that risk/benefit considerations will vary among individuals.

2. *Screening/treatment programs are experiments until benefits and risks have been defined in well-designed studies.* There is broad acceptance for the principle that experimental drugs should be subjected to more rigorous oversight than standard treatment, as risk/benefit ratios are unknown and more likely to be adverse. Moreover, patients cannot meaningfully consent to interventions if there is inadequate information on their benefits and risks. Although drugs, and more recently, devices, have been highly regulated for these reasons, new surgical procedures, laboratory tests, and their attendant treatments have generally not been subjected to high standards of review.

3. *Political factors and zeal can obscure critical thinking.* The rush to institute mass PKU screening was the product of a "PKU lobby," consisting of well-
meaning and passionate advocates for the retarded, including families with personal experience with PKU, as well as scientists and the President of the United
States. The normal scientific caution that accompanies new tests and treatments
was brushed aside, and critics were either dismissed as obstacles in the campaign or their skepticism was suppressed.

4. *Mandatory programs are hard to stop.* The impulse to mandate screening
for PKU was understandable given the rarity of the condition. The normal dif-
fusion of scientific information to the general practitioner is slow, and advances
regarding a disease that affects 1 in 10,000 infants is not likely to attract immediate attention. But the extraordinary step of mandating treatment should create
a special standard for proving its safety and efficacy. As news of the complications and complexities began to trickle in over a decade or more, there was
little enthusiasm to return to the legislatures to admit error or to ask that the
program be reconsidered. Even when the safety and effectiveness of the PKU
had been established, compliance did not necessarily correlate with the presence of mandatory screening: some states with voluntary screening have higher
rates of compliance than those that mandate screening.

Screening for Reproductive Counseling: Sickle Cell Disease

Although the molecular basis of this autosomal recessive disorder has been
understood longer than any other, effective treatment has remained elusive. Inexpensive and accurate tests for heterozygotes have long been available, and
widespread screening was stimulated by the availability of federal funds in the
1970s. Couples found to be carriers had several options: *1)* Abstain from having children; *2)* adoption; *3)* artificial insemination (or later, egg donation) from
a donor known not to be a carrier; *4)* illegitimacy, i.e., natural insemination by a
donor other than the woman's primary partner; *5)* informed "gambling," i.e.,
choosing to have natural children as an informed choice; or *6)* prenatal diagnosis and selective abortion.

Most of these alternatives were either unavailable or unappealing to many
couples who were screened and found to be at risk, but because the tests were
inexpensive and had very low error rates, widespread screening was thought to
offer potential benefits to some clients with little or no risk. As with PKU
screening, the risks began to become apparent after widespread screening, not
as part of prospective studies. They can be classified in two categories: confusion and stigmatization.

CONFUSION Confusion by the clients themselves was common, typically involving a failure to understand the difference between sickle trait (the carrier

state) and sickle cell disease (the homozygous condition) or a failure to under-stand basic elements of probability and reproductive risks. The confusion between trait and disease was aggravated by the reality that sickle trait is asso-ciated with morbidity and even mortality under some conditions. Misunder-standing of probability is a more widespread problem, and is related to the general lack of public education on the subject. This confusion was not due to negligent or apathetic counseling. Experienced and dedicated counselors were surprised and frustrated at their inability to educate effectively.

Confusion could also occur in the minds of others. Many states required sickle screening as a condition of entry into elementary school. This served no apparent public health purpose nor did it offer any clear benefit to prospective students, because the vast majority with sickle cell disease would already have been diagnosed by that age, and those with sickle trait had little to gain from genetic counseling while in elementary school. The muddled motives of these programs can be appreciated from a Massachusetts statute that authorized "tests on every child susceptible to the disease known as sickle cell trait . . ." or a District of Columbia law that required sickle screening as a condition of school entry "to prevent and control the spread of communicable diseases." The Dupont Company was discovered to be discriminating on the basis of sickle trait because of an unproven belief that such persons were at higher risk for workplace-related disability. Life insurance companies denied coverage to ap-plicants with sickle trait, without evidence of shortened life expectancy com-pared with other applicants matched for race and socioeconomic status.

STIGMATIZATION   Stigmatization refers to an undesirable social consequence of being labeled. Like confusion, this can occur within the mind of the person screened or by others.

Self-stigmatization refers to adverse consequences of being labeled despite accurate understanding of the information. Although everyone carries lethal re-cessive genes, ignorance may be bliss and the actual knowledge of it can be distressing and lead to behavioral consequences. The normal inhibitions in sexual relations may be aggravated by the awareness that one is carrying a lethal gene.

Stigmatization by others includes discrimination by employers and insurers. The Air Force Academy excluded African-Americans with sickle trait because of concerns over service-connected disability. This policy was not entirely with-out reason, as persons with sickle trait are at risk for life-threatening sickling at high altitudes, due to low oxygen tensions, although many thought the actual risk for Air Force recruits had been exaggerated. Couples at risk for producing offspring with sickle cell disease do put health insurers at risk for higher costs. A small self-insured employer may be seriously burdened by one such family. Discrimination on the basis of risk has been central to commercial insurance. Most health insurance is purchased by groups, so that individuals are protected from discrimination on the basis of genetic risk. Companies have not found it economically prudent to screen applicants for individual policies, but results from screening tests obtained for other purposes may not be concealed and increasing awareness of such data has led to discrimination.

In addition to insurance and employment problems, screening led to unexpected discovery of illegitimacy. Counselors were often unprepared for this potential calamity, and women were generally unaware that testing could result in such disclosures. Meaningful efforts to obtain informed consent were uncommon.

The net result of federal funding for mass sickle screening, along with mandatory state screening laws, led to a backlash. Because the gene is concentrated in African-Americans in the U.S., screening programs were racially targeted. As persons being screened came to realize that the benefits were unattractive or unavailable, screening was perceived as having more risks than benefits for many individuals. Prenatal diagnosis was not generally available when screening programs were initiated and at their peak. The racial orientation of the programs, along with concerns about the risk/benefit ratio, led to suspicions of genocide.

The problems with sickle screening were not prominent in a national Tay-Sachs program targeted at Jewish couples. This program featured extensive education before screening was offered and rigorous standards for consent and post-test counseling. Follow-up studies showed high levels of satisfaction, with little stigmatization. Some of these differences can be attributed to the higher educational level of the target population; the absence of any medical significance to the carrier status, reducing the risks for confusion; and the availability of prenatal diagnosis. Thalassemia programs in Sardinia and the Greek Cypriot community in Great Britain also had wider acceptance.

In summary, there were several lessons from the sickle experience that should be anticipated in any widespread screening program whose primary purpose is reproductive counseling.

1. As with treatment programs, *screening programs for reproductive counseling are experiments with unknown benefits and risks.* Well-designed pilot studies are needed to demonstrate that pre-test information can be effectively communicated; that laboratory and counseling errors can be minimized; and that post-test counseling is available.

2. *Informed consent* should be a central feature of such programs. Whether any benefits exist for a given client and whether the possible benefits are worth the risks are value judgments that can be made only by the prospective client. Disclosure should include, when appropriate, the possibility of loss of insurance and employment as well the risk of uncovering illegitimacy.

3. *Screening programs may be driven by political considerations.* A major factor in the federal funding of sickle screening was a political promise by President Nixon in anticipation of political support from African-American leaders. Sickle screening did not emerge from the communities most affected nor from advocacy by leaders in medicine. The availability of money attracted physicians and community leaders. As with PKU screening, enthusiasm exceeded considerations of science or public health. In a study in Greece, widespread sickle screening and counseling had no apparent effect on the birth incidence of infants with sickle cell disease.

4. *Justifications for mandatory screening should be scrutinized.* As with PKU screening, screening was mandated prior to demonstrations of need or benefit. These programs eventually were either repealed or unenforced. In addition to the mandatory programs for entry into school, there were premature proposals to screen newborns without careful consideration of risks and benefits. Many years later, well-designed prospective studies demonstrated the effectiveness of early treatment in preventing serious infection in infants with sickle cell disease, although many of these programs have not adequately addressed the problems associated with identifying infants with sickle trait or other unusual hemoglobinopathies.

WHAT IS SPECIAL ABOUT GENETIC SCREENING?

Presymptomatic screening is central to contemporary medical practice, including the routine annual history and physical examination, urinalysis, and multiphasic laboratory screening. The ethical problems identified in the PKU and sickle stories are not unique to genetic screening. All presymptomatic screening presents the possibility for benefits and risks, generally unknown until they have been studied, and is of uncertain value outside a patient's choice based on his or her unique values. It is primarily the tremendous power of recombinant DNA technology that expands the potential of screening. The difference from the past is quantitative, but on such a scale as to raise the possibility of a major change in traditional premises and practices.

Some experts predict that the Human Genome Project will not simply identify the sequence of the human genome but make available to each individual a record of his/her particular genome, including all mutations with accompanying descriptions of the benefits and risks of testing for the associated disorders. The availability of such information would seem incompatible with traditional notions of informed consent. It is almost beyond comprehension that a typical American consumer, with an 8th-grade reading level, could evaluate such an encyclopedia of information and make an informed choice about whether to undergo prenatal diagnosis and selective abortion, or face an even more complex array of choices regarding gene therapy.

These problems are further complicated by the enormous opportunities for profit in genetic technology. The discovery of the gene for cystic fibrosis created an immediate potential market of at least $1 billion. The opportunity for profit has always coexisted in medicine, but the close involvement of practitioners with commercial genetic laboratories is radically different from the health care system of 20 years ago. The rapid growth of complex profitable technology is occurring in a climate of relatively little regulation, so that concerns about quality control are magnified.

Finally, the new technology creates special problems in a country whose citizens are dependent on their employers for health insurance. Such employers are understandably concerned and motivated to reduce the costs of producing goods and services; employees at high risk for expensive illness themselves or their offspring can threaten the economic survival of a business. The ability to screen prospective employees for such risks will certainly be used if it can be shown to be cost effective. Federal law restricts employers from discriminating on the basis of handicap, but it is unclear whether or how much this will limit the ability of employers to use genetic testing to deny employment.

The discovery of the gene for cystic fibrosis is again illustrative. This remarkable breakthrough created immediate hope for prevention or treatment of the most common serious genetic disease in North America. At the very least, it seemed evident to some that pregnant women should be offered the opportunity to be tested, even though the initial mutation discovered accounted for only 70% of abnormal chromosomes. The American Society of Human Genetics and a National Institutes of Health (NIH) workshop recommended that widespread testing not be initiated before pilot studies had demonstrated the safety and efficacy of a screening program. The challenge of effective counseling was complicated by the discovery of more than 150 mutations, collectively accounting for only 85% of affected individuals; by the high costs of a nationwide screening program; and by uncertainty of the public health benefit of such expenditures. At least three federal agencies—the Institute of Medicine, the Office of Technology Assessment, and the Ethical, Legal, and Social Issues Program of the National Center for Human Genome Research—are sponsoring major studies of the policy implications, but screening appears to be expanding despite the absence of studies as to its effectiveness, toxicity, costs, or benefits. Pilot studies funded by NIH had just begun in late 1991.

The controversy surrounding heterozygote screening for cystic fibrosis has been accompanied by disagreement about the justifications for presymptomatic screening of newborns. Colorado began such a program in an uncontrolled fashion years before a prospective controlled study was begun in Wisconsin, and contrary to recommendations of the Cystic Fibrosis Foundation. The Wisconsin study has yet to show any benefits 6 years after the first cohort began receiving presymptomatic treatment.

CONCLUSIONS

The principles that should guide genetic screening—whether for presymptomatic treatment, reproductive counseling, or research—have been well delineated without substantial disagreement for almost 20 years.

1. Screening programs should be thought of as experiments, with unknown benefits and risks, until well-designed pilot studies with clearly stated goals have demonstrated efficacy, safety, and costs.

2. Individuals should have the right to decide for themselves whether or not to be tested. This requires the informed consent of the patient or his or her representative.

3. Mass screening programs are often driven by political considerations or a desire for profit. Policy should include review by those without vested interests, including representatives from the communities most affected.

4. Mandatory programs are extremely difficult to modify, especially vulnerable to political motives, and not necessarily the most effective way to bring clearly beneficial services to the appropriate individuals.

5. Programs of demonstrated efficacy constitute expenditures of limited health care resources, which must be weighed against other potential uses of such funds.

Prenatal Genetic Testing and Screening: Constructing Needs and Reinforcing Inequities*

ABBY LIPPMAN

PRENATAL DIAGNOSIS: A TECHNICAL AND A SOCIAL CONSTRUCTION

Of all applied genetic activities, prenatal diagnosis is probably most familiar to the general population and is also the most used. Prenatal diagnosis refers to all the technologies currently in use or under development to determine the physi(ologi)cal condition of a fetus before birth. Until recently, prenatal diagnosis usually meant amniocentesis, a second trimester procedure routinely available for women over a certain age (usually thirty-five years in North America) for Down syndrome detection. Amniocentesis is also used in selected circumstances where the identification of specific fetal genetic disorders is possible. Now, in addition to amniocentesis, there are chorionic villus sampling (CVS) tests that screen maternal blood samples to detect a fetus with a neural tube defect or Down's syndrome, and ultrasound screening. Despite professional guidelines to the contrary, ultrasound screening is performed routinely in North America on almost every pregnant woman appearing for prenatal care early enough in pregnancy. And although ultrasound is not usually labeled as "prenatal diagnosis," it not only belongs under this rubric but was, I suggest, the first form of prenatal diagnosis for which informed consent is not obtained.

Expansion of prenatal diagnosis techniques, ever widening lists of identifiable conditions and susceptibilities, changes in the timing of testing and the

*Prenatal diagnosis, the focus of much of this paper, is troublesome for all women, users and critics alike. In no way do I intend my remarks about it to reflect on women who have considered or undergone testing; criticism of the technologies is not to be read as criticisms of them. Women considering childbearing today face agonizing issues I was fortunate enough not to have to confront, and I can only admire their resilience and strength.

From the *American Journal of Law & Medicine,* XVII (1991), Parts III (19–36) and V (44–49). Reprinted with permission of the American Society of Law, Medicine & Ethics and Boston University School of Law and the author.

populations in which testing is occurring, and expanding professional definitions of what should be diagnosed *in utero,* attest to this technology's role in the
process of geneticization. But these operational characteristics alone circum-
scribe only some aspects of prenatal diagnosis. Prenatal diagnosis as a social
activity is becoming an element in our culture and this aspect, which has had
minimal attention, will be examined in depth.

Prenatal Diagnosis and the Discourse of Reassurance

Contemporary stories about prenatal diagnosis contain several themes, but these
generally reflect either of two somewhat different models. In the "public health"
model, prenatal diagnosis is presented as a way to reduce the frequency of
selected birth defects. In the other, which I will call the "reproductive autonomy" model, prenatal diagnosis is presented as a means of giving women information to expand their reproductive choices. Unfortunately, neither model fully
captures the essence of prenatal diagnosis. In addition, neither acknowledges
the internal tension, revealed in the coexistence of quite contradictory constructions of testing that may be equally valid: 1) as an assembly line approach to
the products of conception, separating out those products we wish to develop
from those we wish to discontinue; 2) as a way to give women control over
their pregnancies, respecting (increasing) their autonomy to choose the kinds of
children they will bear; or 3) as a means of reassuring women that enhances
their experience of pregnancy.

The dominant theme throughout the biomedical literature, as well as some
feminist commentary, emphasizes the last two of these constructions. A major
variation on this theme suggests, further, that through the use of prenatal diagnosis women can avoid the family distress and suffering associated with the
unpredicted birth of babies with genetic disorders or congenital malformations,
thus preventing disability while enhancing the experience of pregnancy. Not
unlike the approach used to justify caesarean sections, prenatal diagnosis is
constructed as a way of avoiding "disaster."

The language of control, choice and reassurance certainly makes prenatal
diagnosis appear attractive. But while this discourse may be successful as a
marketing strategy, it relates a limited and highly selected story about prenatal
diagnosis. Notwithstanding that even the most critical would probably agree
prenatal diagnosis *can be* selectively reassuring (for the vast majority of women
who will learn that the fetus does not have Down syndrome or some other
serious diagnosable disorder), this story alone is too simplistic. It does not take
account of why reassurance is sought, how risk groups are generated and how
eligibility for obtaining this kind of reassurance is determined. Whatever else,
prenatal diagnosis *is* a means of separating fetuses we wish to develop from

those we wish to discontinue. Prenatal diagnosis does approach children as consumer objects subject to quality control.

This is implicit in the general assumption that induced abortion will follow the diagnosis of fetal abnormality. This assumption is reinforced by the rapid acceptance of chorionic villus sampling (CVS), which allows prenatal diagnosis to be carried out earlier and earlier in pregnancy when termination of a fetus found to be "affected" is taken for granted as less problematic. The generally unquestioned assumption that pre-implantation diagnosis is better than prenatal diagnosis also undermines a monotonic reassurance rhetoric. With pre-implantation (embryo) diagnosis, the selection objective is clear: only those embryos thought to be "normal" will be transferred and allowed to continue to develop. Thus, embryo destruction is equated with induced abortion. In perhaps the most blatant example, Brambati and colleagues have proposed the combined use of *in vitro* fertilization, gamete intrafallopian transfer, chorionic villus sampling and fetal reduction to "avoid pregnancy termination among high risk couples" [sic], and have stated that the "fetus was reduced" when describing a situation in which this scenario actually occurred.

Thus, while no single storyline is inherently true or false, the reassurance discourse appears to mask essential features of genetic testing and screening that are troubling. Reassurance—for pregnant women or for geneticists—notwithstanding, the story is more complex. Prenatal diagnosis necessarily involves systematic and systemic selection of fetuses, most frequently on genetic grounds. Though the word "eugenics" is scrupulously avoided in most biomedical reports about prenatal diagnosis, except when it is strongly disclaimed as a motive for intervention, this is disingenuous. Prenatal diagnosis presupposes that certain fetal conditions are intrinsically not bearable. Increasing diagnostic capability means that such conditions, as well as a host of variations that can be detected *in utero,* are proliferating, necessarily broadening the range of what is not "bearable" and restricting concepts of what is "normal." It is, perhaps, not unreasonable to ask if the "imperfect" will become anything we can diagnose.

While the notion of reassurance has been successfully employed to justify prenatal testing and screening as responses to the problems of childhood disability, we need to question both the sufficiency and the necessity of its linkage to prenatal diagnosis. At best, reassurance is an acquired, not an inherent, characteristic of prenatal diagnosis. Even if testing provides "reassurance," it is of a particular and limited kind. For example, although the fetus can be shown not to have Down syndrome, most disabilities only manifest themselves after birth. Further, it is not the (only) way to achieve a global objective of "reassuring" pregnant women. Indeed, it may even be counterproductive. This becomes clear if one reconstructs the notion of reassurance. Assuming it is an acceptable objective of prenatal care, are there ways to reassure pregnant women desiring "healthy" children that do not lead to genetic testing and control?

Data from the United States Women, Infants and Children program leave little doubt that "low technology" approaches providing essential nutritional, social and other supportive services to pregnant women will reduce the low birth weight and prematurity responsible for most infant mortality and morbidity today. Providing an adequate diet to the unacceptably large number of pregnant women living below the poverty line would clearly "reassure" them that their babies were developing as well as the babies of wealthier women. Similarly, allocation of funds for home visitors, respite care and domestic alterations would "reassure" women that the resources required to help them manage their special needs were readily available without financial cost, should their child be born with a health problem. It would also be "reassuring" to know that effective medication and simplified treatment regimes were available or being developed for prevalent disorders. Reassurances such as these may be all that many pregnant women want. Not only would these alternative approaches provide "reassurance" with respect to (and *for*) fetal disability, they would diminish a woman's feeling of personal responsibility for a child's health, rather than "exacerbate" it as does prenatal diagnosis.

Genes may contribute to the distribution of low birth weight and prematurity in North America, and likely some investigators will seek their location and the order of their DNA base sequences on the human gene map. The social and economic inequalities among women with which they are associated, however, are already well "mapped"; the "location" of women who are at increased risk is well known; the "sequences" of events leading to excessively and unnecessarily high rates of these problems have been well described. From this perspective, *gene* mapping and sequencing may be irrelevant as a source of reassurance in view of the most pressing needs of pregnant women. Even if genes were shown to be related to these problems, it must be remembered that the individuals to whom reassurance will be provided, as well as the concerns chosen for alleviation, rest on social, political and economic decisions by those in power. Such choices require continued analysis and challenge.

Constructing the "Need" for Prenatal Diagnosis

While reassurance has been constructed to justify health professionals' offers of prenatal diagnosis, genetic testing and screening have also been presented in the same biomedical literature as responses to the "needs" of pregnant women. They are seen as something they "choose." What does it mean, however, to "need" prenatal diagnosis, to "choose" to be tested? Once again, a closer look at what appear to be obvious terms may illuminate some otherwise hidden aspects of geneticization and the prenatal diagnosis stories told in its voice.

We must first identify the concept of need as itself a problem and acknowledge that needs do not have intrinsic reality. Rather, needs are socially constructed and culture bound, grounded in current history, dependent on context and, therefore, not universal.

With respect to prenatal diagnosis, "need" seems to have been conceptualized predominantly in terms of changes in capabilities for fetal diagnoses: women only come to "need" prenatal diagnosis after the test for some disorder has been developed. Moreover, the disorders to be sought are chosen exclusively by geneticists. In addition, posing a "need" for testing to reduce the probability a woman will give birth to a child with some detectable characteristic rests on assumptions about the value of information, about which characteristics are or are not of value and about which risks should or should not be taken. These assumptions reflect almost exclusively a white, middle-class perspective.

This conceptualization of need is propelled by several features of contemporary childbearing. First, given North American culture, where major responsibility for family health care in general, for the fetus she carries and for the child she births, is still allocated to a woman, it is generally assumed that she must do all that is recommended or available to foster her child's health. At its extreme, this represents the pregnant woman as obligated to produce a healthy child. Prenatal diagnosis, as it is usually presented, falls into this category of behaviors recommended to pregnant women who would exercise their responsibilities as caregivers. Consequently, to the extent that she is expected generally to do everything possible for the fetus/child, a woman may come to "need" prenatal diagnosis, and take testing for granted. Moreover, since an expert usually offers testing, and careseekers are habituated to follow through with tests ordered by physicians, it is hardly surprising that they will perceive a need to be tested. With prenatal diagnosis presented as a "way to avoid birth defects," to refuse testing, or perceive no need for it, becomes more difficult than to proceed with it. This technology perversely creates a burden of not doing enough, a burden incurred when the technology is *not* used.

A second feature, related to the first, is that women generally, and pregnant women specifically, are bombarded with behavioral directives that are at least as likely to foster a sense of incompetence as to nourish a feeling of control. It is therefore not surprising that a search for proof of competence is translated into a "need" for testing; external verification takes precedence over the pregnant woman's sense of herself. Evidence that the fetus is developing as expected may provide some women with a sense that all is under control (although this suggestion has not been studied empirically to the best of my understanding). Personal experience is set aside in favor of external and measured evidence. Moreover, given that a pregnant woman is more and more frequently reduced to a "uterine environment," and looked upon as herself presenting dangers to the fetus (especially if she eats improperly, smokes, drinks alcoholic beverages, takes medications, etc.), being tested becomes an early warning system to identify whether this "environment" is adequate. Women who share these suspicions and doubt that they can have a healthy baby without professional aid are likely to subject themselves to tests that are offered.

Third, prenatal diagnosis will necessarily be perceived as a "need" in a context, such as ours, that automatically labels pregnant women thirty-five years and over a "high risk" group. Although this risk labeling is, itself, socially rather than biologically determined, women informed that they are "at-risk" may find it hard to refuse prenatal diagnosis or other measures that are advertised to be risk-reducing. Once again, however, this "need" does not exist apart from the current context that created it by categorizing homogeneously those thirty-five and older who are pregnant as "at-risk." Mere identification of one's self as a member of a "high risk" group may influence the interpretation of an absolute risk figure and the acceptance of a test. In this light, the additional screening and testing possibilities generated by genome projects are likely to expand greatly the ranks of those deemed "needy." As the number of factors or people labeled as risks or at-risk increases, so, too, will offers of intervention.

Fourth, as prenatal diagnosis becomes more and more routine for women thirty-five years and older in North America, the risks it seems to avoid (the birth of a child with Down syndrome) appear to be more ominous, although the frequency of Down syndrome has not changed. This, too, may have a framing effect, generating a "need" for prenatal testing among women in this age group. Interestingly, however, this perception may inadvertently influence both the implementation and efficiency of proposed screening programs designed to supplement risk estimates based on maternal age with information from maternal blood samples. Having been socialized during the past fifteen to twenty years to view age thirty-five and over as the entry card to prenatal diagnosis, and convinced that once past this birthday they are "at risk," how will women beyond this age respond when blood test results remove them statistically from those in "need" of prenatal diagnosis? Will there be lingering doubts, and their sequelae, or will it be as easy to remove a risk label as it has been to affix one? What about the younger women who will have become prematurely aged (that is, eligible "by age" for prenatal diagnosis though not yet thirty-five)? As the title of a recent book phrases it, are pregnancy screening and fetal diagnosis *Calming or Harming?* We neither have the data necessary to answer this question, nor do we give priority to studies that would be informative. Instead, we proceed as if calming were a foregone conclusion. Programmatic changes such as these, no less than those subsequent to developments in genomics, underline how risk groups and needs are generated and constructed.

Fifth, on the collective level, prenatal diagnosis is generally presented as a response to the public health "need" to reduce unacceptably high levels of perinatal mortality and morbidity associated with perceived increases in "genetic" disorders. This reduction is of a special kind, in that prenatal diagnosis does not *prevent* the disease, as is usually claimed. Yet, even this "need," ostensibly based on "hard" data demonstrating the size of these problems, is constructed. For example, geneticists say "their" kinds of diseases are increasing as the prevalence of infectious diseases decreases, making genetic intervention seem appropriate. But others construe the same data as evidence of an increase in the "new morbidity" of pediatrics (developmental delays, learning difficulties, chronic disease, emotional and behavioral problems, etc.), the problems of concern in *their* specialty. Clearly, what one counts, emphasizes and treats as "evidence," depends on what one seeks as well as on the background beliefs generating the search. The numbers are then tallied, justifying a "need" to do something.

Moreover, unacceptably high rates of morbidity generate all sorts of "needs." Reducing these solely to biomedical problems hides the range of potential responses that might be considered.

Viewing needs and demands as cultural creations within a social context leads to doubts that assumptions of "free choice" with respect to the actual use of prenatal diagnosis are appropriate. It also clarifies why it is not fruitful to think that there may be a conflict between women who want prenatal diagnosis and critics who do not want them to have it. Not only does this polarization misinterpret the critics' position, it fails to recognize, for example, that prenatal diagnosis cannot really be a choice when other alternatives are not available, or that accepting testing as "needed" may be a way for a woman to justify going through what is a problematic experience for her. Society does not truly accept children with disabilities or provide assistance for their nurturance. Thus, a woman may see no realistic alternative to diagnosing and aborting a fetus likely to be affected.

Parallel to the creation of a woman's "need" for prenatal diagnosis is the development of health professionals' "need" for technological solutions to problems of malformation. Thus, geneticists increasingly choose to use and develop prenatal diagnosis to deal with problems of malformation excluding, if not precluding, consideration of other approaches. They "need" to employ these technologies, and in doing so they establish professional norms about how much is needed. Individual decisions about when a woman needs testing accumulate, and rapidly establish new standards for the profession. The routine use of ultrasound to monitor all pregnancies is probably the most obvious example. Regardless of the driving forces for dependency on this technology, the result is the construction of a particular "need": the basic "need" to know the gestational age of the fetus; the additional "need" to demonstrate that the pregnancy is progressing "normally." And the "needs" grow.

"Needs" for prenatal diagnosis are being created simultaneously with refinements and extensions of testing techniques themselves. In popular discourse— and with geneticists generally silent witnesses—genetic variations are being increasingly defined not just as problems, but, I suggest, as problems for which there is, or will be, a medical/technical solution. With but slight slippage these "problems" come to be seen as *requiring* a medical solution. This again hides the extent to which even "genetic" disease is a social/psychological experience as much as it is a biomedical one. This process is likely to accelerate as gene mapping enlarges the numbers of individuals declared eligible for genetic testing and screening. Given the extent of human variation, the possibilities for constructing "needs" are enormous.

Prenatal Diagnosis and the Social Control of Abortion and Pregnancy

The third element in the prenatal discourse that I will consider here stems from the often told story that testing is an option that increases women's reproductive choices and control. This claim has had much attention in the literature and I will examine it only with respect to how some features of prenatal diagnosis do increase control, but allocate it to someone other than a pregnant woman herself. This is most apparent in the context of abortion.

Without doubt, prenatal diagnosis has (re)defined the grounds for abortion—who is justified in having a pregnancy terminated and why—and is a clear expression of the social control inherent in this most powerful example of geneticization. Geneticists and their obstetrician colleagues are deciding which fetuses are healthy, what healthy means and who should be born, thus gaining power over decisions to continue or terminate pregnancies that pregnant women themselves may not always be permitted to make.

To the extent that specialists' knowledge determines who uses prenatal diagnosis and for what reasons, geneticists determine conditions that will be marginalized, objects of treatment or grounds for abortion. Prenatal diagnosis is thus revealed as a biopolitical as well as a biomedical activity. For example, an abortion may only be "legal" in some countries if the fetus has some recognized disorder, and the justifying disorder only becomes "recognizable" because geneticists first decide to screen for it. Fuhrmann suggests that in Europe, in fact, geneticists significantly influenced legislators establishing limits within which abortion would be at all permissible, by arguing that access to abortion be maintained through a gestational age that reflected when results from amniocentesis might be available. One wonders where limits might have been placed had first trimester chorionic villus sampling been available *before* amniocentesis? Would they have been more restrictive?

Other potential participants in what should be an intensely personal matter for "control" include insurance companies and governments. If either funds genetic screening programs or covers the cost of treatment for conditions diagnosable *in utero,* they may claim a say in determining which tests are carried out, and what action the results entail. Recently circulated reports about a health maintenance organization planning to withdraw medical coverage for a woman who could have avoided the birth of a child with cystic fibrosis if she had "chosen" to abort the pregnancy after the prenatal diagnosis was made, gives substance to concerns about changes in the locus of control. While this kind of abuse of power grabs headlines—and gets discounted as something regulations can prevent—there are more subtle forms of control that achieve the same ends and actually result from seemingly benevolent regulations and public policies. For example, newborn screening for Phenylketonuria (PKU) is carried out in the United States with universal approval. However, in only four states are health insurers required to cover the cost of the special foods children with PKU need. What choices/control does a woman have in this context? What are her options if prenatal diagnosis for PKU is offered? It would not be unreasonable to believe that a pregnant woman who learns that the fetus has the genes for PKU and does not see this as a reason for abortion may feel compelled to terminate her pregnancy because she could not herself finance the special diet her child would require after birth. Such pressures (explicit and implicit) exerted on a woman to abort a pregnancy following the prenatal diagnosis of some problem that makes her unable to keep a pregnancy she wants reveals another way in which social control over abortion may be genetically based.

Policy decisions establish control, too, in the guise of guidelines for seemingly straightforward features of prenatal screening and testing programs. For example, it has been shown that parents' decisions about pregnancy termination for the same chromosome abnormality are influenced by whether or not fetal anomalies are visualized on ultrasound. Even *who* does the counseling associated with prenatal diagnosis can influence what a woman does after learning of a fetal chromosome abnormality; rates of induced abortion are higher when obstetricians relate the results of testing than when geneticists do. Similarly, the interval between prenatal diagnosis counseling and testing is of consequence. This is demonstrated clearly in the reported association between the rates of amniocentesis utilization and the interval between counseling and testing: the shorter the interval, the greater the use. Pressure from state policies establishing when (as well as how) genetic counseling will be provided to screening program participants may be covert, but this does not prevent it from being controlling. In sum, prenatal testing and screening may provide control. But for whom? To what ends? For whose benefit? . . .

CONCLUSION

There are an unlimited number of ways to tell stories about health and disease, and an extensive vocabulary exists for telling them. Yet today, an increasing number of these stories are being told in the same way and with the same language: genetics, genes and genetic technologies. These genetic presentations of health, disease and ways to deal with them are grounded in the political and social context of the storytellers. My concern has been to decipher some of the stories about prenatal genetic screening and testing, and to reveal alternative constructions and interpretations to those already written.

Prenatal testing and screening, as has been repeated throughout this text, are most often presented as ways to decrease disease, to spare families the pain of having a disabled child and to enhance women's choice. The best-selling stories about them speak of reassurance, choice and control. As has also been suggested, this discourse presents a child born with some disorder requiring medical or surgical care as (exhibiting) a "failure." This failed pregnancy theme is reinforced in counseling provided to these families when counselors emphasize how most fetuses with an abnormality abort spontaneously during pregnancy, are "naturally selected," as it were, and how prenatal testing is merely an improvement on nature.

Just as there are several ways to construe reassurance, choice and control, the birth of a child with a structural malformation or other problem, "genetic" or otherwise, can be presented in other than biomedical terms. Is the story claiming that the pregnancy has malfunctioned (by not spontaneously aborting), resulting in a baby with a malformation, any "truer" than the story suggesting that *society* has malfunctioned because it cannot accommodate the disabled in its midst? Social conditions are as enabling or disabling as biological conditions. Why are biological variations that create differences between individuals seen as preventable or avoidable while social conditions that create similar distinctions are likely to be perceived as intractable givens?

While "many people don't believe society has an obligation to adjust to the disabled individual," there is nothing inherent in malformation that makes this so. Consequently, arguing that social changes are "needed" to enable those with malformations to have rich lives is not an inherently less appropriate approach. Actually, it may be more appropriate, since malformation, a biomedical phenomenon, requires a social translation to become a "problem." Expanding prenatal diagnostic services may circumvent but will not solve the "problem" of birth defects; they focus on disability, not on society's discriminatory practices. They can, at best, make only a limited contribution to help women have offspring free of disabilities, despite recent articles proposing prenatal diagnosis and abortion as ways to "improve" infant mortality and morbidity statistics. Thus, as sociopolitical decisions about the place of genetic testing and screening in the health care system are made, it will be important to consider how problems are named and constructed so that we don't mistakenly assume the story told in the loudest voice is the only one—or that the "best seller" is best.

Unarguably, illness and disability *are* "hard" (difficult) issues, and no one wants to add to the unnecessary suffering of any individual. But being "hard" neither makes illness or disability totally negative experiences, nor does it mean they must all be eliminated or otherwise managed exclusively within the medical system. Women's desire for children without disability warrants complete public and private support. The question is how to provide this support in a way that does no harm.

To date, support has been constructed to comprise genetic screening and testing. This construction is, in many ways, a result of the current system of health-care delivery in North America and the economic pressures on it. At a time when cost-containment is a dominant theme and a primary goal of policy makers, identifying those with, or susceptible to, some condition and preventing the occurrence of the anticipated condition seem to "make sense." It coincides, too, with the risk-benefit approach currently applied to most social and environmental problems. It corresponds with middle-class attitudes toward planning, consumers' rights and quality. But while this approach seems to "make sense," it does not suffice as a justification for the use of these technologies. Though it is more than twenty years since the first fetal diagnosis of Down syndrome by amniocentesis, we do not yet know the full impact of prenatal testing and screening on women's total health, power and social standing.

When amniocentesis was introduced, abortion subsequent to a diagnosis of fetal abnormality was presented as a temporary necessity until treatment for the detected condition could be devised. Advocates assumed that this would soon be forthcoming. With time, however, the gap between characterization and treatment of disease has widened. New information from efforts at gene mapping will certainly increase the ability to detect, diagnose and screen, but not to treat. A human gene map will identify variations in DNA patterns. Genes that "cause" specific disease, as well as those associated with increased susceptibility to specific disorders, will be found. Simultaneously, prenatal screening and testing are evolving in a context where a "genetic approach" to public health is gaining great favor. All the variations that will be mapped can become targets of prenatal testing. Which targets will be selected in the quest for improved public health? And who will determine that they have been reached? Given the extraordinary degree of genetic variability within groups of people, what does "genetic health" actually mean—and does it matter?

For society, genetic approaches to health problems are fundamentally expensive, individualized and private. Giving them priority diminishes incentives to challenge the existing system that creates illness no less than do genes. With prenatal screening and testing in particular, the genetic approach seems to provide a "quick fix" to what is posed as a biological problem, directing attention away from society's construction of a biological reality *as* a problem and leaving the "conditions that create social disadvantage or handicap . . . largely unchallenged."

Justice in the domain of health care has several definitions, but only one is generally employed in contemporary choice-and-control stories of genetic screening and testing. In these stories, justice is defined by the extent to which testing and screening programs are available and accessible to all women. Distributive justice is the goal: fair treatment requires access for all.

This definition seems insufficient. Access involves more than availability, even broadly defined. Not all individuals can respond similarly even to universally "available" services and, even if they can, unfairness and injustice may continue. Thus, perhaps we need to introduce other concepts of justice when thinking about prenatal testing and how these programs contribute to, or diminish, fairness in health and health care for women (and others). Do they ensure good for the greatest number (social justice) given all the causes of perinatal morbidity and mortality? Do they recognize and seek to correct past discrimination (corrective justice) given current and historically-based inequities in health? Will they level the playing field for women, for the poor?

One approach to justice is not necessarily better than another. In fact, depending on the circumstances, each one might be seen as "better." We need to keep these multiple routes to fairness in mind as we determine those to whom we wish to be fair and that for which fairness will be sought. For instance, human relationality may be as worthy of guarantees and respect as human autonomy; "individual good" is not always synonymous with "common good," though social responsibility need not become paternalism. There are choices to be made and the choices will reflect our values and ideology. How we choose our culture (by the routes we take) is no less problematic than how we choose our children, and consequences from both will be among our legacies.

Addressing these choices will itself be "hard," and will require we recognize and grapple with disjunction between goals and needs—perhaps even "rights" —on the social and on the individual levels. What seems to be appropriate or best for the individual may not be so for the collectives to which we all belong. We need urgently to address these contradictions now, using our energies to situate, understand and maybe even in some way resolve them, rather than keep them at the periphery of our vision. We must confront the possible need to choose between what is unfortunate and what is unfair in the distribution and reduction of risks to health and well-being. We must also acknowledge how our compassion for an individual's situation may harm women's health in general if addressing private needs dislocates provisions required for the public or solidifies existing inequities in women's position. This disjunction is not unique to genetic screening and testing, but is certainly echoed with force in this area.

This disjunction will make dialogue about the place of prenatal diagnosis in women's health care especially difficult (and, on occasion, tense). However, this only underscores the need to avoid premature closure of discussion and to avoid reducing it to sterile debates between "pros" and "cons." The issue is *not* between experts promoting technology and Luddites trying to retard science. It is not between women who "want" prenatal diagnosis and women who don't want "them" to have it. It is not a dispute between advocates of prenatal diagnosis who are seen as defending women's already fragile rights to abortion and critics who are said to be fueling "right to life" supporters seeking to impose limits on women (and their choices). All of these themes are being played out, but to focus on them is to create false polarities and to trivialize the possible advantages and disadvantages of these technologies when trying to deal with women's health concerns. Moreover, it incorrectly decontextualizes these technologies, severing their essential relatedness to time and place and isolating them from the broader health and social policy agenda of which they are a part.

Consequently, it is imperative that we continue to listen to the stories being told about prenatal testing and screening with a critical ear, situate them in time and place, question their assumptions, demystify their language and metaphors and determine whether, and to what extent, they can empower women. These technologies warrant social analysis. Not to examine repeatedly the tales and their tellers will be to abdicate responsibility to the generations that present and future genetic screening and testing programs will, or will not, allow to be born. A perspective that makes us responsible for the future effects of our current activities, the well-intentioned and the unintended, may stimulate the imaginative re-vision required so that we consider not just "where in the world" we are going with the new genetics, but where we want to go and whether we in fact want genetics to lead us there.

Germ-Line Gene Therapy

LEROY WALTERS AND JULIE GAGE PALMER

ETHICAL ISSUES

An Earlier Stage of the Discussion: *Muller versus Lederberg*

The ethical debate over intentionally introducing genetic changes into the human germ line through advanced biomedical techniques goes back at least to the 1920s and 1930s and the writings of classical geneticists J.B.S. Haldane and H. J. Muller. The discussion was renewed in the late 1950s and early 1960s, with two of the chief protagonists being H. J. Muller and molecular biologist Joshua Lederberg. Muller advocated the improvement of the gene pool through voluntary programs of assisted reproduction—specifically artificial insemination using semen from donors who had what Muller viewed as the best combination of physical, intellectual, and moral qualities. (Egg donation was not a technical possibility in the 1960s, as it is today. Given his general advocacy of women's rights, Muller would surely have approved the equal participation of women in this voluntary program for improving the human gene pool.) At a symposium held in London in November 1962, Joshua Lederberg criticized Muller's proposal for its lack of precision and for the very slow progress that Muller's plan for guided evolution would deliver. In Lederberg's words,

> The recent achievements of molecular biology strengthen our eugenic means to achieve [human survival]. But do they necessarily support proposals to transfer animal husbandry to man? My own first conclusion is that the technology of human genetics is pitifully clumsy, even by the standards of practical agriculture. Surely within a few generations we can expect to learn tricks of immeasurable advantage. Why bother now with somatic selection, so slow in its impact? Investing a fraction of the effort, we should soon learn how to manipulate chromosome ploidy [number of sets of chromosomes], homozygosis [the union of gametes that are identical for one or more pairs of genes], gametic selection, full diagnosis of heterozygotes, to accomplish in one or two generations of eugenic practice what would now take ten or one hundred.

From Chapter 3 in *The Ethics of Human Gene Therapy* by LeRoy Walters and Julie Gage Palmer (Oxford University Press, 1997). Reprinted by permission of the publisher.

Even 30+ years after Lederberg's statement there are many "tricks" that molecular biologists have not yet learned about genes, chromosomes, and cells. The chief trick that remains elusive is guiding new genes to precise locations where they can replace malfunctioning genes. Also, in the 1990s we are less likely to *begin* our discussions of germ-line genetic intervention by thinking of global effects on human evolution. We are much more likely to begin by considering specific diseases and decisions that are likely to be faced by couples who are deciding whether or not to have children. The thinking of those couples will be focused, first and foremost, on the welfare of their children and perhaps on the welfare of their children's children as well.

A Preliminary Question: Should This Issue Be Discussed at All?

In September of 1992 a distinguished physician–scientist, Dr. James V. Neel, appeared before the NIH RAC [National Institutes of Health Recombinant DNA Advisory Committee] to discuss spontaneous and induced germ-line mutation. Dr. Neel argued that it would be premature for the RAC to discuss the scientific and ethical questions surrounding germ-line gene therapy. His precise message, as summarized in a 1993 editorial, was the following:

> The Committee's desire to prepare itself for future developments would under most circumstances be laudable, but for a Committee with this visibility and prestige to begin to consider the subject of germ-line therapy in an organized fashion at this time would send the wrong vibes to the scientific, ethical, and political communities. Such an action might appear to imply the belief that the Committee would be seriously considering this prospect within the terms of office of present Committee members. Given the tremendous issues at stake, and even with the utmost attempt on my part to anticipate the amazing speed of advances in the field of molecular genetics, I could not imagine serious organized discussions of this subject by such a group within the next 20 or 30 years. (Individuals will, of course, express their views as they please.)

Dr. Neel carefully avoids urging individuals, like the present authors, to refrain from discussing the topic of germ-line gene therapy. On the other hand, he clearly thinks that it would be a mistake for public advisory committees like the RAC to engage in anticipatory discussions of this subject. We respectfully disagree. In our view, the years from 1983 through 1988, during which the RAC looked ahead to the first hypothetical somatic-cell gene-therapy proposals, were very profitably devoted to anticipating what the new technology might mean and to developing "points to consider," or very general guidelines, for somatic cell therapy proposals. In a similar way, given the research advances outlined in the earlier part of this chapter, we think that both individuals and public advisory committees would be wise to begin the discussion of this important topic sooner rather than later. If proposals for human application of germ-line gene therapy are delayed because of technical obstacles, or if research moves in unanticipated directions that must then later be taken into account, the risks of premature discussion are low. On the other hand, if a technical breakthrough occurs that makes germ-line gene therapy feasible, the anticipatory discussion of the topic may turn out to have been essential for the calm formulation of rational oversight policies. . . .

Major Ethical Arguments in Favor of Germ-Line Gene Therapy

In this and the following section we will analyze the major ethical arguments for and against germ-line gene therapy. For this analysis we will make the optimistic assumption that germ-line intervention methods will gradually be refined until they reach the point where gene replacement or gene repair is technically feasible and able to be accomplished in more than 95% of attempted gene transfer procedures. Thus, the following analysis presents the arguments for and against germ-line intervention under the most favorable conditions for such intervention.

A first argument in favor of germ-line intervention is that it may be the only way to prevent damage to particular biological individuals when that damage is caused by certain kinds of genetic defects. . . . [O]nly genetic modifications introduced into preimplantation embryos are likely to be early enough to affect all of the important cell types (as in retinoblastoma), or to reach a large enough fraction of brain cells, or to be in time to prevent irreversible damage to the developing embryo. In these circumstances the primary intent of gene therapy would, or at least could, be to provide gene therapy for the early embryo. A side effect of the intervention would be that all of the embryonic cells, including reproductive cells that would later develop, would be genetically modified.

A second moral argument for germ-line genetic intervention might be advanced by parents. It is that they wish to spare their children and grandchildren from either (1) having to undergo somatic cell gene therapy if they are born affected with a genetic defect or (2) having to face difficult decisions regarding possibly transmitting a disease-related gene to their own children and grandchildren. In our first scenario, admittedly a rare case, two homozygous parents who have a genetic disease know in advance that all of their offspring are likely to be affected with the same genetic disease. In the second scenario, there is a certain probability that the parents' offspring will be affected or carriers. An assumption lying behind this second argument is that parents should enjoy a realm of moral and legal protection when they are making good-faith decisions about the health of their children. Only if their decisions are clearly adverse to the health interests of the children should moral criticism or legal intervention be considered.

A third moral argument for germ-line intervention is more likely to be made by health professionals, public-health officials, and legislators casting a wary eye toward the expenditures for health care. This argument is that, from a social and economic point of view, germ-line intervention is more efficient than repeating somatic cell gene therapy generation after generation. From a medical and public health point of view, germ-line intervention fits better with the increasingly preferred model of disease prevention and health promotion. In the very long run, germ-line intervention, if applied to both affected individuals and asymptomatic carriers of serious genetic defects, could have a beneficial effect on the human gene pool and the frequency of genetic disease.

A fourth argument refers to the roles of researchers and health professionals. As a general rule, researchers deserve to have the freedom to explore new modes of treating and/or preventing human disease. To be sure, moral rules set limits on how this research is conducted. For example, animals involved in the preclinical stages of the research should be treated humanely. In addition, the human subjects involved in the clinical trials should be treated with respect. When and if germ-line gene therapy is some day validated as a safe and effective intervention, health care providers should be free to, and may have a moral obligation to, offer it to their patients as a possible treatment. This freedom is based on the professional's general obligation to seek out and offer the best possible therapeutic alternatives to patients and society's recognition of a sphere in which health professionals are at liberty to exercise their best judgment on behalf of their patients.

A fifth and final argument in favor of germ-line gene therapy is that this kind of intervention best accords with the health professions' healing role and with the concern to protect rather than penalize individuals who have disabilities. This argument is not simply a plea for protecting all embryos and fetuses from the time of fertilization forward. Both authors of this book think that abortion is morally justifiable in certain circumstances. However, prenatal diagnosis followed by selective abortion and preimplantation diagnosis followed by selective discard seem to us to be uncomfortable and probably discriminatory halfway technologies that should eventually be replaced by effective modes of treatment. The options of selective abortion and selective discard essentially say to prospective parents, "There is nothing effective that the health care system has to offer. You may want to give up on this fetus or embryo and try again." To people with disabilities that are diagnosable at the prenatal or preimplantation stages of development the message of selective abortion and selective discard may seem more threatening. That message may be read as, "If we health professionals and prospective parents had known you were coming, we would have terminated your development and attempted to find or create a nondisabled replacement."

This argument is not intended to limit the legal access of couples to selective abortion in the case of serious health problems for the fetus. We support such access. Rather, it is an argument about what the long-term goal of medicine and society should be. In our view, that long-term goal should be to prevent disability and disease wherever possible. Where prevention is not possible, the second-best alternative is a cure or other definitive remedy. In cases where neither prevention nor cure is possible, our goal should be to help people cope with disability and disease while simultaneously seeking to find a cure.

Major Arguments Against Germ-Line Gene Therapy

First, if the technique has unanticipated negative effects, those effects will be visited not only on the recipient of the intervention himself or herself but also on all of the descendants of that recipient. This argument seems to assume that a mistake, once made, could not be corrected, or at least that the mistake might not become apparent until the recipient became the biological parent of at least one child. For that first child, at least, the negative effects could be serious, as well as uncorrectable.

Second, some critics of germ-line genetic intervention argue that this technique will never be necessary because of available alternative strategies for preventing the transmission of diagnosable genetic diseases. Specifically, critics of germ-line gene therapy have sometimes suggested that preimplantation diagnosis and the selective discard of affected embryos might be a reasonable alternative to the high-technology, potentially risky attempt to repair genetic defects in early human embryos. Even without in vitro fertilization and preimplantation diagnosis, the option of prenatal diagnosis and selective abortion is available for many disorders. According to this view, these two types of selection, before embryos or fetuses have reached the stage of viability, are effective means for achieving the same goal.

The third argument is closely related to the second: this technique will always be an expensive option that cannot be made available to most couples, certainly not by any publicly funded health care system. Therefore, like in vitro fertilization for couples attempting to overcome the problem of infertility, germ-line gene therapy will be available only to wealthy people who can afford to pay its considerable expense on their own.

The fourth argument builds on the preceding two: precisely because germ-line intervention will be of such limited utility in preventing disease, there will be strong pressures to use this technique for genetic enhancement at the embryonic stage, when it could reasonably be expected to make a difference in the future life prospects of the embryo. Again in this case, only the affluent would be able to afford the intervention. However, if enhancement interventions were safe and efficacious, the long-term effect of such germ-line intervention would probably be to exacerbate existing differences between the most-well-off and the least-well-off segments of society.

Fifth, even though germ-line genetic intervention aims in the long run to treat rather than to abort or discard, the issue of appropriate respect for preimplantation embryos and implanted fetuses will nonetheless arise in several ways. After thoroughgoing studies of germ-line intervention have been conducted in nonhuman embryos, there will undoubtedly be a stage at which parallel studies in human embryos will be proposed. The question of human embryo research was recently studied by a committee appointed by the director of the National Institutes of Health. Although the committee specifically avoided commenting on germ-line intervention, its recommendation that certain kinds of human embryo research should be continued and that such research should be funded by NIH provoked considerable controversy. Critics of the committee's position would presumably also oppose the embryo research that would be proposed to prepare the way for germ-line gene therapy in humans. Their principal argument would be that the destruction or other harming of preimplantation embryos in research is incompatible with the kind of respect that should be shown to human embryos.

Even after the research phase of germ-line genetic intervention is concluded, difficult questions about the treatment of embryos will remain. For example, preimplantation diagnosis may continue to involve the removal of one or two totipotential cells from a four- to eight-cell embryo. While the moral status of totipotential human embryonic cells has received scant attention in bioethical debates, there is, at least a plausible argument that a totipotential cell, once separated from the remainder of a preimplantation embryo, is virtually equivalent to a zygote; that is, under favorable conditions it could develop into an embryo, a fetus, a newborn, and an adult. This objection to the destruction of totipotential embryonic cells will only be overcome if a noninvasive genetic diagnostic test for early embryos (like an x-ray or a CT scan) can be developed. Further, even if a noninvasive diagnostic test is available, as we have noted above, a postintervention diagnostic test will probably be undertaken with each embryo to verify that the intervention has been successful. Health professionals and prospective parents will probably be at least open to the possibility of selective discard or selective abortion if something has gone radically wrong in the intervention procedure. Thus, germ-line genetic intervention may remain foreclosed as a moral option to those who are conscientiously opposed to any action that would directly terminate the life of a preimplantation embryo or a fetus.

The sixth argument points to potential perils of concentrating great power in the hands of human beings. According to this view, the technique of germ-line intervention would give human beings, or a small group of human beings, too much control over the future evolution of the human race. This argument does not necessarily attribute malevolent intentions to those who have the training that would allow them to employ the technique. It implies that there are built-in limits that humans ought not to exceed, perhaps for theological or metaphysical reasons, and at least hints that corruptibility is an ever-present possibility for the very powerful.

The seventh argument explicitly raises the issue of malevolent use. If one extrapolates from Nazi racial hygiene programs, this argument asserts, it is likely the germ-line intervention will be used by unscrupulous dictators to produce a class of superior human beings. The same techniques could be also used in precisely the opposite way, to produce human-like creatures who would willingly perform the least-attractive and the most-dangerous work for a society. According to this view, Aldous Huxley's *Brave New World* should be updated, for modern molecular biology provides tyrants with tools for modifying human beings that Huxley could not have imagined in 1932.

The eighth and final argument against germ-line genetic intervention is raised chiefly by several European authors who place this argument in the context of human rights. According to these commentators, human beings have a moral right to receive from their parents a genetic patrimony that has not been subjected to artificial tampering. Although the term "tampering" is not usually defined, it seems to mean any intentional effort to introduce genetic changes into the germ line, even if the goal is to reduce the likelihood that a genetic disease will be passed on to the children and grandchildren of a particular couple. The asserted right to be protected against such tampering may be a slightly different formulation of the sixth argument noted above—namely, that there are built-in limits, embedded in the nature of things, beyond which not even the most benevolent human beings should attempt to go.

A Brief Evaluation of the Arguments

In our view, the effort to cure and prevent serious disease and premature death is one of the noblest of all human undertakings. For this reason the first pro argument—that germ-line intervention may be the only way to treat or prevent certain diseases—seems to us to be of overriding importance. We also find the third pro argument to be quite strong, that a germ-line correction, if demonstrated to be safe and effective, would be more efficient than repeated applications of somatic cell gene therapy. In addition, the final pro argument about the overall mission of the health professions and about society's approach to disabilities seems to us to provide a convincing justification for the germ-line approach, when gene replacement is available.

Our replies to the objections raised by critics of germ-line intervention are as follows:

1. *Irreversible mistakes.* While we acknowledge that mistakes may be made in germ-line gene therapy, we think that the same sophisticated techniques that were employed to introduce the new genes will be able to be used to remove those genes or to compensate for their presence in some other way. Further, in any sphere of innovative therapy, a first step into human beings must be taken at some point.

2. *Alternative strategies.* Some couples, perhaps even most couples, will choose the alternative strategies of selective abortion or selective discard. In our view, a strategy of attempting to prevent or treat potential disease or disability in the particular biological individual accords more closely with the mission of the health sciences and shows greater respect for children and adults who are afflicted with disease or disability.

3. *High cost, limited availability.* It is too early to know what the relative cost of germ-line intervention will be when the technique is fully developed. In addition, the financial costs and other personal and social harms of preventable diseases will need to be compared with the financial costs of germ-line gene therapy. It is at least possible that this new technology could become widely diffused and available to many members of society.

4. *Use for enhancement.* Prudent social policy should be able to set limits on the use of germ-line genetic intervention. Further, some enhancements of human capabilities may be morally justifiable, especially when those enhancements are health related. We acknowledge that the distribution of genetic enhancement is an important question for policy makers. . . .

5. *Human embryos.* In our view, research with early human embryos that is directed toward the development of germ-line gene therapy is morally justifiable in principle. Further, we acknowledge the potential of a totipotential cell but think that the value of a genetic diagnosis outweighs the value of such a cell. We also accept that, if a serious error is made in germ-line gene therapy, terminating the life of the resulting embryo or fetus may be morally justifiable. In short, there is a presumption in favor of fostering the continued development of human embryos and fetuses, but that presumption can in our view be overridden by other considerations like serious harm to the developing individual or others and the needs of preclinical research.

6. *Concentration of power.* We acknowledge that those who are able to use germ-line intervention will have unprecedented ability to introduce precise changes into the germ lines of particular individuals and families. However, in our view, it is better for human beings to possess this ability and to use it for constructive purposes like preventing disease in families than not to possess the ability. The central ethical question is public accountability by the scientists, health providers, and companies that will be involved with germ-line intervention. Such accountability presupposes transparency about the use of the technology and ongoing monitoring process aimed at preventing its misuse.

7. *Misuse by dictators.* This objection focuses too much attention on technology and too little on politics. There is no doubt that bona fide tyrants have existed in the 20th century and that they have made use of all manner of technologies—whether the low-tech methods of surgical sterilization or the annihilation of concentration camp inmates with poison gas or high-tech weapons like nuclear warheads and long-range missiles—to terrify and to dominate. However, the best approach to preventing the misuse of genetic technologies may not be to discourage the development of the technologies but rather to preserve and encourage democratic institutions that can serve as an antidote to tyranny. A second possible reply to the tyrannical misuse objection is that germ-line intervention requires a long lead time, in order to allow the offspring produced to grow to adulthood. Tyrants are often impatient people and are likely to prefer the more instantaneous methods of propaganda, intimidation, and annihilation of enemies to the relatively slow pace of germ-line modification.

8. *Human rights and tampering.* It is a daunting task to imagine what the unborn and as-yet-unconceived generations of people coming after us will want. Even more difficult is the effort to ascribe rights to human beings. Insofar as we can anticipate the needs and wants of future generations, we think that any reasonable future person would prefer health to serious disease and would therefore welcome a germ-line intervention in his or her family line that effectively prevented cystic fibrosis from being transmitted to him or her. In our view, such a person would not regard this intervention as tampering and would regard as odd the claim that his or her genetic patrimony has been artificially tampered with. Cystic fibrosis was not a part of his or her family's heritage that the future person was eager to receive or to claim.

Would Germ-Line Gene Therapy Be, or Lead to, a Eugenics Program?

We can perhaps best approach this question by imagining a future world in which the global elimination of a genetic disease by means of germ-line gene therapy is technically feasible.

> The year is 2055, and a definitive genetic cure for the mutations that cause cystic fibrosis (CF) has recently been discovered, tested, and perfected. This target-specific mode of gene therapy takes a properly functioning gene to the site of the mutation, splices out and destroys the malfunctioning gene, and replaces it with the properly functioning gene. The new technique can be applied equally well to somatic and germ-line (sperm or egg) cells.
>
> The World Health Organization (WHO) has recently announced a global program to eradicate all CF mutations from the human gene pool. The program is modeled on the earlier campaign to eliminate smallpox. All at-risk persons will be required to undergo testing and, if found to be affected or heterozygous, to accept genetic treatment of both their somatic and reproductive cells. WHO estimates that

the global campaign will succeed within 35 years, at the most, and that the effort, when completed, will save $40 billion annually (in 2050 dollars) in the world health budget.

This hypothetical situation is extrapolated from past and present programs aimed at controlling serious infectious diseases. These programs include the worldwide campaign that eliminated smallpox, as well as state-based programs of mandatory immunization against such diseases as measles and polio.

A first issue raised by this hypothetical is whether it is reasonable to draw an analogy between infectious disease and genetic disease. Proponents of the analogy point to the transmissibility of disease in both cases and argue that the mere direction or mode of transmission—horizontal or vertical—is less important than the spread of disease. Opponents of the analogy point out that, while some infectious diseases are transmitted by intimate behavior, all genetic disease transmission occurs in the context of reproduction, one of the most intensely personal and private spheres of human life.

Second, we are not told in the hypothetical whether a voluntary program of genetic screening and gene therapy for CF has been tried and has failed. If it has not been tried, the burden of proof for the proponent of a mandatory program is heavier. Yet there may be plausible arguments, based on cost or the number of decades required to reach the goal in a voluntary program, for the moral preferability of the mandatory approach in this case and all relevantly similar cases. If a voluntary program has been tried and has failed because of public inertia or unreasonable resistance, a mandatory program might seem to be morally justifiable in this case, even to a civil libertarian, as a reasonable means to a highly desirable end.

Here we as coauthors see no alternative to drawing a sharp, clear moral and public-policy line. In our view, state intervention in reproductive decisions by individuals and couples is virtually always wrong and virtually always counterproductive as a public policy. We would apply this strong preference for voluntary public-health programs to several current technologies, for example, maternal serum alpha-fetoprotein screening to detect neural tube disorders, prenatal testing of HIV-infected pregnant women and postnatal testing of their infants, and newborn screening for genetic disease. In the same way we would apply this preference to the future hypothetical possibility of germ-line genetic intervention. Thus, we would support the *offering* of diagnostic testing and germ-line gene therapy to all adults. In our view, the vast majority of individuals and couples would eagerly participate in such a program, just as the vast majority of parents consent to newborn testing in states where free choice in this matter is respected. However, we regard state intervention to compel people to accept germ-line genetic intervention in their reproduction as a violation of a basic human right.

Would a voluntary germ-line program that aimed to reduce the incidence of one or more genetic diseases in human populations be a eugenics program? Much depends on whether the term *eugenics* is employed as a morally neutral, descriptive term or as a term that already includes in its very meaning a negative moral judgment, like the words "murder" and "rape." The coercive and discriminatory eugenics programs adopted in the United States and Nazi Germany in the first half of the 20th century are rightly condemned as immoral. The question remains, however, whether there is a place for the notion of a morally justifiable eugenics program—one that is strictly voluntary and firmly based on reliable genetic technologies. In our view, the word "eugenics" has been so tainted by the discriminatory, coercive practices of multiple nations in this century that it cannot be rehabilitated. Thus, we would want to use a different and probably more cumbersome formulation to describe such a program, for example, "a voluntary program to reduce the incidence of genetic disease through germ-line genetic intervention."

Finally, we note that the kind of public-health program outlined in this scenario would only be feasible if safe, reliable methods for effecting precise genetic changes in human sperm (or sperm-producing) cells and human egg cells within the bodies of adults are developed. Any technique that depends on in vitro fertilization and in vitro gene repair will be much too expensive to be used on a population-wide basis.

The Continuing Relevance of the "Points to Consider" and General Ethical Principles

The preceding chapter on somatic cell gene therapy discussed seven questions that are currently asked by the NIH RAC as it reviews somatic cell proposals. These questions are contained in a guidance document called the "Points to Consider." The questions can be summarized as follows:

1. What is the disease to be treated?
2. What alternative treatments are available?
3. What is the potential harm of the intervention?
4. What is the potential benefit of the intervention?
5. How will the selection of patients be conducted in a way that is fair to all candidates?
6. How will the voluntary and informed consent of patients (or their parents or guardians) be solicited?
7. How will the privacy and confidentiality of patients be preserved?

In our view, these questions will be relevant to germ-line gene therapy proposals, but their emphasis will shift in important ways. In answering question 2, future researchers may need to discuss not only alternative *treatments* but also alternative strategies to prevent the transmission of genetic disorders to future generations. The options of preimplantation diagnosis and selective discard and of prenatal diagnosis and selective abortion will surely be discussed in this context. Questions 3 and 4 will also be pertinent but with an important shift in emphasis. If germ-line gene therapy is performed on early human embryos, the principal risks will be to the embryo and the embryo's potential descendants, not to the genetic parents of the embryo. Even if the parents have their sperm and egg cells treated in vivo by means of gene therapy, it is more likely that something will go wrong in the offspring than in the parents themselves. Similarly, the benefits of germ-line intervention will accrue primarily to, the genetically repaired embryo and the embryo's future children rather than to the parents. Thus, the focus of the benefit–harm calculus will be expanded to include multiple future generations within a particular family, and both parents and researchers will know that their decisions will have long-term genetic effects.

The third and fourth questions will be broadened in another respect, as well. Some critics of germ-line genetic intervention have raised ethical objections to *ever* employing this technique on grounds of the serious social harm that might ensue. While the same critics have also been concerned about somatic cell gene therapy, their principal focus has been germ-line approaches. Thus, researchers proposing to undertake germ-line gene therapy, or at least the review bodies evaluating such proposals, will need to take into account a much broader range of nonmedical consequences. . . .

The Authors' Conclusion

Ultimately, the moral case for or against germ-line gene therapy must be established by good reasons. In our evaluation of the pro and con arguments and in our discussion of eugenics, we have attempted to indicate why we find voluntary programs of germ-line genetic intervention to be ethically acceptable in principle. We think that this strategy should be employed only when gene replacement or gene repair is a validated technique. In addition, we are hopeful that techniques will be developed for repairing sperm and egg cells in the bodies of prospective parents before fertilization occurs. Finally, we find both the goal of preventing disease in a particular individual and the goal of preventing the transmission of genetic disease to the individual's descendants to be worthy rationales for this intervention.

Index

AIDS. *See also* Epidemics, newly emergent; Tuberculosis
and civil liberties, 88–91, 211–224, 228
as disease of homosexual males and drug-injecting addicts, 212–213
as exception to communicable disease control, 208, 211–224, 217–218
and gene therapy, 342
opposition of gay community to routine testing for, 213–215, 220–222
partner notification and, 211, 216–217
rationale for exempting testing, reporting, and notification, 217–220
testing for and reporting, 5, 211–217
and tuberculosis, 228–229
Alcohol policy. *See also* Drugs (Ilegal); Tobacco policy
and alcohol industry, 142–145
and disease concept of alcoholism, 132, 136–137
Prohibition, 131–132
public health perspective on, 132–149
state prohibitions laws, 62–64
Annas, George, 340
Assisted reproductive technologies. *See also* Infertility
effectiveness and cost of, 323–325
and multiple gestation, 324
Report of Canadian Royal Commission on, 327
risks of, 324–325

Bentham, Jeremy, 13–14. *See also* Ethical theories
Buck, Carrie (*Buck* v. *Bell*), 312–313. *See also* Eugenics

Community. *See also* Provision, communal
and the common good, 21–22, 57–59
and the common life, 68–69
as critique of modern life, 53
definitions of, 53–54, 68
as living together to secure safety and welfare, 68–72
and membership, 68–71
and needs, 68–71
and police (regulatory) power, 59–64
and provision, 68–82
and redistribution, 73–75, 105–109
and social justice, 105–109

Drugs (illegal)
consequences of legalizing or decriminalizing illegal drugs, 160–163
failure of penal approach ("War on Drugs"), 156–160
and libertarian perspective on legalization, 152
public health perspective toward, 152–156
as public problem, 132–133, 150–163

Elias, Sherman, 340
Epidemics, newly emergent. *See also* AIDS
cholera, new variants of, 247–248
and ecosystem instability, 240–250
factors in new epidemics, 240–243
globalization of epidemics, 240–250
hantavirus, 245–247
Equal access to health care principle. *See also* Justice
arguments against equal access, 260–263
defining, 256–257